Psychiatry and
Clinical Neuroscience

Psychiatry and Clinical Neuroscience
A Primer

Charles F. Zorumski, MD

Samuel B. Guze Professor and Head of Psychiatry
Professor of Neurobiology
Chief of Psychiatry, Barnes–Jewish Hospital
Director of the McDonnell Center for Cellular and Molecular Neurobiology
Washington University in St. Louis–School of Medicine

Eugene H. Rubin, MD, PhD

Professor of Psychiatry
Vice-Chair for Education, Department of Psychiatry
Professor of Psychology
Director of Geriatric Psychiatry, Barnes–Jewish Hospital
Washington University in St. Louis–School of Medicine

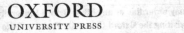

OXFORD
UNIVERSITY PRESS

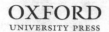

OXFORD
UNIVERSITY PRESS

Oxford University Press is a department of the University of Oxford.
It furthers the University's objective of excellence in research, scholarship,
and education by publishing worldwide.

Oxford   New York
Auckland   Cape Town   Dar es Salaam   Hong Kong   Karachi
Kuala Lumpur   Madrid   Melbourne   Mexico City   Nairobi
New Delhi   Shanghai   Taipei   Toronto

With offices in
Argentina   Austria   Brazil   Chile   Czech Republic   France   Greece
Guatemala   Hungary   Italy   Japan   Poland   Portugal   Singapore
South Korea   Switzerland   Thailand   Turkey   Ukraine   Vietnam

Oxford is a registered trade mark of Oxford University Press in the UK and certain other countries.

Published in the United States of America by
Oxford University Press
198 Madison Avenue, New York, NY 10016

© Oxford University Press 2011

First issued as an Oxford University Press paperback, 2014.

Library of Congress Cataloging-in-Publication Data
Zorumski, Charles F.
   Psychiatry and clinical neuroscience: a primer/Charles F. Zorumski, Eugene H. Rubin.
      p.; cm.
   Includes bibliographical references and index.
   ISBN 978-0-19-976876-9 (hardcover); 978-0-19-936056-7 (paperback)
1. Psychiatry. 2. Neurology. I. Rubin, Eugene H. II. Title.
[DNLM: 1. Mental Disorders—physiopathology. 2. Brain—physiology. 3. Diagnostic Techniques, Neurological.
4. Neurosciences—trends. 5. Psychiatry—trends. WM 140]
RC321.Z67 2011
616.89—dc22 616.89   2010042933

In anticipation of remarkable scientific advances
leading to cures for psychiatric disorders

Foreword

In the minds of many, understanding how the brain works represents the last great scientific frontier in biology, if not science in general. While a fascination with this agenda can be related to brains large and small, the ultimate goal is to understand the workings of the human brain. For herein lies not only the potential to understand and ultimately treat, rationally and effectively, some of the most important diseases afflicting mankind, but also to address social problems that continue to vex scientists and scholars in fields as diverse as anthropology, political science, psychology, sociology, and economics.

Understanding psychiatric diseases must form a cornerstone of any agenda probing the functions of the human brain. In this wonderful new book, Zorumski and Rubin have seized the opportunity to think anew about the brain mechanisms underlying psychiatric disorders and their treatment. This opportunity arose, in part, through developments in cognitive neuroscience that are worth recalling[1].

The term cognitive neuroscience was coined by Michael Gazzaniga and George Miller while riding together in a taxi cab in New York City sometime in the late 1980s (personal communication). Their concept was that understanding human brain function would be enriched significantly if individuals with expertise in the quantitative description of human behaviors (e.g., cognitive psychologists) could be encouraged to join forces with scientists capable of monitoring the functions of the human brain. Their view echoed a plea made almost 80 years before by Sir Charles Sherrington when he suggested that ". . . physiology and psychology, instead of prosecuting their studies, as some now recommend, more strictly apart one from another than at present, will find it serviceable for each to give to the results achieved by the other even closer heed than has been customary hitherto."[2] In this book, Zorumski and Rubin persuasively argue for a much closer relationship between psychiatry and neuroscience.

As a result of the advocacy of Gazzaniga and Miller that was fueled by the rapid emergence of techniques for human functional brain imaging, the James S. McDonnell Foundation and the Pew Charitable Trusts jointly sponsored a program of training and research that created the field of cognitive neuroscience. This program, one of the most successful of its kind ever, has made cognitive neuroscientists an essential component of departments of psychology, psychiatry, neurology, and neurobiology to name just a few of the most active participants. Brain imaging in the hands of cognitive neuroscientists has become the medium for much of the discussion as well as an important means of integrating studies of the human brain into mainstream neuroscience. These developments have appealed to a universal thirst for information about human brain function in health and disease among brain scientists as well as the lay public.

Until recently, work in cognitive neuroscience followed a long tradition in neuroscience of studying responses to stimuli and task performance. In this work, the role of bottom-up versus top-down or feed-forward versus feed-back causality has frequently been discussed, reflecting a debate extending back a century or more on the relative importance of intrinsic and evoked activity in brain function. Recent unexpected discoveries in functional brain imaging research have entered this discussion and will likely be important in shaping future research. These discoveries are important to the ideas put forth by Zorumski and Rubin concerning the role of intrinsic connectivity networks or ICNs in psychiatric diseases. Some historical background to this work will likely enhance the reading of their book.

Since the 19th century and possibly longer, two views of brain function have existed[3]. One view, pioneered by the early work of Sir Charles Sherrington, posits that the brain is primarily reflexive, driven by the momentary demands of the environment. The other view is that the brain's operations are mainly intrinsic, involving the acquisition and maintenance of information for interpreting, responding to, and even predicting environmental demands, a view introduced by a disciple of Sherrington, T. Graham Brown. The former has motivated most neuroscience research including that with functional neuroimaging. This is not surprising because experiments designed to measure brain responses to various stimuli and carefully designed tasks can be rigorously controlled whereas evaluating the behavioral relevance of intrinsic activity[4] can be an elusive enterprise. How do we adjudicate the relative importance of these two views in terms of their impact on brain function?

One means of adjudicating the relative importance of evoked and intrinsic activity is to examine their cost in terms of brain energy consumption. Most know that in the average adult human, the brain represents about 2% of the total body weight yet it accounts for 20% of all the energy consumed, 10 times that predicted by its weight alone. However, far fewer realize that relative to this very high rate of ongoing or 'basal' energy consumption in the resting state[5], the additional energy consumption associated with evoked changes in brain activity is remarkably small, often less than 5%. From these data it is clear that the brain's enormous energy consumption is little affected by task performance. Furthermore, an increasing body of evidence suggests that the majority of brain energy consumption is devoted to functionally significant signaling processes such as glutamate cycling. The challenge is how to study these intrinsic brain processes. Functional brain imaging has provided some intriguing new insights.

A prominent feature of fMRI is the apparent noisiness of the raw blood oxygen dependent or BOLD signal that, for many years, prompted researchers to average their data to increase its signal-to-noise ratio. As first shown by Bharat Biswal and colleagues at the Medical College of Wisconsin, this noise in the BOLD signal exhibits striking patterns of spatial coherence delineating all cortical systems in the human brain and their subcortical connections. This highly organized ongoing activity has been dubbed *a default mode of brain function*.

Not only do spatial patterns of coherence exist *within* brain systems but also *among* systems organized around a hierarchical system of hubs. This satisfies the need to integrate information among systems for the brain to function properly. Of particular interest is that one system in the brain seems to reside at the top of this hierarchical organization. This is a group of cortical areas along the brain's midline in parietal and prefrontal cortices and in lateral parietal and medial temporal cortices as well. This has come to be known as the brain's *default mode network* because it is most active in the resting state and often decreases its activity during the performance of goal-directed tasks. It has been the focus of much attention with regard to psychiatric conditions because of the self-referential nature of its putative functions, as Zorumski and Rubin discuss in detail in their book.

Furthermore, this highly organized ongoing activity appears to transcend levels of consciousness, being present under anesthesia and during sleep. These observations make it unlikely that the patterns of coherence and the intrinsic activity they represent are primarily the result of unconstrained, conscious cognition (i.e., mind-wandering or day dreaming). Rather, they likely represent a fundamental level of functional brain organization adjudicating the delicate balance between maintaining homeostasis yet allowing flexibility needed for learning and memory.

Thus, from resting-state fMRI data, investigators can now interrogate the integrity of the brain's large scale functional organization within and among systems at a level of analysis commensurate with the complex signs and symptoms of psychiatric illness. Remarkably, this can now be done without necessarily resorting to the performance of tasks, a great advantage when comparing patients with diseases impairing performance to normal control subjects.

The recent discovery of the electrical correlates of the fMRI BOLD signal have further expanded our understanding of its importance in brain organization. Emerging from this work is the fact that the BOLD signal represents the lowest end of the brain's electrical frequency spectrum (i.e., frequencies in the range of 0.001 to 0.1 Hz, which are traditionally referred to as slow cortical potentials or SCPs).

Knowing that SCPs and spontaneous fluctuations in the BOLD signal are related provides a bridge to a highly relevant, rich and diverse neurophysiologic literature on low frequency oscillations/fluctuations. For example, current evidence suggests that SCPs represent highly organized fluctuations in cortical excitability whose phase affects both evoked responses and behavioral performance. Entrainment of SCPs (and fMRI BOLD signals) to expected, predictable stimuli is an attractive means of matching predictions instantiated in intrinsic activity with the natural regularities of the environment.

Also, SCPs exhibit a remarkable relationship with other elements of the frequency spectrum of brain electrical activity, including the spiking activity of neurons. These relationships are likely mediated through variations in cortical excitability. This cross-frequency coupling (i.e., nesting) with SCPs serving an overarching coordinating role within and across systems provides a basis for the integration functions in both space and time.

As we move forward, the scope of the inquiry will undoubtedly expand even further into the realm of cell biology where events related to ion channel proteins, synaptic receptors, components of signal transduction pathways, and even cellular redox states exhibit temporal dynamics very similar to the work reviewed above. Integrating across these many levels of analysis will obviously be challenging. Help will come from theoretical modeling approaches where creative work has already begun. Appreciating the richness inherent in brain imaging signals greatly enhances the inferences to be drawn from them regarding the role of intrinsic connectivity networks or ICNs in psychiatric diseases.

The future of psychiatric research and, ultimately, the well-being of patients with psychiatric diseases will depend on tapping into the rich new insights emerging from the work just reviewed. This will require attracting young people who can envision a career in an environment prepared to accept new ways of thinking about disorders of human cognition and emotion. Zorumski and Rubin provide a very attractive road map of the way forward.

Marcus E. Raichle
Washington University School of Medicine
St. Louis, Missouri

Notes

[1] For a more detailed history see *Trends in Neuroscience* (2009) 32:118–126.

[2] *The Integrative Action of the Nervous System* (1906) page 397.

[3] For a more detailed review see *Trends in Cognitive Science* (2010) 14:180–190.

[4] *Intrinsic activity* is ongoing neural and metabolic activity which is not directly associated with subjects' performance of a task. The distinction between intrinsic activity and task-evoked activity applies to brain imaging as well as neurophysiology including events at the cellular level where ion channel protein receptors and the components of signal transduction pathways turn over with half-lives of minutes, hours, days, and weeks.

[5] The resting state is viewed here as a behavioral state characterized by quiet repose either with eyes closed or open, with or without visual fixation. It is understood that during the resting state, subjects experience an ongoing state of conscious awareness largely filled with stimulus independent thoughts (i.e., mind-wandering or day dreaming).

Preface

Psychiatric disorders result from complex dysfunctions of the human mind that alter the aspects of our being that make us most human—our abilities to think, to feel, to care for ourselves and our families, and to work productively. These devastating disorders lead to tremendous suffering for individuals, families, and society. When considered from a public health perspective, psychiatric disorders are leading causes of death and disability. Lists of the top causes of death routinely include heart disease, cancer, diabetes, stroke, pulmonary disorders, and motor vehicle accidents. At first glance, these causes of death may not seem related to psychiatric dysfunction, but upon examining the proximal and potentially treatable factors underlying these causes of death, psychiatric and behavioral problems take center stage, with alcohol and drug abuse, nicotine dependence, depression, and sedentary lifestyles serving as key contributors. Similarly, suicide, which is almost always associated with major psychiatric disorder, claims more than 30,000 lives a year in the United States. Psychiatric disorders are also the leading causes of disability in Western economies, accounting for 40% to 50% of all disabilities in the United States. This staggering percentage reflects the fact that these disorders are common, have an early age of onset, can be chronic, and are associated with severe cognitive, emotional, and motivational dysfunction. Sadly, these statistics regarding death and disability underestimate the toll that mental illnesses take on families and on society, including problems of interpersonal abuse, neglect, homelessness, and violence.

Treatment of psychiatric disorders has advanced greatly over the past 50 years and has helped to relieve a considerable amount of suffering, providing vehicles for de-institutionalization. Unfortunately, current treatments are good but not great from an outcomes perspective, and a substantial minority of individuals with psychiatric illnesses fails to respond to or cannot tolerate available interventions. Compounding the problem, most individuals with psychiatric disorders are not identified as having an illness and thus go untreated. Stigma and socioeconomic disparities in health care contribute significantly to this latter problem.

We highlight these points because we think they underscore the need to advance understanding of the mechanisms that underlie psychiatric illnesses and to use that understanding to develop more effective treatment strategies. From this perspective, it is important to emphasize that psychiatric disorders are problems of the human mind. In turn, the human mind is a product of the human brain. Thus, psychiatric disorders, simply put, are brain disorders. We believe this latter statement is so obvious that it should be beyond misunderstanding and unchallengeable. Yet, as currently practiced, much of clinical psychiatry has little to do with the brain, and many psychiatrists and mental health professionals treat the brain as a "black box" or don't even consider its role at all. Thus, while the defects underlying psychiatric disorders unequivocally reside in brain dysfunction, current practice requires little consideration of how brain mechanisms contribute to symptoms, disorders, and treatments. Most practicing psychiatrists are expert at psychopharmacology and know a lot about how psychiatric medications are thought to work at a neurochemical and receptor level. Many of these same psychiatrists, however, often have little real understanding or concern about what might actually be wrong in the brains of individuals with psychiatric disorders, being content to describe the illnesses as "limbic dysfunctions" or "chemical imbalances." While it is true that the "limbic system" plays a major role in emotional processing and that psychiatric medications affect specific neurochemical systems, these archaic metaphors convey little useful information about the nature of the brain dysfunctions leading to illness and are largely convenient myths bereft of real information content. Furthermore, it is not clear that any current medications actually have anything to do with the fundamental mechanisms involved in the illnesses they are used to treat.

We believe that this situation will change rapidly in the near future. Psychiatry is at a critical time in its history and is poised for major advances. These advances are driven by the advent of highly sophisticated neuroimaging and neurophysiological methods for studying how the human brain functions and how changes in brain function relate to neuropsychiatric illnesses. Coupled with advances in quantitative analytical methods, these approaches are identifying and deciphering the role of specific connectivity networks in the human brain. Furthermore, advances in human brain science are occurring at a time when even more powerful methods are being developed to study the function of individual nerve cells, their synaptic connections, and neural networks in animals, including animal models of stress and illnesses. Findings from current neuroscience research are revolutionizing how we think about brain function and illnesses and represent the scientific underpinnings for what we believe will be a radical change in the future of psychiatry. From our vantage point, it is increasingly clear that psychiatric disorders are problems of distributed and interactive brain networks, not chemical imbalances. Thus, understanding the functional connectivity of the human brain is critical for understanding how these disorders arise. Advances in genetic, cellular, and molecular science are also critical because they point to molecular mechanisms underlying illnesses as well as potential new targets for therapeutic development. Ultimately, understanding how cellular and molecular changes impinge upon network function will be an important step forward. These broadly based scientific advances dictate that psychiatry identifies itself much more directly as a branch of clinical neuroscience—a branch in which network neuroscience becomes the "basic science" of the discipline. We believe that this has major implications for determining how best to train future psychiatrists for clinical practice and implies a much heavier emphasis on principles derived from neurology, primary care, and rehabilitative medicine. This does not obviate the humanistic side of psychiatry, but we believe science and humanism can work hand in hand for the betterment of psychiatric patients.

Our purpose in writing this book is to provide a conceptual framework for describing how advances in neuroscience and genetics will affect psychiatry as a clinical discipline, focusing primarily on major disorders that occur in adults. Thus, the book is not meant to be a textbook of psychiatric or behavioral neuroscience. This effort is drawn from our careers in clinical and cellular neuroscience research as well as more than a half-century of combined experience in teaching psychiatric residents and medical students. It is our belief that systems neuroscience and the study of the brain's intrinsic connectivity networks (ICNs) offer the best hope of a brain-based understanding of clinical symptoms and disorders. We emphasize how this understanding will intersect with advances in molecular and synaptic neuroscience to provide a richer understanding of illness pathophysiology and targets for rehabilitative therapeutic strategies and potentially innovative drug and device design. Neuroscience is advancing rapidly, and future psychiatrists must be prepared to embrace and deal with the changing landscape.

We have written this book with medical students and residents interested in pursuing careers in psychiatry and neurology in mind. In addition, we hope we have achieved a level of discussion that will be instructive for advanced undergraduates contemplating careers in mental health disciplines, including psychology and social work. We also believe that the book will be useful for graduate students in neurosciences and allied fields such as psychology and will be of interest to practicing psychiatrists, neurologists, and mental health professionals as well. Our focus on rehabilitative aspects of psychiatry, broadly defined as efforts designed to help individuals with chronic and relapsing disorders function at the highest levels possible, should also make the book relevant for occupational therapists and specialists in rehabilitative medicine. While some aspects of the work we describe are highly technical and the book presupposes some basic background in neuroscience, we have tried to explain the concepts in a fashion that make them accessible for general audiences interested in understanding how the brain functions and is involved in psychiatric disorders.

Many outstanding scientists and clinicians around the world have contributed to the work described in this book. We have not tried to be comprehensive in our citations or descriptions, but rather we have focused on aspects of the work that we believe are the best understood and most instructive at this point. Where possible we have cited recent review papers or books that discuss the various concepts cogently. This field is evolving rapidly, and rarely a week goes by in which important papers on the topics covered are not published in leading scientific and clinical journals. We recognize that even better and more direct studies will be forthcoming in the future. For these reasons, we have no doubt overlooked the work of some individuals, and for this we apologize. Nonetheless, we believe the story we tell is compelling and represents the tip of a much larger iceberg that will shape the future of psychiatry—a future that looks extremely bright to us.

Charles F. Zorumski
Eugene H. Rubin

Acknowledgments

Numerous colleagues have influenced our thinking about psychiatry and neuroscience. We were privileged to be mentored by the late Eli Robins, Sam Guze, and Leonard Berg during formative stages of our careers. Other key mentors include Gerry Fischbach and John Olney, as well as numerous colleagues, including David Clifford, John Morris, Gene Johnson, Steve Mennerick, Doug Covey, Larry Eisenman, and Yuki Izumi. We are also grateful to be members of the Department of Psychiatry at Washington University in St. Louis. Our institution and department has an extremely creative and collaborative environment, and our colleagues on the faculty have greatly influenced us over the years. We would particularly single out Marc Raichle, Yvette Sheline, Tom Woolsey, Nigel Cairns, and Joel Price for many helpful conversations. In addition, we have benefited from our interactions with numerous members of the Alzheimer's Disease Research Center at Washington University.

We are indebted to the National Institutes of Health (NIH), particularly the National Institutes of Mental Health, Alcohol Abuse and Alcoholism, General Medical Sciences, Neurological Disorders and Stroke, and Aging, for their research funding. Without NIH support, there would be very little biomedical research, and creative thinking would be markedly curtailed. We also appreciate the ongoing support and friendship of Tom and Cherie Bantly and the Bantly Foundation.

In writing this book, we leaned heavily on numerous people for their opinions and critical comments. We are grateful to the team at Oxford University Press, in particular Craig Panner, who has helped us at every step of this project. We also benefited greatly from the input and support of our families, including Teresa, Erik, and Ian Zorumski, Donna Corno, Sue Easterby, Dan and Beth Rubin, and Rachel Silverberg. We are especially indebted to Gene's wife and our colleague, Dottie Kinscherf, for her efforts on this project. As in our prior book, Dottie took on the task of carefully reading, critiquing, and helping us to write and rewrite the entire manuscript.

Finally, we are indebted to our patients as well as our psychiatric residents and medical students at Washington University. Our interactions with them are among our greatest influences and inspirations.

Contents

Psychiatry and
Clinical Neuroscience

1

Psychopathology 101

Psychiatrists diagnose and treat disorders of the human mind and behavior. The premise of this book is that psychiatric disorders are brain disorders and that understanding these complex illnesses at a mechanistic level will require understanding how the brain creates the mind and how changes in the brain result in psychiatric dysfunction. While we are still a long way from this goal, advances in neuroscience, including cellular, molecular, and synaptic studies in animals and neuroimaging studies in humans, are providing important insights and directions for the field by characterizing the structure and operations of specific neural networks at rest and performing specific tasks.

To start this discussion, it is important to consider what is meant by "mind" and "mental disorder." The latter is perhaps easier to describe, with operational definitions provided by the current diagnostic system, DSM-IV. The concept of "mind" is more problematic and is one that has vexed philosophers and scientists for millennia. Because we are interested in understanding how problems of the mind lead to psychiatric disorders, we will attempt to make this discussion more concrete by using a fairly straightforward working definition of mind as provided by leading cognitive neuroscientists. For these scientists, "mind" is the result of processing in specific brain networks that allows humans to do three important things: think, attach meaning or value to things, and set and achieve goals (Table 1-1). These features, more formally called cognition (thinking), emotion (meaning), and motivation (goals), represent what Joseph LeDoux refers to in his book *Synaptic Self* as the "mental trilogy." Importantly, the biology of the brain networks underlying this trilogy is being worked out in considerable detail. We will explore these aspects of mind throughout this book, focusing at the network/systems neuroscience level because we believe this level has the most direct relevance for clinical psychiatry (Figs. 1-1, 1-2, and 1-3). This view is compatible with a recent commentary in which Tom Insel and colleagues from the National Institute of Mental Health state that "mental disorders can be addressed as disorders of brain circuits" (Insel et al., 2010). Throughout this book, we will refer to specific brain regions. Some chapters will have figures or block diagrams with the names of these specific regions. For readers wanting more detail about the location of these various regions, please refer to the appendix.

Our underlying thesis is that all major psychiatric illnesses reflect disturbances in all three aspects of the mental trilogy, resulting in comorbid symptoms across all dimensions of the mind. For example, individuals suffering from major depression

Table 1-1 The "Mind" and Psychiatry

Cognition (thinking)
- Working memory (dorsolateral prefrontal cortex)
- Attention (prefrontal cortex–parietal cortex)
- Executive function (medial prefrontal cortex)

Emotion (meaning)
- Medial prefrontal cortex, subgenual anterior cingulate cortex, amygdala

Motivation (goals)
- Ventral tegmental area, nucleus accumbens, prefrontal cortex

have unequivocal problems with emotion (as manifested by persistent sadness). Depression, however, is much more than persistent sadness, and depressed individuals also experience difficulties with cognition (inability to concentrate and focus attention, for example, as well as recurrent thoughts about death and suicide) and motivation (lack of drive, lack of pleasure, and inability to set and accomplish goals) in addition to neurovegetative symptoms (appetite changes, low energy, and sleep disturbances). It is the combination of these features that results in the profound problems and disabilities associated with this disorder. Similar considerations can be raised for all other major psychiatric disorders.

The features of major depression outlined above are well known to psychiatrists. What is missing from clinical analysis is an understanding of the nature of the defects in brain function that generate these symptoms. Thus, from our perspective, psychiatry seems to have lost its way as a clinical neuroscience discipline. For many clinical psychiatrists, the brain is simply a "black box" and neuroscience seems to play little role in how they think about clinical symptoms, disorders, and dysfunction. To put "brains" back in psychiatry, we need to reconceptualize how we think about psychiatric phenomenology in light of modern neuroscience.

To begin, we will discuss selected aspects of psychiatric symptoms in order to set the stage for discussions about specific disorders, pathophysiology, and treatments.

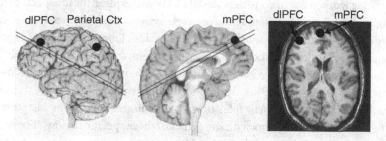

Figure 1-1 Key regions in cognitive processing. The images display key brain structures involved in attention and working memory. Emphasis here is on dorsolateral prefrontal cortex (dlPFC), medial prefrontal cortex (mPFC), and parietal cortex. These are only a few of the major regions involved in complex cognitive processing. The lines through the brain reconstructions indicate the approximate location that is shown in the radiologic image. (Adapted from Damasio, 2005, with permission.)

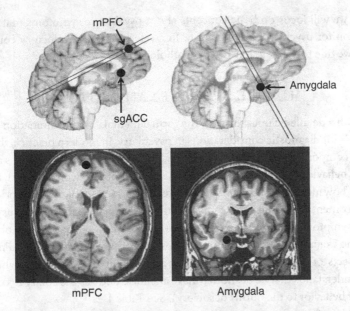

Figure 1-2 Key regions in emotional processing. The images depict key regions involved in emotional processing, including the subgenual anterior cingulate cortex (sgACC), medial prefrontal cortex (mPFC), and amygdala. The lines through the brain reconstructions indicate the approximate locations that are shown in the radiologic images. (Adapted from Damasio, 2005, with permission.)

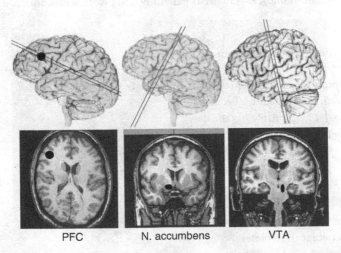

Figure 1-3 Key regions in motivational processing. The images display key brain regions involved in motivational processing, including prefrontal cortex (PFC), nucleus accumbens, and ventral tegmental area (VTA). The areas and networks highlighted in Figures 1-1, 1-2, and 1-3 will be described in greater detail elsewhere in this book. The lines through the brain reconstructions indicate the approximate locations that are shown in the radiologic images. (Adapted from Damasio, 2005, with permission.)

Initially, we will focus on basic concepts about psychiatric symptoms that are the foundation for psychiatric examination. In a reference to introductory courses in college, we title this discussion "Psychopathology 101."

MENTAL STATUS EXAMINATION

Along with a detailed clinical history, the formal mental status examination (MSE) is the basis for diagnostic considerations in psychiatry. In modern practice, there are multiple components to the MSE. These include descriptions of a patient's appearance and behavior, speech (rate, rhythm, and amount of verbal production), form of thought (how ideas flow and whether they are logical, sequential, and goal-oriented), thought content (what the patient talks about; the presence or absence of psychotic or other symptoms), mood and affect (as both reported by the patient and observed during the examination), sensorium and intellect (awareness of surroundings and basic aspects of cognition), and insight and judgment (the degree to which the patient understands that he or she may have an illness and has the ability to conform his or her behavior to the norms of society). See Table 1-2.

Valuable information is gleaned simply from observing and talking with the patient. When assessing appearance and behavior, a psychiatrist notes the level of alertness, grooming, activity (motor agitation and/or retardation), and degree of cooperation with the examiner. This portion of the exam is sometimes underappreciated, but important information is provided by these aspects of behavior. In particular, level of alertness can range across a continuum from fully alert to somnolent (drowsy but arousable), stuporous (arousable with more vigorous stimulation), or comatose (unarousable). Psychiatrists generally don't work with comatose patients,

Table 1-2 Mental Status Examination

General Appearance and Behavior (alertness, grooming, cooperativeness)
Speech (rate, rhythm, amount, inflection)
Form of Thought (goal orientation and flow)
Thought Content (principal themes, delusions, hallucinations, obsessions)
Mood and Affect (sustained and fluctuating emotional themes)
Sensorium and Intellect
- Attention and working memory (digit span, spell word backwards)
- Orientation (person, place, date, circumstances)
- Language (naming, repeating, general usage)
- Memory (recent and remote)
- Fund of knowledge (past presidents, current events)
- Abstraction (similes, proverbs)
- Calculation (serial 7's or 3's, making change)
- Constructional ability (drawing)
Insight and Judgment (awareness of illness, ability to conform behavior)

---

and stupor is relatively rare, although it can be observed in the context of the cata-tonic syndrome and some other disorders.

The sensorium and intellect (SI) part of the examination has multiple compo-nents that describe how a patient perceives and relates to his or her environment (sensorium) as well as aspects of the patient's general intelligence (intellect). This examination includes evaluation of the ability to focus attention and hold items in working memory, as determined by the ability to repeat a string of digits, spell a simple word forwards and backwards (e.g., "world"), or do simple serial calculations (e.g., subtract 3 or 7 from 100 in succession). Also, specific questions are asked to determine whether a patient knows who he or she is, where he or she is, and the cur-rent date and circumstances (referred to under the general heading of "orientation"). Other items evaluated include language function (the ability to name objects, repeat simple phrases, and follow simple commands) and memory function (the ability to recall recent and remote events and to form new memories, as determined typically by the ability to learn and then recall a short list of words after a several-minute delay). Overall fund of knowledge and ability to do simple abstractive reasoning (e.g., by describing how an orange and an apple are alike or interpreting simple prov-erbs like "a stitch in time saves nine") are also assessed. Finally, a patient is asked to perform simple calculations (e.g., the number of quarters in $2.75) and draw simple figures (e.g., the face of a clock or intersecting pentagons). These aspects of the SI examination are usually done in an unstructured fashion, although there are several brief questionnaires that provide quantitative estimates of performance. These include the Mini-Mental Status Examination (MMSE) and Short Blessed Test, for example. It is also important to tailor SI questions to the educational and cultural background of a patient to avoid biased interpretations of intellectual ability.

Some patients exhibit gross abnormalities in the SI examination, and these find-ings are extremely important for understanding their level of function, including understanding their more primary psychiatric symptoms. For example, while psy-chiatric disorders cut across the spectrum of human culture and intelligence, there is evidence that individuals with lower general intelligence are at increased risk for a number of psychiatric disorders, including psychotic illnesses, depression, and sub-stance abuse. Such observations are consistent with a "cognitive reserve" hypothesis of psychopathology, with individuals with lower cognitive capacity being at higher risk for some disorders. Interestingly, some studies suggest that individuals with mania may have higher general intelligence. Deficits in abstract reasoning and decision making (executive function) can be a major factor in determining why a patient may have difficulties keeping emotions and behaviors in check, suggesting a defect in "top-down processing" (higher-order control over emotional systems). Psychiatrists often observe subtle deficits in SI (e.g., minor defects in learning and recall or orientation). These may be difficult to characterize, and at times it is unclear whether the defects reflect longstanding problems or result from current psychiatric distress. Nonetheless, these defects are important to consider when planning a course of treatment for a patient and predicting a patient's reaction to life stressors (e.g., work, school).

THE NATURE OF PSYCHIATRIC SYMPTOMS: INSIGHTS FROM BEHAVIORAL NEUROLOGY

Building on the theme that psychiatric disorders involve problems in cognition, emotion, and motivation, we will now focus on some of the specific symptoms that psychiatrists encounter. Our goal here is not to be comprehensive, but rather to provide a framework for thinking about psychiatric symptoms and their relationship to altered brain function. Our guiding principle is that human cognitive, emotional, and motivational activities require integrated coherence across brain networks. Dysfunction within a given system or disconnections and/or aberrant connections between systems can have profound effects on how information is processed and is communicated.

Studies examining individuals with specific brain lesions have been instructive in helping scientists understand which brain regions contribute to specific functions. For example, damage to the dominant hemisphere (left hemisphere in right-handed persons and about 70% or more of left-handers) results in major problems with speech and language, with the nature of the resulting problem dependent upon the regions involved in the damage. Lesions involving anterior (frontal) speech production regions (called Broca's area) result in marked difficulties in motor aspects of speech (slow, halting speech) but leave language comprehension and reading largely intact. Posterior left-sided lesions, involving regions of temporal cortex (Wernicke's area), result in fluent speech that contains numerous grammatical errors and is nonsensical at times. This form of aphasia is also associated with marked difficulties in language comprehension and defects in repeating words and phrases.

Broca's and Wernicke's aphasias involve specific regions of the dominant hemisphere that must communicate with each other for effective language function. An additional lesson coming from the aphasia field involves the sequelae of lesions that do not directly affect either Broca's or Wernicke's area but instead damage the major connection between the two regions, the arcuate fasciculus. Such lesions result in "conduction aphasia," and individuals with this syndrome have fluent but halting speech along with word-finding problems and marked defects in repeating words and phrases. Speech comprehension remains intact because Wernicke's area is not involved in the lesion, and speech production is fluent because Broca's area is unaffected. The difficulty with repetition is a major defining defect, reflecting the inability to transmit information from Wernicke's area, where language is comprehended, to Broca's area, where motor speech is generated (Fig. 1-4).

The point of this discussion is that symptoms resulting from brain damage can reflect loss of function in primary areas involved in a specific task, or they can be more subtle, reflecting problems of connectivity between brain regions. Both possibilities are likely to be important in psychiatry, but increasing evidence suggests that connectivity problems may be major factors in psychiatric syndromes. Indeed, problems arising from a defect in a primary brain region coupled with disconnection

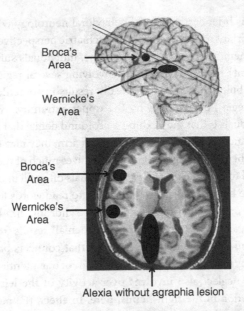

Broca's Area

Wernicke's Area

Broca's Area

Wernicke's Area

Alexia without agraphia lesion

Figure 1-4. Key language areas. The images show key regions in the left hemisphere involved in language processing. The syndrome of alexia without agraphia involves a posterior cerebral lesion that damages the left occipital (visual) cortex and the posterior limb of the corpus callosum. This results in a right-sided visual field defect. Inputs from the left visual field (right occipital cortex) can be processed but have no access to language centers in the left hemisphere because of damage to the corpus callosum. Thus, individuals with this lesion can write but cannot read what they have written. The lines through the brain reconstruction indicate the approximate location that is shown in the radiologic image. (Adapted from Damasio, 2005, with permission.)

from associated regions can result in fascinating but odd symptoms. For example, occlusion of the left posterior cerebral artery results in damage to the left occipital cortex and the posterior part of the corpus callosum (the large fiber tract that provides inter-hemispheric connectivity in that region). Persons suffering this type of stroke exhibit a right homonymous hemianopsia (loss of vision in the right visual field because of left occipital cortex damage), but they can see in their left visual field (because the right occipital cortex is still intact). Interestingly, these persons have intact language function (Wernicke's and Broca's areas are intact), but they cannot read because they cannot see in the right visual field and information from the left visual field cannot be communicated via the corpus callosum to the left angular gyrus (inferior parietal lobule), where visual images are converted to words. Even more bizarrely, although these individuals can write words (the angular gyrus is intact), they cannot read their own writing (called "alexia without agraphia" or "pure word blindness") (see Fig. 1-4). In contrast, damage to the left angular gyrus impairs both reading and writing ("alexia with agraphia"). Thus, understanding strange symptoms as described in these examples requires an understanding of how brain regions contribute to specific tasks AND how those regions are connected to one another to share the information needed to perform a task.

We will end this brief description of behavioral neurology with one other syndrome that is important to consider from a psychiatric perspective: the syndrome of "anosognosia" or hemineglect. In this syndrome, individuals suffer damage to the right (nondominant) hemisphere, usually involving several regions, including the inferior parietal lobule. This damage typically results in some degree of left-sided weakness (hemiplegia), often involving the upper extremity. What is fascinating about these individuals is that they exhibit a profound denial that anything is wrong with their hemiplegic arm. When shown their left arm, they may even report that it doesn't belong to them. Similarly, the neglect involves much of the left side of visual space. When asked to draw a clock, these individuals often fill in only the right side, leaving the left side blank. Similarly, when asked to read words like "woman," they may report seeing only "man." This hemineglect syndrome has been the focus of considerable study, and it now appears that the "denial" results from defective connectivity in a specific ventral attention network that connects parietal and frontal cortices—a pathway that allows us to reset the focus of our attention. Equally important, however, the neglect also involves over-activity of the left hemisphere, not simply loss of function in the right hemisphere. In effect, the person cannot shift attention and the intact left hemisphere (the one generating verbal responses) does not get correct information about the status of the hemiparetic arm. The left hemisphere then appears to make up a story to deal with the lack of coherent input: "That can't be my arm; it must belong to someone else." Importantly, understanding the brain network pathophysiology that produces symptoms of hemineglect also creates potential strategies for therapeutic intervention and rehabilitation. Thus, it would seem that either enhancing activity in the injured right hemisphere or diminishing activity in the over-active left hemisphere might lead to improvement. Indeed, some evidence using transcranial magnetic stimulation and other manipulations (e.g., applications of warm water to the right ear or cold water to the left ear) suggests that this may be true, at least temporarily.

The hemineglect syndrome is just one of many instructive behavioral defects arising from disconnectivity among brain regions. Others include Anton's syndrome (denial of cortical blindness) and the agnosias (inabilities to recognize parts of items or items as wholes when parts are recognized, including problems recognizing faces [prosopagnosia] even when parts of faces can be identified). Other important neuropsychological syndromes involve defects in the ability to carry out higher-order sequences of behavior (e.g., ideomotor apraxia, where an individual cannot pantomime an act, such as how to blow out a match or write with a pen, but may be able to perform the act when the object is in hand). We believe that studies of hemineglect and these other neurobehavioral syndromes are of major importance for psychiatry and highlight how our brains work when they process defective or inappropriate information. One important principle to take away from these studies is that when brain regions receive incoherent data, the dominant hemisphere will often "make up" an answer to make the data coherent; these defects are referred to as "processing errors" by cognitive scientists. We will return to this theme repeatedly throughout the book.

COGNITIVE SYMPTOMS: PSYCHOTIC AND NON-PSYCHOTIC THINKING

Psychiatrists routinely evaluate individuals who have major problems with thought content and perceptions. At the farthest extreme are those individuals described as "psychotic," a term that in its simplest definition refers to the presence of delusions and/or hallucinations. A delusion is a fixed false belief that is outside the cultural context of the individual. Examples include a person believing that he or she is being controlled by external influences (e.g., by an alien force) or is being spied on and monitored by the FBI. Hallucinations are false sensory perceptions that are viewed as arising outside of one's head. Hallucinations can occur in any sensory sphere, but those involving hearing (e.g., hearing your own thoughts out loud or external voices commenting on your behavior) are the most common in psychiatry. A broader view of psychosis would extend beyond delusions and hallucinations to include grossly disorganized speech that is difficult to understand and/or grossly disorganized and erratic behavior (e.g., hoarding trash or being unable to care for one's basic physical needs).

Psychopathologists have sought to characterize delusional thinking further, and it is clear that the content of delusional thinking can have several primary themes, some of which occur conjointly in some patients. For example, the most common delusion is one of persecution, often mistakenly referred to as "paranoid" thinking. (As an aside, the term "paranoid" derives from the Greek word "paranoia" and more accurately refers to delusional, but not necessarily persecutory, thinking.) Persecutory delusions are fixed ideas that some person or agency is trying to inflict harm on the individual. Other common delusions include nihilistic delusions (i.e., the belief that one doesn't exist or is already dead; these include so-called delusions of negation, as highlighted in Cotard's syndrome), grandiose delusions (i.e., the belief that one has special powers and abilities beyond those of other mortals; the fixed belief that one can control the stock market, for example), delusions of depersonalization (that the individual has changed) or derealization (that the world/environment has changed), and delusions of jealousy, which are particularly dangerous for a targeted spouse or loved one. Another fairly common theme is called "referential thinking"; this involves the idea that persons or circumstances are referring specifically to oneself. When such ideas are fixed and clearly false, they are referred to as "delusions of reference." These delusions can sometimes be difficult to distinguish from "ideas of reference," which have a similar theme but lack the unshakability of a delusion. One example of referential thinking is the belief that a group of strangers talking among themselves are specifically talking about you, even though they don't know you.

When considering problems involving thought content, it is important to discern when the thoughts are pathological and when they are less ominous deviations from normal. When delusions are dramatic and florid, there is usually no problem making this distinction. However, one can view human thought content across a spectrum of flexibility and veracity. Fluid and adaptable thinking could be viewed as one end of the spectrum. Moving along the spectrum from flexible toward delusional, one could consider problems that arise from "preoccupations"—thoughts on a particular theme that are recurrent and persistent. Examples might include being repeatedly concerned about problems related to work or one's family, but in a way that reflects life circumstances and is not unusual or bizarre. Further along the spectrum would be "overvalued ideas," concepts that are false as judged by a person's culture but are nonetheless strongly believed. Examples might include a belief that the U.S. government was the perpetrator of the Sept. 11, 2001, terrorist attacks. Some might agree with the concepts, but others, in the same culture, would see the ideas as highly improbable. Importantly, overvalued ideas are not as rigidly believed as fixed and false delusions, which represent the farthest end of the spectrum.

It might be a good idea at this point to discuss "obsessions," which are recurring and persistent ideas, thoughts, impulses, and images that are difficult for a person to clear from consciousness. In contrast to delusional thinking, however, the individual recognizes the obsessions as abnormal and struggles against them. Obsessions are associated with considerable anxiety and are often, but not always, accompanied by "compulsions," habitual motor acts and rituals performed to diminish this anxiety (e.g., repeated hand washing or showering because of thoughts about contamination).

Another factor to consider when discussing what defines a symptom as pathological is the notion that many symptoms observed in psychiatric patients are also observed in the general population. For example, some studies indicate that up to one third of people report significant feelings of suspiciousness and even persecutory ideas about work, the government, and other agencies or individuals, including ideas of reference about coworkers and others. Similarly, some studies indicate that about one fourth of the population has significant obsessions, including persistent ideas about harm and disease, recurrent thoughts about cleanliness and contamination, symmetry and order, and hoarding behaviors and counting rituals. Given that psychotic and obsessional disorders together occur in less than a few percent of the population, this suggests that odd thinking by itself is not a marker for psychiatric illness. This raises an important question that we will deal with later in the book: what elements of brain function result in specific psychiatric symptoms? We will argue that the human brain generates abnormal ideas and perceptions regularly; these are the "errors" in cognitive function described previously. However, "normal" brains correct these errors so they do not lead to persistent problems or dysfunction.

How does the brain generate delusional/pathological thinking? This is an area of active investigation, and current work suggests that defects in the ability to focus attention and to reason abstractly are likely to contribute. Also, habitual thinking patterns, including attributional biases (i.e., assigning causality on the basis of preconceived ideas), are involved. Importantly, delusions appear to involve more than just errors in cognition; there is also an emotional component in which negative emotions (dysphoria, irritability) combine with altered executive processing (as manifest by jumping to conclusions and faulty logic) to result in the aberrant thoughts. The jump from bad ideas and faulty logic to delusions may, in the words of Paul Fletcher and Chris Frith, involve disturbances in updating inferences about the world so that individuals accept evidence for a belief (sometimes extremely strained or vague evidence) and reject evidence against that belief. It is also important to consider what has been learned from studies of hemineglect about how our brains handle information and the notion that when incomplete or defective information is processed, the brain may "fill in the blanks" and create answers that may or may not have a basis in reality. This is seen routinely when our brains interpret gestalt perceptual images, visually filling in lines and figures where none are present. In effect, our brains are extremely effective at pattern completion, relying on memory and habitual modes of processing to deal with, sometimes inappropriately, new information or situations. Similarly, if there are defects in connectivity between emotional and perceptual systems, the brain can make up a solution to deal with the discrepancy. Some cognitive neuroscientists, like V. S. Ramachandran, suggest that this may be what happens in Capgras syndrome, where a person develops the delusional idea that a loved one has been replaced by an identical double. When the perception of the familiar person is not accompanied by the expected emotion, the brain (left hemisphere) simply makes up a story to explain the discrepancy (e.g., "That person looks like my wife, but I have no feelings for her. Therefore she cannot be my spouse; she must be an identical double"). Interestingly, variants of this phenomenon are seen following damage to the nondominant hemisphere and can involve the belief that one is in a place that is identical to a known place but located somewhere else (called "reduplicative paramnesia").

In addition to delusions, psychotic thinking is often accompanied by hallucinations, false sensory perceptions. Again, one can consider that these symptoms exist across a spectrum of abnormalities. On one end are normal sensations and perceptions. Next along the spectrum are more complex phenomena like synesthesias (experiencing a sensation from one sensory modality in another modality; e.g., "hearing" the color red). Other alterations in perception include illusions (mistaken interpretation of a real sensory input; for example, seeing a shadow as a demon) and true hallucinations. Once again it can be difficult to determine whether a given symptom is pathological, and the genesis of these altered perceptions is a matter of active study. For example, there is evidence that synesthesias involve spillover or blending of areas in sensory cortex, and it is this mixed sensory representation that results in a visual input (e.g., the color red) being experienced (e.g., "heard") in a second sensory modality. Interestingly, certain hallucinogenic drugs like LSD that alter serotonin neurotransmission are notorious for causing synesthesias, but these experiences also occur in otherwise normal individuals; artists, for example, are thought to have a higher incidence of synesthesia compared to the general population. Similarly, there is considerable interest in determining whether auditory hallucinations reflect altered perceptions of one's self relative to the environment and misinterpretation of one's own inner thoughts as being the product of an external agent. Some individuals experience "pseudohallucinations," which are sensations arising from internal processing that lack the substance of a normal perception (e.g., hearing voices inside one's own head as opposed to hearing voices coming from the outside in a true hallucination). Pseudohallucinations are not thought to reflect psychosis but may, instead, reflect heightened awareness of internal processing driven by an intense emotional state. Again, a defective ability of the brain to correct errors in processing may underlie some of these symptoms, particularly illusions and hallucinations. Altered brain wiring can contribute also, as indicated by lessons learned from the synesthesia literature. It is also important to understand that what we may consider to be a simple sensation is often a highly processed piece of information, reflecting not only the primary sensation but also current emotional, motivational, and cognitive states. Thus, even things we think are primary perceptions are subject to considerable error and misinterpretation.

DISTURBANCES IN THE FORM OF THOUGHT

Speech and language are critical for our ability to communicate effectively with others, and disturbances in speech and language, particularly the form that thought takes when it is put into language, often go hand in hand with some of the disturbances in thought content described previously. At times, defects in the form of thought reflect the defective logic that produces a delusion (e.g., illogical speech that reflects a delusional belief: "I am a man and Jesus Christ was a man; therefore, I am Jesus Christ"). At other times, defects in speech may be so profound on their own as to interfere with a person's ability to express ideas coherently. When assessing patients with these types of thought disorder, it is important to determine whether the defects reflect a type of aphasia resulting from damage to or dysfunction of the dominant cerebral hemisphere. The fluent but at times meaningless verbal output of patients with Wernicke's aphasia can have features akin to the verbal production of some patients with severe psychosis, perhaps providing a first-level indication of brain regions involved in the psychiatric dysfunction.

Psychiatrists use many terms to describe defects in both the flow (form) of thought and the use of specific words and phrases. Nancy Andreasen has helped to bring this into focus by providing systematic definitions of commonly used terms, definitions that help engender a common clinical language for discussing defects in form of thought and their associations with illnesses. As described by Andreasen and others, "formal thought disorders" can be positive or negative. Positive thought disorders include speech that is tangential (wanders markedly off target in response to a question), derailed (wanders off target during spontaneous discourse), illogical (conclusions don't follow premises), or incoherent (individual sentences don't make sense). Other positive thought disorders include circumstantiality (overly inclusive speech that only eventually gets to the point) and flight of ideas (a speeded-up/pressured version of derailment that is typically associated with mania). Examples of negative thought disorder include poverty of speech (diminished overall verbal output), poverty of content (adequate output but no significant message), blocking (thoughts go blank in the process of explaining something), and loss of goal (losing track of where one is going with a comment).

These disturbances occur at the level of sentences and paragraphs. There are also defects that appear at the level of words or phrases. Examples include using the wrong word (semantic paraphasia), mispronouncing words (phonemic paraphasia), making up words (neologisms and word approximations), and using the same words or phrases repeatedly (perseveration). Other rarer manifestations include clang associations (basing the next comments on the words or sounds last spoken) and echolalia (repeating and mimicking the exact words of the examiner). The latter is sometimes associated with echopraxia (mimicking the movements of the examiner).

In general, severe disturbances of the form of thought are most common in individuals with psychotic illnesses, particularly schizophrenia and mania. However, just as with the thought content and perceptual disturbances described previously, problems in speech and logic can be observed in non-psychotic individuals. The marked circumstantiality observed in some patients with obsessive-compulsive disorder is one example, as is the poverty of speech and content in some depressed individuals. Carol North has examined the concept of "non-psychotic thought disorder" in some detail and found that speech and language difficulties can be a frequent occurrence in individuals with somatization disorder (hysteria) and personality disorders. She observed that these individuals often use speech that is highly circumstantial, vague, and meandering; is accompanied by all-or-none logic (e.g., repeatedly using terms like "always" or "never"); and is overly generalized (e.g., "everybody" or "nobody"). Such speech is reminiscent of the poverty of content described by Andreasen and raises questions about defects in the logic used by these individuals. Importantly, when deciding whether speech in a given individual is pathological, context seems to be critical. For example, some politicians are extremely good at controlled poverty of content and tangentiality, but this is highly dependent on context. It is also important to determine whether defects in speech and language are state or trait dependent—that is, do the defects represent longer-standing problems in logic and speech ("trait" phenomena) or an acute state such as psychosis or mood disturbance?

DISTURBANCES IN EMOTIONS

Emotions reflect the way our brains attach meaning to the things we do, and disturbances in emotions, as manifest by problems with mood and affect, accompany all psychiatric disorders. For this discussion, we will define "mood" as the long-lasting and prevailing emotional state of the individual and "affect" as the more changeable and fluctuating aspects of emotions. Other definitions are sometimes used by psychiatrists; for instance, mood might refer to what is reported by the patient and affect to what is observed during clinical examination.

In this discussion, we will focus on what is being learned about the neurobiology of emotions from both cross-cultural studies of humans and studies in animals. Emotions are important because they provide neural mechanisms by which information can be rapidly (and unconsciously) processed and acted upon. This can have huge survival benefits; for example, because of prior experience, one might be frightened by a sound or a perceived movement and take defensive action well before becoming consciously aware of what is going on. The initial processing involves subcortical structures, including the amygdala and related parts of the brain; only secondarily and later does neocortex add conscious awareness. Thus, in many ways our emotions are survival modules, and our primary emotions are of evolutionary importance. It is important to keep this in mind as we think about the defects in emotions that occur in psychiatric disorders.

Based on work by cultural psychologists and anthropologists, humans are thought to have six (or possibly seven) primary emotions: happiness, sadness, fear, anger, surprise, and disgust. Contempt is sometimes included, and other scientists add anticipation (hope) and acceptance. These, particularly the first six, are considered to be primary emotions because they are observed across human cultures and because humans of different cultures use similar facial expressions to convey a particular emotion. Humans also express a variety of social emotions, such as pride and affiliation, but these may be derivatives of the primary emotions.

Interestingly, many of these emotions or their derivatives are observed in animals, including rodents. Jaak Panksepp, a leader in the field of emotional evolutionary biology, has described seven emotional systems that are mediated by specific brain pathways. These include joy (playfulness), panic (separation distress), fear, rage, seeking (exploration), lust (sexual drive), and nurturance (maternal care). Some of these systems (fear, rage, and perhaps joy and panic) seem to map clearly onto the primary human emotions; others may be related, or possibly inverse, emotions. For example, contempt may be the inverse of nurturance and disgust the inverse of the appetitive emotion of lust in animals. Seeking may be related to surprise—perhaps reflecting an assessment of the novelty or "information content" in the environment—although surprise seems to have more of an alerting function and seeking more of an exploratory function. Disgust is a particularly interesting emotion to consider. At a base level, disgust helps us avoid poisons or noxious substances (and people). At another level, it may be the emotion that helps us set our moral compass—in other words, the level of emotion beyond which we won't perform an act, providing a so-called "gut" feeling that something is right or wrong. Indeed, work in human cognitive neuroscience indicates that our first and most rapid processing of a moral judgment involves our emotional systems, including the brain regions involved in disgust.

At first glance, it appears that psychiatric disorders largely involve the primary negative emotions (sadness, fear [anxiety], and anger). Aaron Beck describes this as a negative emotional bias in psychiatric disorders. Mania may be an exception, but even here manic euphoria can be short-lived and give way to more persistent irritability and rage. The neural systems underlying the primary emotions are being worked out in considerable detail, and because of the apparent overlap in animal and human emotions, it is possible to extrapolate cautiously across species. Fear is the emotion mapped out in greatest detail, and it is clear that the amygdala and its extended connections play a critical role. The role of the amygdala in fear processing makes it possible to consider whether anxiety disorders reflect defects in amygdala function and/or in more distributed emotional networks that interface and interact with networks underlying cognition and motivation.

DISTURBANCES IN MOTIVATION: THE ROLE
OF SALIENCE AND PERSONALITY

Psychiatry has developed fairly sophisticated ways to describe disturbances of thinking and emotion, but it deals much less effectively with descriptions of defects in motivation. Several things seem clear, however. Motivation involves, at least in part, a distributed neural network that uses dopamine as a key modulator and involves the midbrain ventral tegmental area (where dopamine neurons reside), the ventral striatum (nucleus accumbens), and regions of frontal cortex. This is closely related to the brain's "reward" processing network and is an evolutionarily old system, meaning that similar systems are found in lower animals such as rodents. This system also appears to be important in helping us determine the "salience" of things we encounter in our lives; that is, whether something is worthwhile or is worth our time. In addition, this network helps with error detection and correction. Psychiatric disorders have major effects on this system. For example, almost all known drugs of abuse act directly or indirectly on this dopamine system and, in effect, acutely hijack the system, leading to psychological addiction. The long-term consequences of this drug-induced hijacking of the motivational system may be one reason that chemical dependency problems are so difficult to treat and other psychiatric disorders are more difficult to treat when patients also are abusing drugs or alcohol. Other psychiatric disorders, such as schizophrenia and depression, can also disrupt motivation or lead to aberrant motivation.

The motivation system is closely linked to emotional systems, and the emotion Panksepp calls "seeking" may be a significant component of this link. Also, some evidence suggests that the neural systems underlying personality traits in humans also contribute to determining how the motivational system functions. For example, C. Robert Cloninger has proposed that personality has two principal components: temperament and character. *Temperament* reflects the basic tendencies of people to be motivated by their environment and has four dimensions: novelty seeking (akin to Panksepp's seeking), harm avoidance, reward dependence, and persistence. Importantly, these temperament traits appear to reflect activity in specific neural circuits that feed into the nucleus accumbens (ventral striatum) motivational system. Individuals vary across these dimensions, and things that motivate different individuals reflect assessments of novelty, threat, and reward. The *character* dimensions are more modifiable aspects of personality that reflect the degree to which individuals are cooperative, self-directed, and self-transcendent (able to see beyond themselves). Cloninger views personality disorders as problems primarily involving character (particularly cooperativity and self-directedness), while the individual's temperament profile determines the form that the personality disorder takes.

DISTURBANCES IN MEMORY

Memory is a critical component of cognition and plays a major role in determining who we are and how we behave. It is an aspect of our being that makes us unique as

Table 1-3 Types of Human Memory

Working Memory
- Current thoughts

Explicit (Declarative) Memory
- Episodic (events)
- Semantic (facts)

Implicit Memory
- Procedural (skills)
- Emotional
- Conditioned
- Habits

individuals, and some form of altered memory function accompanies many, if not all, psychiatric disorders. It is important to understand that there are multiple types of memory and that different forms of memory involve distinct, but sometimes overlapping, brain regions (Table 1-3). *Declarative memory* refers to the encoded record of our personal experiences, events, and spatial/cognitive maps. It has two subcategories: episodic memory (the record of our personal experiences) and semantic memory (facts not necessarily based on experience; recalling that Jefferson City is the capital of Missouri, for example). The hippocampus plays a key role in the formation of declarative memories, although other cortical and subcortical regions also contribute. Declarative memory is similar to what is called "explicit memory" by some cognitive scientists. In contrast, "implicit memories" involve motor (procedural) skills, conditioned experiences, habits, priming, and emotions. Skill learning (procedural memory), in contrast to declarative memory, involves primary motor systems, including the dorsal (motor) striatum, cerebellum, and supplementary motor cortex. The striatum (both dorsal and ventral aspects) also appears to participate in habit formation and thus may be a key structure involved in the generation of the stereotyped behaviors exhibited in many psychiatric disorders. Habits are overlearned implicit behaviors that many animals, including humans, often revert to under stressful circumstances. *Emotional memories* involve the amygdala, although the hippocampus also contributes to this form of learning, particularly with regard to the context (place, time, and events) associated with an emotional experience. In fact, whenever context (particularly place) is involved in a memory, the hippocampus is likely to be involved.

As the terms "explicit" and "implicit" suggest, memories can be processed consciously and unconsciously. When we become conscious of our thoughts, that information resides in *working memory*, a cognitive function involving a distributed neural network including dorsolateral prefrontal cortex and parts of parietal cortex and hippocampus. The contents of working memory are the things you are thinking about right now. Working memory has limited capacity and is relatively short-lived; to maintain items in working memory, they need to be updated repeatedly. There are several clinical tests used to assess working memory. Among others, these include digit span (the number of digits a person can repeat immediately), the Wisconsin Card Sorting Test, and the "n-back test," in which an individual is asked to respond whenever he or she hears an item that was presented one (one-back) or more (n-back) items previously in a list. Working memory is said to have a "7 ± 2" capacity; that is, we can store about 7 items in working memory at any given time (the number of digits in a typical phone number).

There are multiple steps in generating a declarative memory trace in the brain, and problems with memory can occur at any step in the process. Initially, an item must be perceived and comprehended. That perception is then stored as a short-term trace in the hippocampus before being converted to a more durable memory trace in neocortex. Over time, the item is consolidated in memory and subject to modification by subsequent learning. When the item is recalled, several steps are also involved. These include recognizing that the item is needed, isolating the memory trace in cortex, and using the item in the new context. The processes involved in memory processing seem most easily disrupted during the initiation phase, when the short-term trace is being formed in hippocampus, and soon after registration in cortex. This follows a phenomenon called Ribot's Law, which states that new memories are lost before old memories, a type of memory disturbance observed in dementing illnesses like Alzheimer's disease. Loss of short-term memory is sometimes referred to as "anterograde amnesia," a defect in learning new information. A clear example of anterograde amnesia is observed in alcohol-induced "blackouts" during which an individual is awake and alert (although intoxicated) and performs complex activities but later has no recollection for what was done or said during the period of the blackout. "Retrograde amnesia" refers to the loss of previously stored memories, again following Ribot's Law. There are other types of amnestic syndromes observed clinically. These include "global amnesia," where an individual experiences a loss of recollection for most or all prior events; such memory disturbances have been observed with bilateral defects in cerebral blood flow and are usually transient.

Some psychiatric disorders are associated with complaints of complex memory loss, often involving specific portions of an individual's life, particularly those that are emotionally charged. This has sometimes been referred to as "hysterical (or con-version) amnesia." The neural mechanisms underlying such defects are unclear but likely include a large emotional component. A major consideration in assessing dis-turbances in memory, particularly in individuals with psychiatric disorders, is to realize that human memory is not a truth-generating device. Our memories reflect an amalgam of factual events and our internal emotions, thoughts, and motivations at the time the memories are formed or recalled. Also, as memories are used, they are subject to new learning and modification; thus, over time, many memories change and are only a partial reflection of the actual events that occurred. These issues are extremely important to keep in mind when considering the role of memory problems in psychiatry and have been highlighted cogently by Daniel Schacter in his book *The Seven Sins of Memory*. Schacter emphasizes that common memory problems involve both omissions and commissions. Omissions include blocking, absent-mindedness, and transience, aspects of memory processing that result in our not being able to recall items that we believe we should be able to recall. Commissions, on the other hand, include several forms of bias, misattributions, persistence, and suggestibility, aspects of memory that cause us to recall things incorrectly from a factual standpoint. Biases include mistakes made because of hindsight (interpreting the past in terms of how things turned out), stereotypes (interpreting the past in terms of cultural and personal beliefs), and changes in ourselves (seeing the past as we currently view things). All of these defects severely limit the accuracy of our recollections. However, these types of memory defects are not pathological in their own right; they simply reflect the way the human brain handles information. To paraphrase Michael Gazzaniga, the way our brains process information largely ensures that human memory is faulty; we are always "self-concerned interpreters" of incoming information, and this fact biases the data we store and the information we recall. Humans even have the ability to "recall" events that never actually occurred. Psychiatrists and psychologists have sometimes forgotten this fact with disastrous consequences, as evidenced by subsequent family and societal problems. A recent example of this phenomenon was the "recovered memories" fiasco of the 1990s, in which well-intentioned but naïve therapists encouraged patients to "remember" events, often of a sexual abuse nature, that were later shown to have never happened. Humans are highly suggestible, and what they report as a memory is usually the "truth" as far as they can recall. These recollections, however, are not necessarily the observable "truth" that would be reported by an unbiased neutral observer.

Points to Remember

Psychiatric disorders are dysfunctions of the human mind and the human brain.

Major psychiatric disorders reflect disturbances in all aspects of the mind, including thinking (cognition), emotion (meaning), and motivation (goals).

Understanding the nature of psychiatric symptoms and the processes by which they arise in the brain is a necessary step in developing a meaningful pathophysiology of psychiatric illnesses.

Lessons from behavioral neurology about the ways complex symptoms and syndromes can arise from specific brain lesions and interruption in connections between brain regions can provide a framework for thinking about psychiatric symptoms and disorders.

Disturbances of thought content, speech, and language are commonly seen in psychiatry. Psychiatric disorders largely reflect negative emotional biases, and personality features can contribute to defects in motivation.

The normal human brain makes errors in perception, thinking, emotional processing, and memory. Failure of the brain to correct these errors and perpetuation of the errors may be a significant factor contributing to mental illnesses.

SUGGESTED READINGS

American Psychiatric Association. (1994). *Diagnostic and statistical manual of mental disorders* (4th ed.). Washington, DC: American Psychiatric Association.

Hamilton, M. (1976). *Fish's clinical psychopathology.* Bristol: John Wright & Sons.

Heilman, K. M., & Valenstein, E. (2003). *Clinical neuropsychology* (4th ed.). New York: Oxford University Press.

Schacter, D. L. (2001). *The seven sins of memory: How the mind forgets and remembers.* Boston: Houghton Mifflin.

Strub, R. L., & Black, F. W. (1989). *Neurobehavioral disorders: A clinical approach.* Philadelphia: F. A. Davis Company.

OTHER REFERENCES

Andreasen, N. C. (1979). Thought, language, and communication disorders. I. Clinical assessment, definition of terms, and evaluation of their reliability. *Archives of General Psychiatry, 36,* 1315–1321.

Andreasen, N. C. (1979). Thought, language, and communication disorders. II. Diagnostic significance. *Archives of General Psychiatry, 36,* 1325–1330.

Beck, A. T. (2008). The evolution of the cognitive model of depression and its neurobiological correlates. *American Journal of Psychiatry, 165,* 969–977.

Bell, V., Halligan, P. W., & Ellis, H. D. (2006). Explaining delusions: A cognitive perspective. *Trends in Cognitive Sciences, 10,* 219–226.

Bentall, R. P., Rowse, G., Shryane, N., Kinderman, P., Howard, R., Blackwood, N., et al. (2009). The cognitive and affective structure of paranoid delusions. *Archives of General Psychiatry, 66,* 236–247.

Bloch, M. H., Fanderos-Weisenberger, A., Pittenger, C., & Leckman, J. F. (2008). Meta-analysis of the symptom structure of obsessive-compulsive disorder. *American Journal of Psychiatry, 165,* 1532–1542.

Budson, A. E., & Price, B. H. (2005). Memory dysfunction. *New England Journal of Medicine, 352,* 692–699.

Cloninger, C. R. (2004). *Feeling good: The science of well-being.* New York: Oxford University Press.

Damasio, A. (1999). *The feeling of what happens: Body and emotion in the making of consciousness.* San Diego, CA: Harcourt.

Damasio, H. (2005). *Human brain anatomy in computerized images* (2nd ed.). New York: Oxford University Press.

Devinsky, O. (2009). Delusional misidentifications and duplications. *Neurology, 72,* 80–87.

Fletcher, P. C., & Frith, C. D. (2009). Perceiving is believing: A Bayesian approach to explaining the positive symptoms of schizophrenia. *Nature Reviews Neuroscience, 10,* 48–58.

Freeman, D., Garety, P. A., Bebbington, P. E., Smith, B., Rollinson, R., Fowler, D., et al. (2005). Psychological investigation of the structure of paranoia in a non-clinical population. *British Journal of Psychiatry, 186,* 427–435.

Fullana, M. A., Mataix-Cols, D., Caspi, A., Harrington, H., Grisham, J. R., Moffitt, T. E., et al. (2009). Obsessions and compulsions in the community: Prevalence, interference, help-seeking developmental stability and co-occurring psychiatric conditions. *American Journal of Psychiatry, 166,* 329–336.

Gazzaniga, M. S. (2008). *Human: The science behind what makes us unique.* New York: HarperCollins.

Greene, J. (2003). From neural "is" to moral "ought": What are the moral implications of neuroscientific moral psychology? *Nature Reviews Neuroscience, 4,* 847–850.

Hamilton, M. (1976). *Fish's schizophrenia* (2nd ed.). Bristol: John Wright & Sons.

He, B. J., Snyder, A. Z., Vincent, J. L., Epstein, A., Shulman, G. L., & Corbetta, M. (2007). Breakdown of functional connectivity in frontoparietal networks underlies behavioral deficits in spatial neglect. *Neuron, 53,* 905–918.

Insel, T., Cuthbert, B., Garvey, M., Heinssen, R., Pine, D. S., Quinn, K., et al. (2010). Research domain criteria (RDoC): Toward a new classification framework for research on mental disorders. *American Journal of Psychiatry, 167,* 748–751.

Kandel, E. R. (2006). *In search of memory: The emergence of a new science of mind.* New York: WW Norton & Company.

LeDoux, J. (2002). *Synaptic self: How our brains become who we are.* New York: Viking Press.

North, C. S., Osborne, V. A., Vassilenko, M., Kienstra, D. M., Dokucu, M., Hong, B., et al. (2006). Interrater reliability and coding guide for nonpsychotic formal thought disorder. *Perceptual and Motor Skills, 103,* 395–411.

Panksepp, J. (2004). *Affective neuroscience: The foundations of human and animal emotions.* New York: Oxford University Press.

Ramachandran, V. S., & Blakeslee, S. (1998). *Phantoms in the brain: Probing the mysteries of the human mind.* New York: William Morrow.

Tulving, E. (2002). Episodic memory: From mind to brain. *Annual Review of Psychology, 53,* 1–25.

2

Depression and Dementia
An Introduction to Systems Neuroscience and Psychiatry

How will a conceptual understanding of neurosciences, genetics, epigenetics, and gene–environment interactions help us better understand psychiatric disorders? On the surface, current clinical diagnosis and management of psychiatric disorders may not appear to require understanding concepts such as "the central reward system" or "central nervous system (CNS) plasticity." Nonetheless, we believe that psychiatrists and other mental health professionals must be equipped with knowledge to adapt to a changing landscape in diagnosis and treatment. Over the next several decades, we believe that brain research will have a major impact on how we think about psychiatric disorders and how we develop treatment strategies, aiming at more mechanism-based therapies and rehabilitative strategies targeted toward correcting specific defects in brain function. Thus, a firm knowledge base in the neuroscientific underpinnings of the field will be required in order to adapt to a changing clinical environment. This may not be obvious to current psychiatrists or students entering the field, but it will become clear as emerging advances in neuroscience take root.

The purpose of this chapter is to describe how a conceptual understanding of clinically relevant basic sciences, including neuroscience and genetics, will be essential for understanding tomorrow's diagnostic systems and treatments. For illustrative purposes, we will focus on two groups of disorders: major depression and the dementias. Depressive disorders are among the most common illnesses that psychiatrists treat. Alzheimer's disease is the most common cause of dementia and one of the best-characterized neuropsychiatric illnesses in terms of neural mechanisms. The scientific advances in understanding molecular, cellular, and systems neuroscience mechanisms in Alzheimer's disease are highly instructive and can lead to better ways to conceptualize the mechanisms contributing to primary psychiatric disorders.

SOME BASIC CONCEPTS ABOUT SYSTEMS NEUROSCIENCE AND PSYCHIATRY

Certain evolutionarily ancient brain regions such as the amygdala and nucleus accumbens (parts of the "limbic system") are primarily involved in processing and integrating information related to emotion and motivation. These regions receive information about our external and internal worlds and generate responses that help us quickly assess a situation by attaching meaning to the incoming information. Other interconnected brain regions, particularly those in the more recently evolved areas of neocortex, are primarily involved in cognitive processing and allow us to think consciously and to plan and execute decisions. In these examples, a collection of specific brain regions are directly connected to each other and constantly talking with each other, forming a brain system (or network). Some brain structures belong to several brain systems—for instance, the hippocampus is involved in emotional processing as well as cognitive and motivational brain systems. On the other hand, individual brain systems do not operate in isolation. The emotional processing brain systems, for example, require cognitive processing brain systems in order for a person to become conscious of emotions (called "feelings" in the words of Antonio Damasio), learn from emotions, and even control emotions via top-down processing. Thus, emotional systems interact closely with cognitive systems that involve brain regions such as the prefrontal cortex, parietal cortex, and temporal cortex.

In addition to the emotional and cognitive processing systems, pathways related to reward and motivation are involved in determining and regulating a person's feelings and actions. People change their behaviors depending on how rewarding a particular behavior is and the perceived costs associated with the behavior. If we like the way something feels, we take steps to prolong that feeling. If we enjoy the taste of a certain food, we want to eat more of it. If we do well in the stock market, we want to continue investing in stocks. Interestingly, if we suddenly do poorly in the stock market, we may have a response that is out of proportion to our loss. Such decisions are often emotionally and not cognitively driven. Bad outcomes or perceived bad outcomes can have a big impact on behavior and tend to trigger centers in the brain that process negative emotions such as fear and anxiety. Sometimes this is appropriate and we take defensive action, but at other times it is inappropriate and leads to bad decisions and interpersonal problems.

The symptoms associated with clinical depression involve abnormal functioning of systems underlying emotional processing, cognition, and reward. While we classify these disorders as "mood problems," it is important to realize that defects occur across all aspects of the mind, including cognition and motivation. When these systems aren't working in concert, the human brain reacts with a range of symptoms that can include sadness, decreased interest in everyday surroundings and activities, poor concentration and inattention, appetite and sleep changes, poor energy and motivation, and, at times, lack of will to live and suicidal thoughts. A depressive syndrome does not reflect abnormalities in one or a few brain structures or in one or a few neurotransmitter systems; it reflects a complex and distributed multi-network problem. This is discussed in more detail in Chapter 5.

There are likely to be many different reasons for malfunctions in these brain systems. Some people have a genetic makeup that makes it hard to perturb these particular brain networks; such people are highly resilient and not prone to depression, even in the face of adverse life circumstances. Others have brains that are wired in such a way that even slight perturbations can lead to significant disruption and, therefore, to changes in behavior. There is little doubt that genes contribute significantly to the predisposition to becoming depressed. Some families have higher risks for depression than other families. These risks may involve small effects of many common genes or possibly larger effects of rarer genetic variants. Various factors that disrupt brain systems are discussed in Chapter 9.

DEPRESSION

The DSM-IV diagnosis "major depression" refers to a broad and heterogeneous category of disorders and is a term that is somewhat parallel to the term "cancer." When told that a friend has cancer, we want to know what kind of cancer because that can have a huge impact on treatment and life expectancy. Similarly, when a patient has a history of depression, clinicians should want to know what kind of depression, because the answer to this question has a huge impact on treatment decisions and the likely course of the illness. Our current diagnostic system lumps many types of dysfunction under the heading of "major depression." While this simplifies clinical practice, it creates major difficulties for understanding the underlying biology of the disorders and for devising the most effective treatment strategies for individual patients. We will give a few examples of the heterogeneity below.

Some patients with depression seem to have a "pure" form of the illness—a type of depression that runs in their families and seems to be independent of other psychiatric illnesses or major environmental stressors. A young adult with this type of "pure" depression may experience the onset of severe depressive symptoms over a period of several weeks that interfere with school, work, and relationships. This person's family history may reveal a similar illness in close family members who might each have responded well to the same therapeutic approach—for example, bupropion in combination with cognitive behavioral therapy. In such cases, it is likely that the patient will respond to the same treatment as well. The particular group of genes that this person inherited may result in fragility in the smooth functioning of the neural systems involved in emotional processing and mood regulation. In theory, bupropion and psychotherapy help to re-establish healthy activity, connectivity, and interactions of these systems, leading to clinical improvement.

There are data strongly suggesting that individuals with these types of highly familial major depressive disorders have significant changes in brain structure and function. For example, a recent study by Brad Peterson and colleagues at Columbia University demonstrated that there is substantial thinning (more than 25% thinning) in certain areas of the right parietal cortex in persons whose families have multigenerational major depression. This right-sided cortical thinning in areas involved in cognition correlated with problems in focusing attention and visual memory (cognitive defects) and familial risk for depression (an emotion-based illness). These recent findings build upon earlier work in familial depression demonstrating structural changes in areas of subgenual anterior cingulate cortex that are part of an emotional processing network, changes that include a loss of glial cells in the region. These findings suggest that some of the genetic abnormalities predisposing to depression may be associated with significant structural changes in the brain. Such changes influence the connectivity within and across specific brain systems, and it is likely that these changes in connectivity contribute to risk for mood disorder. As we will discuss in subsequent chapters, it is currently unclear how the changes in brain structure and function arise and whether they are actually causal changes or the consequence of illness, although studies in children and adolescents increasingly suggest that at least some of the brain changes antedate significant clinical symptoms. The important point is that these changes are associated with a specific form of depression and are not necessarily found in other forms of depression.

A different clinical scenario might involve a patient who developed cocaine dependence as a teenager. This patient was seen in the emergency room on several occasions with severe, short-lived depressive symptoms time-linked to coming off cocaine highs. Each time, his symptoms were dramatic and involved significant suicidal ideation, but resolved over several hours without specific intervention. After several years of cocaine addiction, the patient again was seen in the emergency room with severe depressive symptoms, but this time the symptoms did not resolve as quickly as before when he came off his high. His clinical presentation included a full spectrum of depressive symptoms, including thoughts of suicide. He was admitted to the hospital, but his depressive symptoms persisted for several days. With resolution of his suicidal thoughts, the patient was transferred to a residential treatment program for management of his chemical dependency. After 3 weeks of cocaine abstinence and group therapy, depressive symptoms resolved. Although he continued to have a strong desire to use cocaine, he began to develop insight into his addiction and the connection between his cocaine dependence and his mood symptoms. He stayed clean for 3 months before relapsing. During those 3 months, he did not experience depressive symptoms.

This person demonstrates two types of depressive syndromes that are every bit as severe as the symptoms observed in the individual with familial major depression. The earlier presentations to the emergency room resulted from pharmacologic withdrawal from cocaine. This withdrawal acutely disrupted one or more of the neural systems related to mood regulation; it likely involved abnormal function of the dopamine transmitter system that is involved in motivational processing and is a prime target for drugs of abuse like cocaine. The disruption was acute and time-linked to the short-term effects of coming off the cocaine high. While severe, the depressive symptoms lasted for only several hours. This syndrome would not qualify for a diagnosis of major depression, but it does illustrate that perturbation of neural systems can acutely cause a depression-like picture. The longer-lasting depressive picture that occurred several years later was likely related to a longer-term dysregulation of the patient's central reward system as a result of persistent cocaine dependence. In this case, the depressive syndrome lasted several weeks but gradually resolved after several weeks of behavioral treatment and abstinence from cocaine.

In earlier terminology championed by Eli Robins and Sam Guze at Washington University-St. Louis, this more persistent depressive syndrome would be referred to as a "secondary depression." This means that the depression occurred subsequent to the onset of an addictive disorder and thus was "secondary" in time to the cocaine dependence. Importantly, cocaine dependence was already running its course prior to the onset of persistent mood symptoms and was thus having a significant impact on brain networks, including those involved in mood regulation and cognition. Note, however, that the term "secondary depression" does not imply causality; it indicates only that the depressive syndrome occurred at some point in time after the onset of drug abuse. In contrast, a "primary" depression is one that arises in the absence of a preexisting psychiatric or serious medical disorder. We believe this distinction is useful conceptually because it helps to differentiate subtypes of depression, including separating depression in the context of cocaine dependence from the highly familial ("primary") mood disorder described previously. This also highlights the possibility that the neural pathways leading to depression and dysfunction may be different. In the examples presented, the "primary" depressions likely involve prominent changes in emotional processing systems (e.g., abnormal function and perhaps cell loss in subgenual cingulate cortex, neocortex, and amygdala), while the "secondary" depression occurred in the context of cocaine-induced changes in motivation/reward systems. We would further argue that treatments for the different types of depression should be tailored to the underlying brain dysfunction. Failure to recognize this may be a contributing factor to the overall weak remission rates observed in recent large-scale clinical effectiveness trials such as STAR*D, where early age of onset and high psychiatric and medical comorbidity were predictors of worse outcomes.

Although the cocaine-dependent patient's depressive symptoms resolved, his craving for cocaine did not, and he returned to the use of cocaine several months after discharge from the residential treatment center. Several years later, he once again was hospitalized for treatment of depressive symptoms and cocaine addiction. This time, however, his depressive symptoms did not resolve after several weeks of abstinence. After another month of treatment for his drug addiction in a residential facility, he was able to remain abstinent for years; however, his depressive symptoms were more persistent. Eventually, this depressive disorder responded to a combination of medications, psychotherapy, and lifestyle changes, including diet, exercise, and abstinence from drugs. Based on what we are learning about the biology of drug addiction, it is likely that this patient's long-term substance dependence led to structural and functional changes in his central reward system as well as in his emotional processing and cognitive systems. Such changes required pharmacologic, psychological, and lifestyle interventions to help the neural systems regain function.

Contrast these two scenarios with the depressions frequently observed in individuals with bipolar disorder, an illness characterized by episodes of both mania and depression. Although a person with bipolar depression is likely to have abnormalities in brain systems that overlap with those involved in the previous two cases, these abnormalities result from neural mechanisms that cause bipolar disorder, an illness that typically runs in families and at times presents with depression and psychotic features. The causes of bipolar disorder are not known, but mood stabilizers, as opposed to antidepressants, are the initial drug category of choice for treatment. Appropriate treatment might involve a mood stabilizer coupled with antipsychotic medication and, when appropriate, talk therapy and education about the importance of good sleeping habits and other routines that help circadian rhythms stay on track. Interestingly, there is evidence that bipolar disorder tends to worsen over time in some individuals, with more frequent episodes of illness and shorter periods of wellness between episodes. This led Robert Post and colleagues to propose that a "kindling" or behavioral sensitization phenomenon occurs in these individuals, and they conducted trials of anticonvulsant medications as "anti-kindling" mood stabilizers. It also appears that conventional antidepressant medications may worsen the course of bipolar disorder, leading to greater instability in some individuals. Thus, it is likely that the brain biology of bipolar disorder differs from the depression scenarios outlined previously. Note also that bipolar disorder is a form of "primary" mood disorder that probably shares some, but not all, mechanisms with primary major depression. For example, subjects with bipolar disorder have shrinkage and cell loss in subgenual cingulate cortex, but they clearly have illness features that differ from non-bipolar mood disorders.

These are only a few of the different "types" of depression routinely encountered in clinical practice. Other examples include depressions arising in the context of personality disorders (e.g., borderline personality disorder or somatization disorder) or serious medical illnesses (e.g., cardiac illnesses, cancer, or diabetes). The symptoms of these disorders are all similar, but the underlying brain mechanisms are likely to be different. Furthermore, appropriate treatments are likely to vary as a function of the cause of the syndrome, not the clinical phenotype. Patients in our examples usually experienced weeks of the symptoms listed in DSM-IV; however, the triggers for their symptoms were different and even changed over time within the same individual depending on other variables (e.g., the duration of cocaine abuse). From a neuroscience perspective, clinical symptoms result from abnormal functioning of specific brain networks. Treatments, on the other hand, fall into two broad categories: rehabilitative treatments and cause-based treatments. Rehabilitative treatments are not specific to the etiology of the illness; they decrease symptoms by influencing the brain in a manner that bypasses or minimizes the dysfunctional system. For instance, certain psychotherapies teach people methods to minimize depressive symptoms by training them to think differently. This new learning may establish or re-establish brain circuits that promote clinical improvement. A cause-based treatment would directly fix the broken circuitry. Current antidepressants and mood stabilizers are not cause-based therapies. Rather, these drugs likely work by enhancing function in certain dysfunctional systems even though the primary defects in the malfunctioning circuits aren't actually fixed. The key point we want to emphasize is that DSM-IV "major depression" is an extremely heterogeneous set of disorders. We don't yet know whether the neural circuitry involved in depression is the same or different across illness subtypes. What seems highly likely is that the neural pathways leading to depression can vary according to subtype, and this has practical implications for how we think about diagnosis and treatment. We believe that lumping all depressions together makes no more sense than lumping all cancers or dementing illnesses together. To make these latter points more vivid, we will turn our attention to recent advances in understanding the pathobiology of dementing illnesses—advances that graphically highlight how brain network dysfunction drives clinical presentation, while effective treatment strategies target causal molecular mechanisms.

DEMENTIAS

Much progress has been made in understanding Alzheimer's disease. In contrast to primary psychiatric disorders, the term "Alzheimer's disease" refers to a specific pathology-based diagnosis that cannot yet be definitively confirmed until examination of the brain at autopsy. Thus, when Alzheimer's disease is suspected clinically, it is diagnosed as "dementia of the Alzheimer's type" (DAT), reflecting uncertainty about the underlying pathological process. The clinical phenotype and course of DAT are well described, and the structural abnormalities in the brain underlying Alzheimer's disease are well characterized. Another well-defined dementia is known as behavioral variant frontotemporal dementia (bvFTD). Recent studies of DAT and bvFTD are providing information that is clarifying the relationship between clinical presentation (phenotype) and cause (molecular mechanisms). In this section, we will briefly review the clinical picture of both dementias. In addition, we will discuss recent information pertaining to two brain networks—the *default* system and the *emotional-salience* system—and the ways in which these neural networks appear to contribute to illness. Core neural systems like these are called "intrinsic connectivity networks" (ICNs) by some neuroscientists, and these ICNs appear to process specific types of information. Measuring biomarkers in individuals thought to show indications of a dementing illness can also provide information that is likely to have a direct impact on treatment. We believe that the information learned from clinical phenotypes, neural systems, and causes of these two dementias has substantial implications for understanding other psychiatric disorders. While we note that the descriptor "ICN" is used by some by not all neuroscientists, we prefer this terminology and will use it throughout the book. Others refer to these networks as "resting state connectivity networks" or "functional connectivity networks."

Dementia of the Alzheimer's Type

DAT is characterized by gradual deterioration in many brain functions, including memory, thinking, executive function (decision making), learning, and personality. It is a disorder that becomes increasingly common with aging: about half the population over age 85 exhibits symptoms of DAT. The brains of persons with DAT have characteristic structural changes that involve the accumulation of two polypeptides (proteins): beta-amyloid and hyperphosphorylated *tau*. Beta-amyloid accumulates outside of cells and forms a visible microscopic structure called an amyloid plaque. *Tau* is a protein involved in the function of microtubules that are involved in the efficient trafficking of molecules within neurons. Hyperphosphorylated *tau* accumulates inside neurons and destroys their ability to transport materials from the cell body to distant parts of the cell (synaptic terminals). The accumulated *tau* forms pathological "tangles" inside neurons. Both plaques and tangles eventually interfere with neuronal function and intercellular communication. Interference with function leads to neuronal loss and the clinical symptoms of DAT.

Certain specific brain regions appear to be involved earlier than others in the course of DAT, and this information provides clues about how clinical symptoms develop and evolve. These brain regions include the hippocampus, areas near the hippocampus such as the entorhinal cortex, and neurons in the precuneus, a region of neocortex located toward the back of the brain near the posterior cingulate gyrus (see Appendix for structural brain maps that indicate the anatomical location of these areas). These structures overlap with brain regions that make up a neural network called the "default" system, which is a collection of broadly distributed brain regions that are functionally connected. Using neuroimaging techniques such as positron emission tomography (PET) or functional magnetic resonance imaging (fMRI), investigators have shown that brain activity in each of the structures involved in the default system correlates highly with each other (Fig. 2-1 and Table 2-1). This default ICN is most active when a person isn't focusing on a particular task (hence the name "default" network). At such times, structures in the default system are all humming together in correlated activity and processing largely internal (intra-self) information, including memories, emotions, and overall state of well-being (Table 2-2). Interestingly, the default system uses a lot of energy when other regions of the brain are "resting," and the regions of the default ICN are among the most energy-demanding areas in the human brain. It appears that the heavy energy demand in the default system makes these brain regions particularly susceptible to the earliest damage in DAT. Furthermore, there is evidence that the demands of ongoing synaptic activity may be a key factor rendering these regions vulnerable to amyloid deposition, and current thinking highlights synaptic dysfunction as a

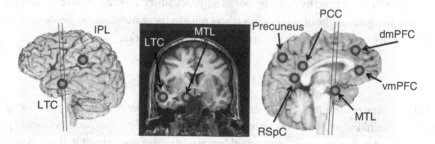

Figure 2-1 Key nodes of the default mode network. The figure depicts key structures involved in the default mode network as defined by Marc Raichle, Randy Buckner, and others. The highlighted regions include the lateral temporal cortex (LTC), inferior parietal lobule (IPL), precuneus, retrosplenial cortex (RSpC), posterior cingulate cortex (PCC), dorsomedial PFC (dmPFC), ventromedial PFC (vmPFC), and medial temporal lobe (MTL), including the hippocampus. The lines through the brain reconstructions indicate the approximate location that is shown in the radiologic image. (Adapted from Damasio, 2005, with permission.)

Table 2-1 Default Network: Key Structures

Medial temporal lobe
  Hippocampus
  Entorhinal and parahippocampal cortex
Lateral temporal cortex
Dorsomedial prefrontal cortex
Ventromedial prefrontal cortex
Posterior cingulate, precuneus, and retrosplenial cortex
Inferior parietal lobule

---

prime driver in the pathogenesis of Alzheimer's disease. The key point is that the regions involved early in DAT appear to be the same regions involved in a specific brain network. It is logical to propose that malfunction of this network drives at least the early clinical manifestations of DAT. A principle evolving from this work is that when dysfunction/degeneration occurs within a specific network, it tends to spread within the network, perhaps as a result of coordinated neural activity within the system.

Behavioral Variant Frontotemporal Dementia

bvFTD is much less common than DAT. It also tends to occur in younger people, with age of onset typically between 50 and 60 years. The most obvious symptoms involve profound changes in social behavior. For example, a well-mannered person may gradually demonstrate behaviors that are grossly inappropriate, like telling obscene jokes in public settings or becoming overly friendly and even sexually inappropriate with strangers. These new-onset behaviors are embarrassing to family and friends but are not usually recognized by the individual. Other changes may accompany these inappropriate behaviors, including changes in eating habits, sex drive, and speech. Cognitive tasks become more difficult, and changes in memory and thinking similar to those found in persons with DAT develop.

A recent report by William Seeley and colleagues suggested that the brains of people with bvFTD demonstrate a breakdown in a specific ICN known as the "emotional-salience system" (Table 2-3 and Fig. 2-2). This system involves several limbic and cortical brain regions that help to process emotions and meaning (Table 2-4). The cause

Table 2-2 Default Network: Internally Focused Functions

Autobiographical memories
  Encoding and retrieval
Mood and motivation state
Mental simulations
  "Remembering" the future
Social interactions
  Conceiving perspectives of others (theory of mind)

Table 2-3 Emotional-Salience Network: Key Structures

Frontal and anterior insula cortex
   Anterior cingulate cortex
   Orbital fronto-insular cortex
   Frontopolar cortex
Temporal polar cortex
Extended amygdala
Ventral striatopallidum
   Ventral tegmental area/substantia nigra
Hypothalamus and periaqueductal gray

of the breakdown in the emotional-salience system may involve abnormalities in specific proteins. These include a protein called TDP-43 (TAR DNA-binding protein 43), another that is an abnormal form of *tau*, and yet another called FUS (fused in sarcoma). The form of *tau* involved in bvFTD differs from the hyperphosphorylated *tau* seen in DAT. It is important to note, however, that on rare occasions, the protein abnormalities associated with DAT, leading to the formation of plaques and tangles, can cause the clinical syndrome of bvFTD. This suggests that amyloid and hyperphosphorylated *tau* can, in some individuals, selectively attack the emotional-salience system instead of the default system. Interestingly, such patients have a

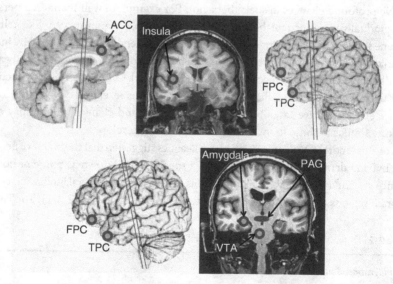

Figure 2-2 Key nodes of the emotional-salience system. The figure depicts key structures involved in the emotional-salience network as defined by William Seeley and colleagues. Highlighted regions include the anterior cingulate cortex (ACC), insular cortex, frontopolar cortex (FPC), temporal polar cortex (TPC), amygdala, periaqueductal gray area (PAG), and ventral tegmental area (VTA). The lines through the brain reconstructions indicate the approximate locations that are shown in the radiologic images. (Adapted from Damasio, 2005, with permission.)

Table 2-4 Emotional-Salience Network Function

Conflict monitoring
Interoceptive awareness
Autonomic nervous system processing
Reward processing

clinical syndrome that is indistinguishable from bvFTD caused by TDP-43, FUS, or the non-DAT form of *tau*. Why would the emotional-salience system be more vulnerable to plaque and tangle pathology in some individuals (resulting in bvFTD) while the default system is more vulnerable in other individuals (resulting in DAT)? We don't yet know, but a key finding seems to be that once pathology attacks a particular ICN, it seems to percolate throughout that ICN and lead to characteristic clinical features that reflect the function of the ICN.

Importantly, in both DAT and bvFTD, the phenotype of the dementia (i.e., the clinical manifestation of the disorder) appears to be defined by the specific neural networks that are being disrupted. The clinical phenotype does not always define the biochemical cause of that disruption. Most but not all persons with DAT have amyloid plaque and *tau* tangle pathology. There are now brain-imaging techniques that are able to demonstrate amyloid accumulation in humans during life (using Pittsburgh Compound B [PIB] to label amyloid, for example), and this work has the potential to allow earlier identification of individuals at high risk for DAT and perhaps early intervention. Studies using PIB are already demonstrating changes in resting-state default-mode connectivity in elderly individuals who are cognitively normal. How and whether these early changes drive a progression to dementia will be an important consideration going forward. In addition, DAT appears to be associated with decreased levels of amyloid and increased levels of *tau* in cerebrospinal fluid (CSF), changes that can be assessed by lumbar puncture, a relatively simple clinical procedure. These changes, like amyloid deposition in the brain, may occur prior to the onset of clinical symptoms. We are not far away from the time when physicians will be able to use imaging procedures and CSF biomarker studies to determine whether a phenotypic DAT is associated with amyloid plaques in the brain and diminished CSF amyloid. This information will allow physicians to determine whether an individual's DAT is likely caused by amyloid and abnormal *tau*. When such changes are identified prior to any symptoms, it may be possible to delay or prevent the development of clinical DAT. In fact, treatments are currently being tested that are directed at eliminating the initial accumulation of pathological levels of amyloid (i.e., the proposed cause of the disorder). If amyloid accumulation is the proximal cause of the destruction of the default system (something that is still not certain), then the clinical manifestations of the illness may be halted or perhaps even prevented by decreasing amyloid formation or by increasing its elimination. This cause-based mechanistic treatment is in contrast to current symptomatic treatments for DAT. Support and education can help families and patients handle the illness better—a form of rehabilitative treatment. Cholinesterase inhibitors may influence one brain system that allows for short-term stabilization of symptoms, but these medications certainly do not treat the actual cause of the disorder.

It should also be possible to apply imaging and biomarker procedures to people with bvFTD and use the results as the basis for rational treatments. For example, if a patient with bvFTD shows amyloid plaques on imaging and decreased amyloid in the CSF, it is likely that the etiology of that patient's bvFTD is amyloid-based instead of being caused by the other proteins more typically associated with bvFTD. This would suggest that anti-amyloid therapy would be helpful in this particular patient with bvFTD, something that could not have been predicted on the basis of the clinical picture alone. In this example, the clinical phenotype would be bvFTD; however, the imaging and biomarker modifiers would suggest that the etiology of this particular case of bvFTD involves amyloid and hyperphosphorylated *tau*. Eventually, it may be possible to measure levels of other abnormal proteins in CSF or plasma, such as TDP-43. With such measurements, physicians will have a more specific understanding of the cause of the clinical syndrome. The clinical phenotype predicts the current and future clinical course of the illness, but the biomarker data suggest the underlying pathology.

Will these types of advances ever be applicable to the depressive disorders or other psychiatric illnesses? We clearly know the clinical phenotype in depression. As more is learned about the different causes of depression, we should be able to be more specific in terms of treatments. Akin to DAT and bvFTD, the clinical phenotype will be determined by the specific brain networks involved in the primary pathophysiology, while the cellular, synaptic, and molecular mechanisms leading to abnormal function will likely be the targets for specific treatment approaches. One can also imagine that specific rehabilitative efforts (i.e., behavioral, lifestyle, and psychotherapeutic strategies) could be directed toward restoring function in the disrupted brain networks involved.

Similarly, progress in understanding DAT and bvFTD should lead to optimism about understanding disorders such as schizophrenia and bipolar disorder. For physicians to understand the clinical ramifications of this progress, we suggest that psychiatrists and mental health professionals must understand the neuroscience underlying these advances. We will continue to develop this theme throughout this book.

Points to Remember

The clinical phenotype (i.e., signs and symptoms of a disorder) reflects the nature of the neural networks that are involved in the illness.

There are many causes of dysfunction in specific neural networks. Borrowing from advances in the dementing illnesses, it appears that specific clinical disorders and pathology can attack specific brain systems. The reason that certain brain systems are vulnerable to attack is not yet clear. Networks with high activity and high energy utilization may be particularly vulnerable in illnesses like DAT.

The more specific the knowledge of a particular cellular and molecular cause, the more specific the pharmacologic treatment can be.

Understanding basic principles of neural networks, molecular sciences, and clinical diagnoses will be essential for keeping up to date with specific treatments.

SUGGESTED READINGS

Buckner, R. L., Andrews-Hanna, J. R., & Schacter, D. L. (2008). The brain's default network: anatomy, function and relevance to disease. *Annals of the New York Academy of Science, 1124,* 1–38.

Kertesz, A. (2008). Frontotemporal dementia: A topical review. *Cognitive and Behavioral Neurology, 21,* 127–133.

Koob, G. F., & Volkow, N. D. (2010). Neurocircuitry of addiction. *Neuropsychopharmacology Reviews, 35,* 217–238.

Morris, J. C. (2006). Alzheimer's disease and mild cognitive impairment. In J. C. Morris, J. E. Galvin, & D. M. Holtzman (Eds.), *Handbook of dementing illnesses* (2nd ed., pp. 191–208). New York: Taylor & Francis.

Morris, J. C. (2006). Dementia update 2006. In J. C. Morris, J. E. Galvin, & D. M. Holtzman (Eds.), *Handbook of dementing illnesses* (2nd ed., pp. 475–503). New York: Taylor & Francis.

Price, J. L., & Drevets, W. C. (2010). Neurocircuitry of mood disorders. *Neuropsychopharmacology Reviews, 35,* 192–216.

Rabinovici, G. D. & Miller, B. L. (2010). Frontotemporal lobar degeneration: Epidemiology, pathophysiology, diagnosis and management. *CNS Drugs, 24,* 375–398.

Seeley, W. W., Crawford, R. K., Zhou, J., Miller, B. L., & Greicius, M. D. (2009). Neurodegenerative diseases target large-scale human brain networks. *Neuron, 62,* 42–52.

OTHER REFERENCES

American Psychiatric Association. (1994). *Diagnostic and statistical manual of mental disorders* (4th ed.). Washington, DC: American Psychiatric Association.

Buckner, R. L., Sepulcre, J., Talukdar, T., Krienen, F. M., Liu, H., Hedden, T., et al. (2009). Cortical hubs revealed by intrinsic functional connectivity: Mapping, assessment of stability, and relation to Alzheimer's disease. *Journal of Neuroscience, 29,* 1860–1873.

Buckner, R. L., Snyder, A. Z., Shannon, B. J., LaRossa, G., Sachs, R., Fotenos, A. F., et al. (2005). Molecular, structural and functional characterization of Alzheimer's disease: Evidence for a relationship between default activity, amyloid and memory. *Journal of Neuroscience, 25,* 7709–7717.

Craig-Schapiro, R., Fagan, A. M., & Holtzman, D. M. (2009). Biomarkers of Alzheimer's disease. *Neurobiology of Disease, 35,* 1288–1140.

Damasio, A. (1999). *The feeling of what happens: Body and emotion in the making of consciousness.* San Diego, CA: Harcourt.

Damasio, H. (2005). *Human brain anatomy in computerized images* (2nd ed.). New York: Oxford University Press.

Duyckaerts, C., Delatour, B., & Potier. M.-C. (2009). Classification and basic pathology of Alzheimer disease. *Acta Neuropathologica, 118,* 5–36.

Fagan, A. M., Roe, C. M., Xiong, C., Mintun, M. A., Morris, J. C., & Holtzman, D. M. (2007). Cerebrospinal fluid tau/β-amyloid$_{42}$ ratio as a prediction of cognitive decline in nondemented older adults. *Archives of Neurology, 64,* 343–349.

Josephs, K. A. (2008). Frontotemporal dementia and related disorders: Deciphering the enigma. *Annals of Neurology, 64,* 4–14.

Palop, J. J., & Mucke, L. (2010). Amyloid-β-induced neuronal dysfunction in Alzheimer's disease: From synapses toward neural networks. *Nature Neuroscience, 13,* 812–818.

Peterson, B. S., Warner, V., Bansal, R., Zhu, H., Hao, X., Liu, J., et al. (2009). Cortical thinning in persons at increased familial risk for major depression. *Proceedings of the National Academy of Sciences (USA), 106,* 6273–6278.

Post, R. M. (2007). Kindling and sensitization as models for affective episode recurrence, cyclicity and tolerance phenomena. *Neuroscience and Biobehavioral Reviews, 31,* 858–873.

Rush, A. J. (2007). STAR*D: What have we learned? *American Journal of Psychiatry, 164,* 201–204.

Sheline, Y. I., Raichle, M. E., Snyder, A. Z., Morris, J. C., Head, D., Wang, S., et al. (2010). Amyloid plaques disrupt resting state default mode network connectivity in cognitively normal elderly. *Biological Psychiatry, 67,* 584–587.

Snider, B. J., Fagan, A. M., Roe, C., Shah, A. R., Grant, E. A., Xiong, C., et al. (2009). Cerebrospinal fluid biomarkers and rate of cognitive decline in very mild dementia of the Alzheimer type. *Archives of Neurology, 66,* 638–645.

Sperling, R. A., Laviolette, P. S., O'Keefe, K., O'Brien, J., Rentz, D. M., Pihlajamaki, M., et al. (2009). Amyloid deposition is associated with impaired default network function in older persons without dementia. *Neuron 63,* 178–188.

3

Systems Neuroscience and Psychiatry
Basic Principles

THE BRAIN IS COMPLEX BUT NOT HOPELESS

A major difficulty in understanding the mechanisms underlying psychiatric disorders is that these illnesses affect the most complicated organ in the human body and alter the most complicated aspects of that organ, the features of the human brain that make us most human. We are only at the beginning of understanding how the brain is organized and how it generates thought, emotion, and motivation. Thus, psychiatry is at a much more primitive stage of scientific development than neurology, although there are clear areas of overlap between the two disciplines. Indeed, there are areas in neurology that are at least as poorly understood as those in psychiatry, including the cognitive (dementing) illnesses outlined in Chapter 2 and several disorders considered part of behavioral neurology, such as the various forms of epilepsy and traumatic brain injury. Interestingly, these are areas where neurology and psychiatry have a great deal of overlap.

It is an understatement to say that the brain is complicated. Reasonable estimates indicate that human brains have at least 100 billion (10^{11}) neurons. These cells handle input, create output, and are the workhorses for brain computations. In turn, each neuron may have 100,000 (10^5) or more connections (synapses) with other neurons, resulting in a total number of about 10^{15} to 10^{16} direct neuronal connections, a staggering and largely incomprehensible number by any definition. Complicating this further, glial cells, the cells that are typically thought to provide support for neurons, outnumber neurons by about 5 to 10:1. Glial cells, particularly astrocytes, are more than passive participants in brain function, however. They provide energy for neurons and work with neurons to regulate how the chemicals that mediate transmission between neurons are stored, processed, and released. Also, through a process called gliotransmission, glial cells can release neurotransmitters and modulate neuronal activity. Thus, they also participate in the computational work of the brain.

The task of understanding how this huge number of cells and connections works to produce thought, emotion, and behavior is daunting. Perhaps because of this complexity and because the clinical aspects of psychiatry deal with "softer" and less well-defined aspects of clinical neuroscience, most psychiatrists seem to use indirect and metaphorical concepts in discussing how the brain contributes to psychopathology. By "softer" we don't mean to imply that psychiatric problems aren't real, only that they are less directly tied to specific hard-wired brain pathways and have much less well-defined brain pathology. These are features that typically make neurology a more tractable and, from a psychiatric perspective, less interesting field of study.

To deal with brain complexity, some psychiatrists (we hope a diminishing minority) abdicate the effort and treat the brain as a "black box." In such a conceptual approach, input arrives, gets processed in some mysterious fashion by the "black box," and results in observable output (speech, behavior, mood, etc.). These psychiatrists and other mental health professionals focus on the outputs and what to do about outputs that result in dysfunction; little thought is given to the processing that occurs within the brain. Such approaches can result in a host of well-intentioned but ill-conceived ideas about how to explain thinking and behavior, including ego psychology, repressed memories, and certain approaches loosely based on behaviorism, among others. The major problem with the "black box" approach is its lack of grounding in how the brain produces thought, emotion, and behavior.

An alternative approach that many "biological psychiatrists" use is to describe brain function, illness, and treatments in chemical terms, treating the brain as a "chemical organ." The advantage of this approach is that it deals with the fact that neurons and glia use neurochemicals to send and receive messages. Also, it takes advantage of the fact that psychopharmacological treatments manipulate the activity of well-known neurotransmitter systems and can lead to beneficial responses. Examples of neurotransmitters familiar to psychiatrists include glutamate, the major fast excitatory transmitter in the human brain; gamma-aminobutyric acid (GABA), the major fast inhibitory transmitter; and the biogenic amines (dopamine, norepinephrine, and serotonin). The biogenic amines have become household names and are important modulators that help to coordinate activity within and across regions of the brain; they are also major targets of many psychoactive drugs. The "chemical organ" approach has led to some interesting, although not always correct, hypotheses about the causes of psychiatric disorders. Examples include the "dopamine theory of schizophrenia," the "catecholamine theory of depression," and the "serotonin theory of depression and anxiety." A weakness of this approach is that these theories don't explain very effectively how the brain actually generates behavior, thought, and emotions. Furthermore, this approach is prone to overly simplistic explanations for illnesses, including the archaic ideas that psychiatric disorders result from "chemical imbalances" or are the product of "leaky synapses," concepts that sound more profound than they actually are.

Our premise is that psychiatrists must become better versed in systems and network neuroscience and better acquainted with the ways in which neural systems generate thinking, emotions, and motivation in order for the field to take advantage of the promise modern neuroscience offers for psychiatric patients. Understanding the brain at this level will dovetail with the chemical organ hypothesis outlined previously as a means to understand how brain systems operate and are connected. An issue for conveying and conceptualizing this information is the level of detail necessary for psychiatrists to know. Brain wiring diagrams that map the connections among brain regions can be extremely arcane and can lead to the hopeless idea that "everything is connected to everything." While at one level this seems to be true, we believe that an intermediate strategy dealing with how neurons function and with how key circuits operate can help to overcome intellectual despair. A mounting body of evidence concerned with the operations and pathophysiology of intrinsic connectivity networks (ICNs) is a great place to start.

NETWORK THEORY AND BRAIN SYSTEMS

Before delving into ICNs, it is important to understand a bit about modern network theory and how biological systems are thought to be organized. Such background provides a conceptual foothold for thinking about how neural systems work. This discussion takes us into the science of "small-world" and "scale-free" networks; principles derived from this work seem to apply to a variety of biological networks ranging from genes and proteins to neuronal connections and higher-order neural systems. Perhaps even more surprising, these same network approaches have relevance for describing human social interactions and for understanding how problems like epidemics, cigarette smoking, and obesity cluster and spread within human populations.

To understand how a network operates, it is important to describe several parameters: the system structure (how it is organized and wired together), system dynamics (how it changes over time and reacts to perturbations), control methods (how the system regulates itself or is regulated by other systems), and the overall design methods (how it is modified and grows). Although the application of network theory to brain systems is still relatively new, it is providing a lot of insights into psychiatric and neuropsychiatric illnesses.

Early work on network organization was based on mathematical principles that were developed in the 1950s by Paul Erdos and colleagues and dealt with the structure of "regular" networks. In such a network, each node has about the same number of connections as any other node. A "node" is an individual point of connection within a network; for example, a single person in a social network, a neuron in a synaptic network, or a brain region in a higher-order neural system. The regular network model works well for describing some networks like the U.S. highway system, where each major city has about the same number of major roads coming in and going out. The problem is that biological and human social networks are more complicated, and nodes can vary greatly with respect to how many connections they have, how their connections are organized, and how strong the connections are.

Network science was advanced by social scientists in the 1960s and 1970s who found that human networks have a high degree of local clustering as in a regular network, reflecting individuals who are closely affiliated, but also exhibit shortcuts between clusters that allow for effective information transfer. This is the essence of "small-world" connectivity outlined by Stanley Milgram, showing that humans have a high degree of relatedness to each other. This is famously known as "six degrees of separation," a phenomenon indicating that all humans are connected to one another via their social ties; none of us is more than about six contacts away from persons in

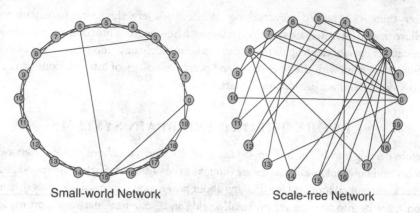

Small-world Network **Scale-free Network**

Figure 3-1 Small-world vs. scale-free networks. The left graph depicts the connectivity of a small-world network in which a few longer-range connections are interposed within a regular network. The right graph shows a scale-free network in which there are a few highly connected nodes along with some long-range connections. (Models provided by Larry Eisenman, Washington University in St. Louis.)

the most remote parts of the planet. Thus, a friend of a friend of a friend of your personal friend and so on can connect you to quite distant areas of our planet.

Duncan Watts and Steven Strogatz pursued these concepts further in the 1990s by analyzing several well-characterized real-world networks, including the connectivity of cells in the nervous system of the roundworm, *Caenorhabditis elegans*. They found that the *pattern* of connections in these networks followed a "small-world" topology in which there was a high degree of clustering with a few long-range connections that allowed certain clusters to have significant impact on other clusters. This topology is intermediate between completely regular and completely random connectivity. Such "small-world" networks, as they are called, are described by their *path length* (a measure of the distance between any two nodes) and *clustering coefficient* (a measure of the relatedness or connectedness of a local neighborhood of nodes). The "small-world" phenomenon occurs when there is a significant drop in path length resulting from a few long-range shortcuts in networks that are otherwise very highly clustered at a local level (Fig. 3-1). Importantly, the long-range connections don't have to be very strong in order to have a major impact on network function. Mark Granovetter described this cogently in the 1970s in his studies of how humans use their social network to perform tasks. When seeking a new job, for example, it is typically a person's weaker connections to people who are more peripheral in his or her social spheres who help the most, largely because these connections differ from and complement those of closer associates. Granovetter referred to this as the "strength of weak ties," a notion that current research in neuroscience is showing may have as much relevance to brain function as to human social networks.

Albert-Laszlo Barabesi and colleagues extended this work by examining the *distribution* of connections in biological and social networks. They proposed that real networks have a "scale-free" type of connectivity. Here, the distribution of connections follows a "power law" in which most nodes in a system have only a few connections, but a few nodes in the network have a lot of connections. Thus, the distribution of the number of connections that nodes have is a rapidly decreasing function of the number of nodes in the network, and there is no true "average" number of connections within the network with which to create a measure to "scale" the network (hence they are called "scale-free"). This is in distinction to a "normal distribution" of connections described by a "bell-shaped curve"; here the majority of nodes would have about the same number of connections and, therefore, there would be a true "average" number of connections.

Importantly, a scale-free topology is characteristic of self-organizing systems and results in a network in which there are *hubs* of connectivity (much like the map of U.S. airline routes, where a few cities, like New York and Los Angeles, are highly connected, while most others, like Topeka and Omaha, have only a few routes coming in and out) (see Fig. 3-1). This type of distribution is sometimes referred to as the "80–20 law"—that is, 20% of nodes have 80% of the connections. This is also referred to as the Pareto Principle (economics) or Zipf's Law (linguistics) when used to describe the distribution of wealth in a population or words in a written text, respectively. A scale-free connectivity distribution is found in many biological and social systems, including the U.S. power grid, the Internet, and the nervous system of *C. elegans*. It also has major implications for network dynamics and may predict how a network develops and grows. For example, network growth is thought to result, at least in part, from preferential attachment of new nodes to highly connected existing nodes. In effect, the "rich get richer," in Barabesi's terms. Such a system is highly robust because attacks on individual nodes rarely disrupt network function; this is because most nodes have only a few connections and aren't critical to network function. In contrast, damage to a few highly connected nodes can greatly disrupt the network. Thus, scale-free networks are very tolerant to damage to most individual nodes but can experience cascading failures if enough major nodes are disrupted.

This work on small-world and scale-free networks is relevant to systems neuroscience. These types of connectivity appear to be extremely important for understanding how ICNs are organized in the brain and may be important for explaining why certain brain structures seem to show up in multiple systems, resulting in the important but frustrating idea that "everything is connected to everything." Current data support the idea that the brain is organized into circuits that are a series of closed loops rather than a hierarchy. These brain networks have small-world properties that are important for efficient information flow. It is less clear that the scale-free topology pertains, although some brain regions are more heavily connected than others and have hub-like properties, including power law connectivity. We will use both the small-world and scale-free perspectives in our discussion, but we readily admit that this is an evolving area of science. We believe that these concepts are also important for understanding why the brain is as robust as it is and why, with rare exceptions, the brain doesn't "crash" like a computer. Interestingly, however, recent studies have examined how dysfunction of nodes in one network of an interdependent set of networks can have a negative influence on non-damaged networks. These observations may be relevant for understanding why psychiatric disorders result in

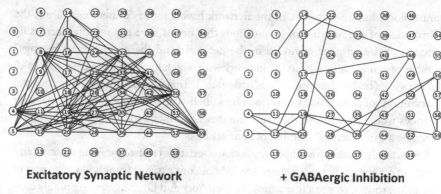

Excitatory Synaptic Network   **+ GABAergic Inhibition**

Figure 3-2 Effects of inhibition on a neural network. This figure displays correlations in neuronal firing in a culture of rat hippocampal neurons using multi-electrode array (MEA) recordings. The small numbered circles in the figure represent recording electrodes. Lines in the graph depict neurons that fire in a coordinated (correlated) fashion. As shown in the diagram on the left, some "nodes" are highly connected (e.g., #59). When GABAergic inhibition is added to the network, correlated firing is diminished and the pattern of connectivity changes dramatically, as depicted in the diagram on the right. (Data provided by Larry Eisenman, Washington University in St. Louis.)

dysfunction across multiple neural systems. Recent work has also examined how "stress" affects network development and topology, and results suggest that milder stresses on a system help to drive initially random networks toward scale-free connectivity as a means of becoming more robust and self-sustaining. Unfortunately, greater and more persistent stress can cause disintegration of connectivity and a breakdown of the system as highly connected hubs are damaged. We will return to the theme of stress and network function in a later chapter. Also, in neuronal networks different forms of synaptic transmission (excitatory vs. inhibitory) can have a significant impact on network topology and activity. Figure 3-2 shows results from an experiment that highlights the impact of manipulating fast GABA-mediated inhibition in a network of cultured hippocampal neurons.

ORGANIZATION OF THE BRAIN

To discuss how brain systems contribute to psychiatric disorders, it is important to have a "big picture" understanding of how the brain is organized. For this discussion, we will again borrow from Joseph LeDoux and his book *Synaptic Self*. LeDoux described several basic concepts that are important for psychiatrists to understand. Some of these concepts may seem self-evident and even trivial, but they have profound implications for later discussions of ICNs and their roles in psychiatric symptoms and illnesses.

When viewed from a high level, the brain is organized as a collection of parallel processing systems. These parallel systems all perceive and act upon the same information, the world of the individual human being. This may seem trivial, but because there are many parallel systems processing information simultaneously, mismatches in how and when information is processed in one brain system relative to another can lead to major distortions in "reality." This is clearly a fundamental defect in the disconnection syndromes described in Chapter 1. There is debate about how many processing systems exist in the brain, but the number is relatively large—at least 15, depending on how subsystems are categorized. For example, we receive separate inputs from each of our five primary senses (vision, hearing, taste, smell, and touch). Added to this are systems for balance, arousal, attention, language, memory, spatial information, emotions, reward, neuroendocrine control, and so on. There are also multiple systems for generating outputs (e.g., motor systems and language output systems). At the simplest level, the primary sensory systems provide basic perceptions about the world. It is important to realize, however, that these "perceptions" are actually complex experiences and do not usually reflect only one sensory input in one specific modality. At the minimum, there is often more than one system involved in an experience, and the actual perception is flavored by both internal and external information, including emotions and memories. This makes it debatable whether there even is such a thing as a simple pure perception.

How to coordinate activity flexibly across these various parallel systems to generate a coherent picture of reality is a major challenge for the brain. One way the brain accomplishes it is through activity-dependent changes in the structure and function of synapses within and between parallel systems, a process referred to broadly as "plasticity." A key driver for brain plasticity seems to be the temporal correlation of incoming information—that is, information perceived by different systems as occurring at the same time has a big impact on whether those systems act in unison. The brain's fast excitatory synapses that use glutamate as a neurotransmitter are very good at detecting activity that occurs in close temporal correlation. Coincident activity in neurons that are sending and receiving information (called presynaptic and postsynaptic neurons, respectively) results in a strengthening of the connections between those neurons, a process known as "Hebbian plasticity" after the psychologist Donald Hebb, who proposed such changes as the basis for certain types of memory. It is now clear that many brain synapses undergo Hebbian plasticity, and this process is the basis of the adage that "neurons that fire together wire together." Through this type of plasticity, brain regions have the ability to hook themselves together based on mutual coincident experiences. In contrast, temporally discoordinated activity leads to a weakening of connections between neurons and brain systems (called anti-Hebbian plasticity). The mechanisms underlying both of these forms of brain plasticity have yielded important insights into the molecular and structural biology underlying memory processing and offer potential targets for correcting dysfunction in a number of major neuropsychiatric disorders. We will deal with some of these mechanisms and opportunities later in this book.

In addition to changes resulting from plasticity, the brain also uses several classes of neurotransmitters and neuromodulators to help coordinate activity within and across systems. Neurotransmitters can be classified in several ways. For example, certain transmitters (e.g., glutamate and acetylcholine) are "excitatory" because they depolarize neurons and make it easier for them to fire action potentials, the electrical signals that promote fast intracellular communication within neurons and fast intercellular communication between neurons. Other transmitters (e.g., GABA and glycine) are "inhibitory" because they make it harder for neurons to fire action potentials. Other schemes classify transmitters according to chemical structures (e.g., biogenic amines, amino acids, peptides).

To understand coordination of activity in the brain, it is also helpful to think about neurotransmitters based on the time course over which they work, as described by Bertil Hille and other physiologists. In this scheme, transmitters are said to be "fast" or "slow." Fast transmitters (glutamate and GABA, for example) are released from presynaptic neurons at high concentrations and act rapidly for brief durations (millisecond time scales) on receptors that open ion channels in the cell membrane of the postsynaptic (receiving) neuron. Ion channels are typically multi-subunit protein pores that open or close in response to a transmitter (or in some cases to a change in the electrical gradient across the cell membrane, or both). These pores let ions enter or exit the cell, changing the electrical gradient across the cell membrane in the process. Glutamate opens cationic channels that allow positively charged ions (sodium, potassium, and calcium) to move across the membrane; this results in depolarization (excitation). GABA works on anionic channels that let negatively charged ions (chloride and some other anions) move across the membrane; this usually, but not always, results in hyperpolarization (inhibition). In general, it is the effect on membrane potential that defines a transmitter as excitatory or inhibitory. The fast transmitters provide the moment-to-moment action in the brain, in effect giving lots of "bang for their buck." Table 3-1 presents a summary of how fast and slow transmitter systems are organized.

In contrast, slow transmitters are typically present at lower concentrations in synaptic areas and act more diffusely, providing a way to organize and coordinate activity within and across brain regions. These transmitters also act on a different class of receptors that couple to chemical second-messenger systems. The effects of these slow transmitters often occur in a multi-step process that involves binding of transmitter to its receptor and activation of a linking protein (called a G-protein because of the involvement of guanine nucleotides) that couples the receptor to an

Table 3-1 Fast and Slow Neurotransmitters

Glutamate/GABA (Fast)	Biogenic amines (Slow)
Fast signal (<100 ms duration)	Slow, persistent signal (sec)
Vesicles docked at active zones and are primed	Vesicles may release from active zones and elsewhere
Release: requires high local Ca^{2+}	Release: sustained low Ca^{2+} elevation
Rapid removal (diffusion, transporters; microsec)	Slow removal (transporters; sec)
Point-to-point transmission	Spillover (paracrine effects)
Synaptic, discrete	Volume transmission
Receptors: low affinity ligand-gated ion channels (LGICs)	Receptors: high affinity G-protein-coupled (GPCRs)

intracellular messenger system. The G-protein helps to activate specific enzymes that produce further chemical changes in the receiving cell; for example, activation of adenylate cyclase and production of cyclic AMP or activation of phospholipase C and production of inositol trisphosphate (IP3) and diacylglycerol. Importantly, these slow transmitters produce effects that can last seconds to even minutes or longer, resulting in longer-lasting effects on cellular function and excitability. The chemical events these transmitters initiate lead to further cascading and amplifying chemical events in the cell, which eventually can promote or inhibit the expression of genes in the cell nucleus. Gene expression can then direct the synthesis of receptors, cell growth, and other structural changes that have long-term influences on cell communication.

These slow transmitters also act diffusely, since one presynaptic cell may simultaneously release its transmitter at multiple locations along an extended and branching axon, including releasing transmitter in different brain regions. Under the influence of a slow transmitter, the receiving cell is placed in a state that makes it more or less responsive to an incoming message from a fast transmitter. This provides an opportunity to coordinate activity across synapses and across regions of the brain. In effect, these slow transmitters "set the tone" for nerve cells and regions, establishing the background against which faster inputs have their impact. Examples of slow transmitters include many of the neuromodulators altered by psychotropic drugs (e.g., dopamine, serotonin, and norepinephrine). It is important to note that many fast transmitters also act on their own transmitter-specific slow receptors to provide yet another source of modulation of their own fast activity. For example, glutamate, GABA, and acetylcholine act on "metabotropic" or G-protein-coupled receptors (GPCRs) in addition to their fast ligand-gated ion channels. The term "ligand" refers to a chemical that binds to a receptor, and "gating" is a term that refers to the ability of an agent to open or close an ion channel. Figure 3-3 presents a diagram of the structure of neurotransmitter receptors.

Once activity is coordinated across brain regions, it must be integrated in some fashion to make it useful for higher-order processing as well as for driving output. It appears that regions of high connectivity, particularly those in neocortex, play a key role in pulling this information together while adding their own computational dimension to the processing. These areas are called "convergence zones" in LeDoux's terminology and include the parahippocampal, posterior parietal, and prefrontal cortices. These regions receive multimodal inputs and are like the highly connected nodes in the scale-free networks described previously. These regions of high connectivity allow synthesis of inputs into more complex representations. LeDoux describes these regions as being able to turn "perceptions" into "concepts," reflecting cognitive synthesis and higher-order processing. Importantly, areas of very high connectivity in neocortex can also influence lower centers in the brain, providing yet another form of coordination across regions in which high-level abstract thinking that is synaptically removed from direct sensory experiences can influence its own subsequent input via "top-down processing," a form of feedback (and even conscious) control. This type of cognitive control may be unique to humans (or at least high-level

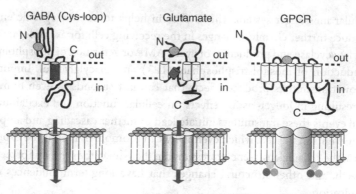

Figure 3-3 Three classes of neurotransmitter receptors. The diagrams depict the proposed structure of three major classes of neurotransmitter receptors: ionotropic GABA-A receptors (which belong to the Cys-loop family along with nicotinic acetylcholine receptors and glycine receptors), ionotropic glutamate receptors (which include AMPA, kainate, and NMDA-type receptors), and the broad family of G-protein-coupled receptors (GPCRs). The bottom set of diagrams depict how multiple subunits are thought to contribute to ion channel function in the case of the ionotropic receptors and how dimerization and linkage to G-proteins are thought to contribute to GPCR activity. (The diagrams are courtesy of Steve Mennerick, Washington University in St. Louis.)

primates) and is a way by which abstract thoughts can influence sensations, emotions, motivations, and memories.

The convergence zones also provide input to an area of brain called the hippocampus, which is critical for the formation of new memories. The hippocampus is an evolutionarily old part of the brain that is called "archicortex" because it has a three-layered structure that is distinct from the six-layered appearance of neocortex. This region handles a wide array of information, including high-level inputs from association cortices that provide data about place and time, emotional inputs from the amygdala and other regions, and information about our own internal state of body and brain function. Using Hebbian plasticity, the hippocampus puts these pieces of information together to form new memories. In effect, this region helps us to process novelty, associations, and context while generating short-term memory traces that allow us to remember things. In turn, the hippocampus sends its processed data back to association cortices and other brain regions where more enduring memory traces are generated. Because the hippocampus deals with both novel and previously processed information, it is capable of taking old memories and turning them into something new. This provides a great deal of flexibility for what and how we remember, but it also provides an avenue by which memory processing may be highly influenced by both our past and current states. Also, our ability to project ourselves into the future is based, in large part, on our memories. Thus, the hippocampus is also critical for planning future endeavors. Because of its high degree of connectivity and the nature of its inputs, the hippocampus represents what LeDoux refers to as a "superconvergence zone" and appears to play a role in many major neuropsychiatric disorders, including major depression, bipolar disorder, schizophrenia, and stress-related disorders. It is an area that is critical for new declarative memory formation.

Loss of hippocampal function by any mechanism leads to catastrophic effects on cognitive function, just like loss of key nodes in any scale-free network can lead to cascading network failure.

These basic principles set the stage for thinking about ICNs, the brain networks that play key roles in processing high-level information and in generating symptoms of psychiatric disorders. ICNs have been identified largely based on correlated BOLD (blood oxygen level-dependent) signals observed in functional magnetic resonance imaging (fMRI) studies. The BOLD signal measures the ratio of oxygenated and deoxygenated hemoglobin resulting from local activity in brain regions (as detected by changes in the magnetic properties of hemoglobin). The signal is thus a hemodynamic response involving local changes in cerebral blood flow and oxygen consumption. Its physiological correlates are uncertain but thought to reflect local field potentials (LFPs), electrical signals of integrated neural activity in a brain region. Studies using BOLD have revealed coherent low-frequency fluctuations in the activity of specific brain regions occurring at rates of about 0.01 to 0.1 cycles per second (Hertz [Hz]). Thus, these correlations of function occur on a time frame of tens of seconds, much slower than the millisecond time frame associated with action potential firing and fast synaptic transmission. These slowly fluctuating signals are highly correlated across linked regions of the brain and allow the generation of connectivity maps of activity. A simple way to think about this is that the connected brain regions seem to "hum" together in coincident activity, and it may be this "humming" (and its associated connectivity) that drives higher-order processing in the brain. What generates this slow coordinated activity is not yet clear, but neuromodulators provided by neurons and glia likely contribute. Although the details of how neurotransmitters contribute to brain networks and mental processing are still uncertain, we present a summary of some current thinking in Table 3-2.

A number of major ICNs have been described, and more will undoubtedly be discovered in the future. In Chapter 2, we discussed the default network that appears to process self-related information when the brain is not focused on doing other tasks and the emotional-salience system involving limbic networks. Other currently recognized ICNs include distributed neural systems regulating spatial attention (probably consisting of at least two frontoparietal networks in the nondominant hemisphere), language (a perisylvian network in the dominant hemisphere), face

Table 3-2 Fast and Slow Transmitters: Role in Behaviors

Glutamate/GABA (Fast)	Biogenic amines (Slow)
Millisecond thoughts	Arousal
Volitional behaviors	Attention
Encoding and retrieving memories	Mood
	Reward
Targets for anticonvulsants, neuroprotectants, anxiolytics, antidepressants	Targets for antidepressants, anxiolytics, antihypertensives

Table 3-3 Mind and ICNs

Cognition (thinking)

  Working memory network (dorsolateral prefrontal cortex–parietal)

  Attention/reorienting networks (frontoparietal)

  Prefrontal executive network

  Spatial navigation network (frontoparietal)

  Language networks (perisylvian)

  Face and object recognition networks (inferotemporal)

Emotion (meaning)

  Extended amygdala processing network

  Emotional-salience network

  Explicit memory network (limbic)

Motivation (goals)

  Ventral tegmental area–ventral striatal motivation network

  Reward processing network

---

and object recognition (an inferotemporal network), decision making (a prefrontal executive network), and cognitive control (at least two frontoparietal networks). We will return to some of these ICNs and how they may be involved in mind and mental illness later in the book. Table 3-3 presents a summary of some currently identified ICNs and how they might be conceptualized as contributing to the tripartite functions of the human mind. For those interested in structural correlates, please see the Appendix as well as Figures 2-1 and 2-2.

How do the brain systems involved in emotions and motivation fit into this organizational scheme? Similar to the hippocampus, these systems are evolutionarily ancient and likely evolved to help humans survive by providing ways to assess an environment rapidly and to navigate that environment successfully. They can operate independently and don't require neocortex or hippocampus to function effectively. While these systems usually work in conjunction with cortex and hippocampus, they have the ability to take over control when triggered. Anyone who has experienced the emotion of rage can attest to this. Rage can clearly override reasoning and result in aggressive actions that are sometimes beneficial to the individual, but often are regretted when cortex kicks back in and assesses what happened. Simply put, a person does not need a cortex to experience intense primary emotions. These systems are an important part of life and their activity does much to flavor our experiences and memories, both good and bad. Using a combination of fast and slow transmitters, emotional and motivational networks use their connectivity to help coordinate broadly distributed brain regions and functions, including activity in higher-order processing centers in neocortex.

"BIG PICTURE" PRINCIPLES OF BRAIN FUNCTION

We will return to neural systems and ICNs shortly. The discussion to this point is designed to provide a background about overall brain organization and how it can be conceptualized when thinking about psychiatric symptoms and syndromes. We will end this part of the discussion by describing several additional principles of brain function, again focusing on high-level concepts that help us think about how brain systems are organized, how they operate, and how they may go awry in illnesses.

For this discussion, we borrow from some of the principles cogently described by Read Montague is his book *Why Choose This Book?* First, the brain is a highly effective processing device. While it is not a "computer" in the usual sense of the term, it is sometimes useful to think about how the brain stacks up against modern computers. In such an analysis, it is clear that although the brain is slow relative to even the simplest personal computers, it readily performs tasks that sophisticated electronic devices struggle with; face recognition and complex pattern completion are two examples. The brain's slow speed is actually a bit of a blessing because fast computers require a lot of power (energy) and generate a lot of heat through wasted effort. In fact, the brain is extremely demanding from an energy standpoint, requiring about 20% to 25% of cardiac output to maintain function while representing only about 2% to 3% of human body weight, an impressive energy demand by any metric. Perhaps even more impressive, however, is the fact that the brain doesn't overheat, except under extreme circumstances. In part, its slow speed relative to a computer helps with heat dissipation: slower devices don't heat as much as fast devices. It is important for psychiatrists to recognize that the brain requires a lot of energy and doesn't work well when it is deprived of energy or fatigued. This is probably easiest to observe when a person's brain is engaged in top-down processing; for example, when higher-order cognition is used to override and control more primitive functions, like emotions. Fatigue and lack of rest are notoriously bad for emotional control and can contribute to a lot of poorly thought-out behaviors.

Second, the brain is an efficient processing device because it takes shortcuts to save energy and effort. When confronted with an ambiguous or uncertain stimulus, the brain will often fill in missing details to make the situation coherent. This can occur with ambiguous sensory inputs (e.g., gestalt figures) or more complex situations (e.g., social encounters). As described by Montague, brain computations are imprecise and the brain must compress a lot of information to save space and energy. This is great for computing efficiency, but it means that the brain is not necessarily a "truth-generating device." It creates and uses schemes and patterns to deal with internal and external realities, and this approach leads to biases in how information is processed and interpreted. Again, think about how efficient emotions can be for sizing up a situation rapidly—but how wrong they can be at times.

This brings us to a third general principle: the brain creates a person's "realities." Psychiatrists routinely deal with this fact across the broad spectrum of psychiatric disorders. That the brain serves as a creator of "reality" may be most obvious in the psychotic disorders, where misperceptions, misinterpretations, and just plain logical errors can lead to fixed, bizarre, and false beliefs about how the world works. Yet for individuals with psychosis, that is reality as they perceive it. Similarly, certain psychotherapies, like cognitive behavioral therapy (CBT), are designed to help patients understand and correct their misperceptions about the world and their lives. Again, for depressed patients their negative bias about the world is their reality, but it is not necessarily the reality of a neutral observer. While the idea that the brain creates reality may be easiest to see in psychiatric disorders, this phenomenon is not unique to people with illness; in fact, it occurs in all of us. Once one wanders into the realm of interpretation and belief, it becomes clear that many humans have interesting, but not necessarily factual or logical, interpretations of reality. Think about politics and religion, for example. Humans believe all kinds of odd things and often hold those beliefs with extreme conviction regardless of circumstances or consequences. The difference between a firmly held opinion and a delusion may be a quantitative, not a qualitative, distinction, and some observers have made a distinction between psychotic and non-psychotic "delusions."

If the normal brain creates reality and makes mistakes, what conceptually separates those with psychiatric illnesses from those who do not suffer from these disorders? One difference may lie in having enough cognitive and emotional flexibility to correct the "errors" that our brains routinely make. All humans are subject to bad moods, bad ideas, and bad social interactions, but only a minority develops serious psychiatric illnesses. Most people find a way to correct misperceptions and mood changes, consciously or unconsciously. Montague has argued that error correction is critical for information processing in the brain and results, in part, from a strategy in which the brain uses goals (motivation) and expectations to guide its computations and outputs. Goals and expectations are internally generated and can be modified to accommodate new experiences. Our brains compare the outcomes of "reality" as we perceive and experience it to those internal expectations and goals, and generate error signals when expectations are not met. The neurotransmitter dopamine seems to play a critical role in this process, and relative changes in the firing of midbrain neurons that produce dopamine appear to reflect whether an outcome meets expectations. Behavior and thinking is then biased to help deal with any perceived mismatch; the latter computation appears to involve regions of rostral anterior cingulate cortex that are connected to key nodes within the dopamine-ventral striatum system. This sets up a type of "reinforcement learning" that allows the brain to update and correct its "virtual world" and to try to align its expectations with reality for more efficient goal-directed behavior. The role of dopamine in this important error-correction process may be one of the major reasons why changes in dopamine-mediated transmission seem to play such a key role in major neuropsychiatric disorders.

Finally, reinforcement learning, and learning in general, is a reflection of brain plasticity. All human brains are "plastic," capable of experience-dependent learning and memory. We described this previously as Hebbian synaptic plasticity and discussed its role as an organizing principle in neural systems function. This "plastic" attribute of the brain cannot be overemphasized. If brains were not plastic, there would be no hope for psychiatric patients. We would argue that every treatment used in psychiatry works via brain plasticity, and the fact that neural circuits can adapt and be reconfigured based on experience is critical for achieving optimal illness outcomes. Thus, in our view psychiatrists must become experts in understanding brain plasticity and in taking advantage of plasticity, broadly conceptualized, for therapeutic purposes.

BASIC PRINCIPLES OF ICNs

To illustrate general concepts about ICNs, including how they are identified, we will review the evolution of our understanding about an ICN we have already mentioned: the default system. While we focus on the default system, it is important to understand that many of the principles outlined pertain to other ICNs. In Chapter 2 (Table 2-1 and Fig. 2-1), we presented an overview of key structures and functions of this network. We now want to focus on how ICNs like the default system are identified based on functional neuroimaging studies.

Using positron emission tomography (PET) and BOLD functional magnetic resonance imaging, Marc Raichle and colleagues demonstrated that certain brain regions display highly correlated activity when examined over relatively long (10 second or longer) intervals. The brain exhibits this correlated activity when a person is resting and not attending to any particular tasks. The discovery that this "resting" activity is highly correlated between *specific* widely dispersed brain areas was surprising and new. The areas involved in this resting intrinsic activity came to define the "default mode network." When a person attends to a task and actively starts to pay attention to something specific, activity in the default network decreases and activity in brain regions that make up attentional systems and systems involved in performing the actual task increases. This has led some cognitive scientists to conceptualize neural networks as being "task-dependent" or "task-independent." In fact, in early studies it was the repeated observation of regions with consistent task-dependent *decreases* in activity that led Raichle and colleagues to believe that they were likely dealing with an important brain network that was more active at rest than when doing tasks. Later analyses demonstrated the presence of high activity and coherence in the resting state among these same structures. It turns out that the correlated fluctuations in the dispersed brain regions making up the default network occur whether a person is awake, resting, or even undergoing anesthesia. Coherent activity in this system also persists in light sleep, but during deep (slow-wave) sleep there is a decoupling of some regions with diminished involvement of prefrontal cortex, possibly reflecting a shift in interregional excitation and inhibition. These latter findings suggest that the default network may contribute to the experience of conscious awareness and that network connectivity can be dynamic and even state-dependent. Figure 3-4 presents a diagram of some of the key brain regions that make up the default network.

Importantly, some of the regions in the default ICN are more functionally connected than others, although most loci within this network are actually hubs themselves. There also may be subsystems within the main default ICN, reflecting

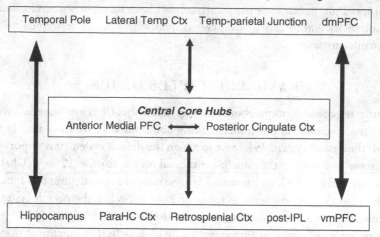

Dorsomedial PFC System: self referential processing

Temporal Pole   Lateral Temp Ctx   Temp-parietal Junction   dmPFC

Central Core Hubs
Anterior Medial PFC ←——→ Posterior Cingulate Ctx

Hippocampus   ParaHC Ctx   Retrosplenial Ctx   post-IPL   vmPFC

Medial Temporal Lobe System: envision self in future

Figure 3-4 Default net subsystems. The diagram depicts key regions in the default mode network. As currently conceptualized, the network appears to include a dorsomedial prefrontal cortex (dmPFC) system that processes self-referential information and a medial temporal lobe system that deals with memory processing and future-oriented thinking. These subsystems interact with hubs in a central core that include the anterior medial PFC and the posterior cingulate cortex. Other abbreviations: ParaHC Ctx (parahippocampal cortex), post-IPL (posterior inferior parietal lobule), vmPFC (ventral medial prefrontal cortex). (Adapted from Andrews-Hanna et al., 2010.)

differences in degrees of connectivity. To determine how regions are functionally connected, researchers examine the activity in a specific brain structure of interest and compare that structure's activity to activity in other brain regions over time. The area of primary interest in such an analysis is called the "seed" region. For instance, the posterior cingulate cortex (PCC), a portion of neocortex behind the corpus callosum, is a key hub region of the default system (see the Appendix for a map of brain regions). To determine how it is connected to the other areas in the default system and to other brain systems, functional imaging data are examined with the PCC as the center of attention. Connected regions are identified on the basis of activity that correlates positively with changes in PCC; other regions of the brain resonate out of sync with the seed region and may even be "anti-correlated," indicating that their activity changes in the opposite direction. Similar analyses are conducted with other seed regions in the brain, and this allows determination of their intrinsic functional connectivity. Using different seed regions for these analyses, investigators are able to develop high degrees of statistical confidence in identifying key structures involved in a network of interest.

As noted, the strength of the various connections within an ICN varies and is determined by the magnitude of the statistical correlation of activity between the regions of interest. For example, in Figure 3-4, the connections between the PCC and the anterior medial frontal lobe are strong because these two regions have a higher degree of correlation, and hence they are more closely coupled than some of the other regions. As noted above, brain regions in a particular ICN sometimes have strong negative correlations with other brain regions. This suggests that some ICNs are turned off (or at least are less active) at times when other ICNs are active. For instance, activity in the default ICN is negatively correlated with activity in frontoparietal ICNs involved in attention. Importantly, and one of the principles of interest to psychiatry, changes in the pattern and degree of connectivity within and across ICNs can vary over time with learning, physiological state (e.g., sleep stage), and neuropsychiatric illnesses (to be discussed in subsequent chapters).

From this discussion, it is apparent that changes in correlated activity as a function of doing specific tasks are important in determining how an ICN is defined. Thus, the scientific marriage of functional neuroimaging with cognitive neuroscience has been extremely important in helping scientists identify specific brain ICNs and how they compute information. An increasing number of ICNs have been described. These networks are involved with various functions, including attentional processing, speech processing, memory processing, motivation, and so on. Certain brain regions contribute to several different networks. Several networks are likely to work together, allowing higher-order information processing. Over the next several years, there will continue to be an explosion of information regarding the normal and abnormal functioning of ICNs.

It is also increasingly evident that certain brain regions are critical hubs in several ICNs. These hubs are the highly connected nodes mentioned earlier in our discussion of small-world and scale-free networks, and are areas that integrate a variety of types of information and help to coordinate higher levels of cognitive, emotional, and motivational processing. These are called "convergence zones" in LeDoux's terminology. Several of these hubs are also part of the default system. This is consistent with the likelihood that the default system is important in helping to coordinate many aspects of brain function.

In summary, ICNs are identified as brain regions that resonate (hum) together to accomplish specific functions. Some regions within a particular ICN are hubs and are more highly connected than other regions. These hubs can be involved in several ICNs, leading to the opportunity for coordination of information flow within and across brain networks. Activity in certain functional systems is specifically turned down when another system is working, and vice versa. Studies that map brain activity across a range of cognitive, emotional, and motivational tasks can help to identify ICNs and can give us better understanding of the specific regions that contribute to performing various tasks. Some areas, such as the hippocampus and amygdala, appear to be involved in multiple ICNs that are relevant to behavior and to psychiatric disorders. Such regions are particularly important to understand both in terms of their roles in various systems and in terms of how they process information and contribute to overall brain connectivity. Also, their roles in memory processing may be important in how network connectivity changes dynamically over time as a result of learning and new experiences.

Points to Remember

Psychiatric disorders are brain disorders. To make sense of psychiatric symptoms and dysfunction, it will be increasingly important to conceptualize psychiatric symptoms and dysfunction in terms of brain function.

We believe that the best hope for understanding the symptoms and clinical presentations of psychiatric disorders from a neuroscience perspective is at the levels of systems biology and network function. Understanding how neural circuits operate and what functions they perform can help in devising diagnostic and therapeutic strategies, including important rehabilitative strategies that can help to repair or work around defective brain regions.

Many biological networks have a small-world and scale-free organization. Current evidence indicates that the brain has small-world connectivity that underlies efficient information processing. It also has highly connected hubs and modularity that may give it some scale-free properties as well. Such organization provides a framework for understanding how these networks function and how dysfunction may attack and propagate within a network.

Understanding the brain as a computational device has implications for diagnosis and treatment in psychiatry. An important consideration is how the brain generates errors and how healthy brains correct those mistakes without becoming persistently dysfunctional.

SUGGESTED READINGS

Barabási, A.-L. (2002). *Linked: The new science of networks*. Cambridge, MA: Perseus Publishing.

Kandel, E. R. (2006). *In search of memory: The emergence of a new science of mind*. New York: WW Norton & Company.

LeDoux, J. (2002). *Synaptic self: How our brains become who we are*. New York: Viking Press.

Montague, R. (2006). *Why choose this book? How we make decisions*. New York: Dutton Press.

Power, J. D., Fair, D. A., Schlaggar, B. L., & Petersen, S. E. (2010). The development of human functional brain networks. *Neuron, 67*, 735–748.

OTHER REFERENCES

Andrews-Hanna, J. R., Reidler, J. S., Sepulcre, J., Poulin, R., & Buckner, R. L. (2010). Functional-anatomic fractionation of the brain's default network. *Neuron, 65*, 550–562.

Attwell, D., & Laughlin, S. B. (2001). An energy budget for signaling in the grey matter of the brain. *Journal of Cerebral Blood Flow and Metabolism, 21*, 1133–1145.

Buckner, R. L. (2010). The role of the hippocampus in prediction and imagination. *Annual Review of Psychology, 61*, 27–48.

Buldyrev, S. V., Parshani, R., Paul, G., Stanley, H. E., & Havlin, S. (2010). Catastrophic cascade of failures in interdependent networks. *Nature, 464*, 1025–1028.

De Bruijn, E. R. A., de Lange, F. P., von Cramon, D. Y., & Ullsperger, M. (2009). When errors are rewarding. *Journal of Neuroscience, 29,* 12183–12186.

Deco, G., Jirsa, V. K., & McIntosh, A. R. (2011). Emerging concepts for the dynamical organization of resting-state activity in the brain. *Nature Reviews Neuroscience, 12,* 43–56.

Hille, B. (2001). *Ion channels of excitable membranes* (3rd ed.). Sunderland, MA: Sinauer Associates Inc.

Esser, S. K., Hill, S., & Tononi, G. (2009). Breakdown of effective connectivity during slow wave sleep: Investigating the mechanism underlying a cortical gate using large-scale modeling. *Journal of Neurophysiology, 102,* 2096–2111.

Fox, M. D., & Raichle, M. E. (2007). Spontaneous fluctuations in brain activity observed with functional magnetic resonance imaging. *Nature Reviews Neuroscience, 8,* 700–711.

Friston, K. J. (2009). Modalities, modes and models in functional neuroimaging. *Science, 326,* 399–403.

Horovitz, S. G., Braun, A. R., Carr, W. S., Picchioni, D., Balkin, T. J., Fukunaga, M., et al. (2009). Decoupling of the brain's default mode network during deep sleep. *Proceedings of the National Academy of Sciences (USA), 106,* 11376–11381.

Kitano, H. (2002). Systems biology: A brief overview. *Science, 295,* 1662–1664.

Lewis, C. M., Baldassarre, A., Committeri, G., Romani, G. L., & Corbetta, M. (2009). Learning sculpts the spontaneous activity of the resting human brain. *Proceedings of the National Academy of Sciences (USA), 106,* 17558–17563.

Linden, D. J. (2007). *The accidental mind: How brain evolution has given us love, memory, dreams, and God.* Cambridge, MA: Belknap Press.

Mesulam, M. (2009). Defining neurocognitive networks in the BOLD new world of computed connectivity. *Neuron, 62,* 1–3.

Raichle, M. E. (2008). A brief history of human brain mapping. *Trends in Neurosciences, 32,* 118–126.

Raichle, M. E. (2009). A paradigm shift in functional brain imaging. *Journal of Neuroscience, 29,* 12729–12734.

Szalay, M. S., Kovacs, I. A., Korcsmaros, T., Bode, C., & Csermely, P. (2007). Stress-induced rearrangements of cellular networks: consequences for protection and drug design. *FEBS Letters, 581,* 3675–3680.

Thompson, R. H., & Swanson, L. W. (2010). Hypothesis-driven structural connectivity analysis supports network over hierarchical model of brain architecture. *Proceedings of the National Academy of Sciences (USA), 107,* 15235–15239.

Watts, D. J. (2003). *Six degrees: The science of a connected age.* New York: WW Norton & Company.

Woolsey, T. A., Hanaway, J., & Gado, M. H. (2008). *The brain atlas—a visual guide to the human central nervous system* (3rd ed.). Hoboken, NJ: John Wiley & Sons.

Zhang, D., & Raichle, M. E. (2010). Disease and the brain's dark energy. *Nature Reviews Neurology, 6,* 15–28.

Zhang, Q., & Haydon, P. G. (2005). Roles for gliotransmission in the nervous system. *Journal of Neural Transmission, 112,* 121–125.

Zorumski, C. F., Isenberg, K. E., & Mennerick, S. (2009). Cellular and synaptic electrophysiology. In B. J. Sadock, V. A. Sadock, & P. Ruiz (Eds.), *Kaplan and Sadock's comprehensive textbook of psychiatry* (9th ed., pp. 129–147). Baltimore, MD: Lippincott Williams and Wilkins.

4

Brain Networks and the Human Mind

Armed with background information about intrinsic connectivity networks (ICNs), we will now consider how brain systems are thought to create the mind and how dysfunction within and across brain networks may contribute to psychiatric symptoms and psychiatric disorders. For this discussion, we will continue to use the definition of "mind" outlined in earlier chapters and championed by Joseph LeDoux in his book *Synaptic Self*. According to LeDoux, the mind is the result of activity in brain circuits that allows humans to do three things: think (cognition), attach value to things (emotions), and set and achieve goals (motivation). It is our premise that all major psychiatric disorders involve defects in each of these three aspects of mind but that dysfunction in a given aspect of mind does not necessarily imply that there is specific pathology localized to that system. Rather, effective processing in interlinked systems depends upon appropriate and accurate inputs from other networks, and pathology in one system can result in dysfunction in another. Two examples cited earlier highlight this. First, in disconnection syndromes such as hemineglect, the lack of appropriate input from a damaged system results in peculiar interpretations by the remaining undamaged systems. This concept that healthy brain regions may make peculiar interpretations when confronted with problematic input from other regions seems to be a basic principle underlying the way the brain works. Second, illnesses like Alzheimer's disease may initially result from a preferential attack on a specific ICN early in their course, although clinical manifestations, even at very early time points, involve more widespread defects in cognition, emotion, and motivation. These latter concepts have been extended recently in studies examining connectivity in brain networks that have sustained damage from focal lesions. It appears that damage that is confined to a single network (e.g., a cognitive control network) results in dysfunction and altered connectivity in intact nodes within the damaged system but does not result in rearrangements within a closely related but undamaged network. Nonetheless, interactions between the two networks are altered because of defective processing within the damaged system.

COGNITION (THINKING)
Working Memory and Prefrontal Cortex

There is little doubt that human cognition is extremely powerful. It gives us the ability to process distinct inputs from the external world and to combine these inputs with our personal internal world, including evaluation of our current state of well-being and memories. Such integration requires coordinated activity in regions of the brain that are highly connected, the "convergence zones" in LeDoux's terminology. For us to become aware of what we are thinking, we must hold those thoughts "on-line" in conscious awareness. Thus, it is no surprise that the brain has networks devoted to this process. Cognitive scientists refer to this as "working memory." While working memory does not result from activity in a single brain region, the prefrontal cortex (PFC), particularly the dorsolateral PFC (dlPFC), plays a major role. When we are consciously thinking about something (like what we had for lunch today or what we have to do this evening), dlPFC is dealing with this information.

Working memory may represent the most basic aspect of what it means to think consciously. This function has several key features. First, working memory is not a storage device. Rather, it seems to be a series of operations that pulls information from multiple sources and keeps track of that information while it is being used—a kind of "scratch pad" processing. Second, working memory has limited capacity, and it must be continuously updated for a person to remain conscious of current thoughts and stay on track with a task. It is estimated that working memory can hold about five to nine items at a time. In psychology, this is referred to as the "seven plus or minus two" (7 ± 2) rule, and it is thought to be the cognitive basis for the use of seven-digit phone numbers and the fact that humans are not particularly efficient at handling multiple tasks at the same time, given that most tasks have multiple sub-components. Recent work has shown that even though humans believe they are good at multitasking, individuals who are frequent multitaskers, particularly those who use multiple types of media, are actually highly distractible and have more difficulty completing tasks than people who try to do fewer things at a given time using a more limited repertoire of media. In part, this distractability reflects overloading of working memory and the way our PFCs seem to work naturally. Although working memory capacity is limited, it can be frequently updated, and this updating may be important for the ability to maintain a stream of thoughts while "thinking." How working memory is continually updated is a matter of active study; some evidence suggests the importance of inputs acting on NMDA-type glutamate receptors and the involvement of dopamine D1 receptors as a filtering device. Persistent neural activity in dlPFC is also likely to contribute.

How Does the Brain Select Thought Content?

While the network involved in working memory is critical for conscious thinking, the brain must figure out how to choose the content of our thoughts—how to select what to include in our thinking and what to exclude. It appears that at least two other ICNs play a major role in this process—the default-mode ICN and an ICN (or ICNs) regulating attention. Working memory is closely associated with attention networks and appears to involve at least two essential operations that draw upon this association: a mechanism for "selecting" items that engages the rostral superior frontal sulcus, posterior cingulate cortex, and precuneus, and an "updating" operation that involves the caudal superior frontal sulcus and posterior parietal cortex. This latter system helps to change the focus of our attention (see the Appendix for locations of key brain regions).

As described in Chapter 3, functional imaging studies indicate that human brains are never really idle or at rest. When we are not engaged in an active task, certain regions of the brain are very active in terms of metabolism and blood flow; this is one of the primary reasons the brain uses so much energy. Task-dependent energy use is a relatively small contributor (5% or less) to overall brain energy demand compared to this baseline activity. When a person's attention is directed to a task of interest, activity in the regions with high baseline use diminishes while brain activity in the regions required for the specific task increases. When we shift away from the focused attention required for a specific task to a more "relaxed" brain state, activity in the brain regions required for the task decreases and the background activity once again increases. Various functional imaging studies examining how humans process different types of information have found the same set of brain regions to be involved in this high baseline (background) activity. As mentioned in Chapters 2 and 3, this led Marc Raichle and colleagues to refer to this brain network as a "default system." The default-mode network involves a distributed collection of connected brain regions that includes the ventromedial PFC, the posterior cingulate and retrosplenial cortices, the precuneus and parts of the ventromedial temporal lobe, the hippocampus, and the inferior parietal lobule (see Fig. 2-1). Importantly, some of these same default regions overlap with the working memory system; this is not surprising given that when we are awake we are usually thinking about something, even when not doing a specific task.

When we focus attention on a task (e.g., doing a math problem or reading this sentence), we must engage working memory and shift out of the default state into a mode that engages the ICNs required to perform the job at hand. A key component of this attention-shifting process is an ICN that Maurizio Corbetta refers to as a "reorienting system." In the visual system, this involves cortical circuits in the right (nondominant) hemisphere that link frontal and parietal lobes. It consists of at least two pathways: a *ventral* circuit that interrupts current thinking and resets attention to the new task and a *dorsal* pathway that selects the new objects of attention and links them with ICNs appropriate for the needed computations. Figure 4-1 presents a diagram of the dorsal and ventral reorienting networks.

The ventral path acts like a type of "circuit breaker" that allows us to change our cognitive focus and shift our attention. It is triggered by task-relevant stimuli and allows us to switch from the internal focus of the default system to operations that address specific external demands. The dorsal pathway helps to select the specific items of focus and to evaluate the nature of the external variables in order to determine the content of working memory that relates to the specific stimulus at hand. In other words, the dorsal system seems to prioritize external (world) demands while the default system prioritizes internal (self) information. Perhaps because of the limited capacity of working memory, we usually don't perform both of these tasks at

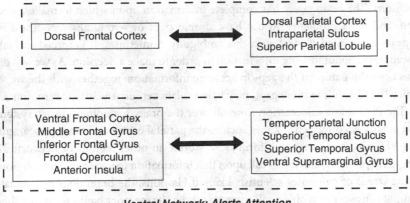

Figure 4-1 Attention and frontoparietal reorienting networks. The diagram depicts key brain structures thought to be important in reorienting and attention networks as described by Maurizio Corbetta and colleagues.

the same time, or at least we don't perform both efficiently at the same time. Put another way, daydreaming doesn't usually help with getting one's job done.

PFC Does More than Working Memory

In addition to its roles in working memory and attention, the PFC is also critical for many other cognitive tasks, including planning and decision making, drawing inferences, determining cause-and-effect relationships, and making predictions about things, people, and events by determining regularities and patterns. These are some of the so-called "executive" functions of the brain and represent the highest-order levels of cognitive processing.

Using this executive function analogy, Elkhonon Goldberg has described the PFC as the "chief executive officer" (CEO) of the brain. As is true of corporate CEOs, this analogy indicates that the PFC is probably not the site where all jobs (computations) are performed or even the site with the skills needed to solve a given problem. Rather, the PFC knows "who" in the organization has the abilities required for a given task and refers the "job" to those regions for processing. The results are then fed back to PFC for further analysis, evaluation, and decision making. The various subdivisions of the PFC are among the most highly connected regions of the brain—convergence zones where inputs from many sources are combined, integrated, and then used to signal other brain regions in order to generate responses. The great expansion in size and connectivity of the PFC over the course of human evolution is thought to be one of the major contributors to the advanced cognitive capabilities exhibited by humans compared to other species.

Pursuing the CEO analogy further, some view one of the primary functions of the PFC to include handling the uncertainties that accompany most situations and decisions. The brain rarely has complete information upon which to make a decision, and most problems do not have simple right or wrong answers. The PFC appears well suited to deal with this ambiguity. Sometimes, it is forced to make assumptions about missing information in order to make a decision. As we will discuss later, the nature of the gaps in accurate information, together with the way in which the PFC fills in these gaps, may help explain certain psychiatric symptoms.

The PFC draws information from all over the brain, including sensory systems and other key convergence zones such as the parietal cortex and the hippocampus. The PFC also has access to information "stored" in other regions of neocortex in long-term memory, and it can call upon that information to generate new solutions. In the words of computer scientists like Jeff Hawkins, the brain does not actually compute answers to problems. Rather, it searches its memory banks to "remember" solutions—even to "remember" solutions to new and ambiguous situations. Others refer to this as the ability of the PFC to "remember the future." Although the future really doesn't mean anything to our stored memories, the PFC, often working in conjunction with the hippocampus, tries to utilize prior information and apply it to new situations.

One can imagine that the various functions of the PFC make this brain region extremely complicated in terms of its internal anatomy and its inputs and outputs. To avoid getting lost in too much detail, we will use a simple scheme that divides the PFC into three major subsections: lateral, medial, and ventral. Lateral PFC, particularly the dorsolateral aspect, appears to contribute significantly to working memory; it is most developed in higher-order primates and humans. The medial PFC includes anterior cingulate cortex and is involved in decision making and selecting outputs to be implemented. This may be the true "executive" region of the brain. The ventral (orbital) PFC is coupled to the brain's emotional-processing systems; it provides a way for emotions to affect decision making and, in turn, helps to regulate emotions. The PFC has diverse efferent (outflowing) connections throughout the brain that allow generation of a complex array of responses. Table 4-1 and Figure 4-2 present a description of subregions within the PFC and their proposed cognitive functions.

One of the key PFC connections is a close coupling with specialized ICNs for language in the dominant (usually left) cerebral hemisphere. This coupling to sophisticated language ICNs is most highly developed in humans, and it provides humans with the ability to think in terms of language. Language provides the basis for generating conceptual metaphors, analogies, and categories—types of thinking that allow humans to move beyond simple perceptions into the realm of complex concepts. Interestingly, many of these higher-order abstractions are tied to the operations of simpler sensory systems, leading us to express abstract ideas (like affection and love) in sensory terms (warm, hot, cold). This type of abstraction is so natural for us that we largely take it for granted, and it pervades many of our abstract ideas, including concepts in math and science (e.g., the idea that numbers are points on a line or values of positions in a game). Understanding human thought often requires deciphering the

Table 4-1 Frontal Cortex: Subdivisions and Proposed Functions

Dorsolateral prefrontal cortex (dlPFC)
- Working memory
- Top-down control of attention, emotions, and impulses
- Reasoning and dealing with ambiguity

Anterior cingulate cortex (ACC)
- Conflict monitoring

Dorsomedial prefrontal cortex (dmPFC)
- Error detection
- Reality monitoring

Ventromedial prefrontal cortex (vmPFC)
- Emotional regulation
- Self-reflection

Orbitofrontal cortex (OFC)
- Affective value of stimuli and reward expectation
- Impulse control

metaphor being used to express a concept. In some psychiatric disorders, defects in this type of abstraction can result in "concrete" (rigid) thinking and problems in communication. Psychiatrists sometimes try to assess this by having patients interpret simple analogies or proverbs. Misunderstanding the metaphor or abstraction can lead to a total inability to understand the message an individual is trying to communicate.

In addition to generating responses via interactions with language ICNs, the PFC has the ability to direct other regions in their responses. This is referred to generically as "top-down processing," reflecting the fact that this mode of control uses the highest levels of the brain to regulate more primitive systems, like emotions, motivation, and motor function. For the PFC to exert top-down control, several ICNs have evolved that utilize different time scales in order to accomplish PFC-mediated cognitive control. One such ICN involves a frontoparietal system that provides a means

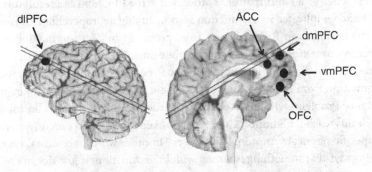

Figure 4-2 Key regions of frontal cortex. The diagram shows the approximate locations of key regions of the PFC that are listed in Table 4-1. See Table 4-1 for abbreviations. (Adapted from Damasio, 2005, with permission.)

for rapidly altering focus and adjusting control (not unlike the operations involved in attention). A second ICN involves the opercular regions of the PFC and the cingulate cortex; this cingulo-opercular system plays a role in more persistent control by providing stable maintenance over the duration of a task. (The frontal "operculum" is the most posterior part of the inferior frontal gyrus and includes Broca's speech area in the dominant hemisphere.) Both of these systems take advantage of structures in the PFC that are involved in working memory as well as other regions involved in decision making. There is also evidence that the cerebellum, a structure primarily involved in motor function, may participate in mediating interactions between the frontoparietal and cingulo-opercular control systems. This latter observation is an indication of how complex neural circuitry can be and how defining a brain region as "motor," "sensory," or "cognitive" can be a bit arbitrary and function-dependent.

These two cognitive control systems utilize a number of strategies to regulate function. Two examples are referred to as "proactive" and "reactive" strategies. Proactive strategies bias attention, perception, and action toward a goal, while reactive strategies respond only when they detect a need for changes, a type of error correction. Interestingly, age may affect which strategy is used for cognitive control, with older persons being more reactive and younger persons being more proactive. It also appears that individuals can be taught to adapt and change their preferred mode of control, and this may provide a target for psychotherapy and rehabilitative strategies. It is important to emphasize that top-down control over emotions and motivation can be extremely difficult and energy-demanding. The more primitive centers of the brain are not designed for this type of control, and it is clear that they can generate responses and behaviors independent of the PFC. As noted by LeDoux, this may be a reason that knowing and doing the right thing can be difficult. Figure 4-3 presents a diagram highlighting how several forms of top-down processing are thought to operate.

PFC and Neuropsychiatric Disorders

Complex higher-order information is processed in the PFC, and as a result this brain region is often implicated in dysfunction accompanying neuropsychiatric disorders. While abnormalities in PFC function (e.g., problems in decision making or top-down control over emotions) may suggest abnormalities in the PFC itself, this may not necessarily be the case. Rather, the PFC may perform poorly because it receives misinformation from other regions or because it is disconnected from key inputs and outputs. Problems with input or output to the PFC may result in clinical symptoms. For this reason, Elkhonon Goldberg has likened defects in executive function to nonspecific physical symptoms like "fever." In other words, abnormal executive processing says that something is wrong with brain function; it just doesn't tell you what is wrong or where the primary problem is located.

Difficulties in dealing with ambiguity may be one of the earliest manifestations of PFC dysfunction in psychiatric illnesses. Ambiguous or confusing information,

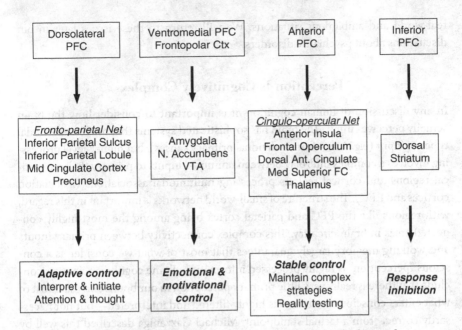

```
┌──────────────┐   ┌──────────────────┐   ┌──────────────┐   ┌──────────────┐
│ Dorsolateral │   │ Ventromedial PFC │   │   Anterior   │   │   Inferior   │
│     PFC      │   │  Frontopolar Ctx │   │     PFC      │   │     PFC      │
└──────────────┘   └──────────────────┘   └──────────────┘   └──────────────┘
        ↓                   ↓                      ↓                  ↓
┌──────────────────┐  ┌────────────┐  ┌──────────────────────┐  ┌──────────┐
│ Fronto-parietal  │  │  Amygdala  │  │  Cingulo-opercular   │  │          │
│       Net        │  │ N. Accumb. │  │        Net           │  │  Dorsal  │
│ Inferior Parietal│  │    VTA     │  │  Anterior Insula     │  │ Striatum │
│     Sulcus       │  │            │  │  Frontal Operculum   │  │          │
│ Inferior Parietal│  │            │  │  Dorsal Ant. Cingulate│ │          │
│     Lobule       │  │            │  │  Med Superior FC     │  │          │
│ Mid Cingulate    │  │            │  │  Thalamus            │  │          │
│     Cortex       │  │            │  │                      │  │          │
│   Precuneus      │  │            │  │                      │  │          │
└──────────────────┘  └────────────┘  └──────────────────────┘  └──────────┘
        ↓                   ↓                      ↓                  ↓
┌──────────────────┐  ┌────────────┐  ┌──────────────────────┐  ┌──────────┐
│ Adaptive control │  │ Emotional &│  │    Stable control    │  │ Response │
│ Interpret &      │  │ motivational│ │ Maintain complex     │  │inhibition│
│ initiate         │  │  control   │  │     strategies       │  │          │
│ Attention &      │  │            │  │   Reality testing    │  │          │
│ thought          │  │            │  │                      │  │          │
└──────────────────┘  └────────────┘  └──────────────────────┘  └──────────┘
```

Figure 4-3 Top-down processing: prefrontal cortex and control networks. The diagram depicts some of the key PFC regions and networks providing top-down control over mental processing. Included are the adaptive control and stable-set control networks discussed in the text and described by Steve Petersen and colleagues. See the Appendix for location of key structures.

for example, may lead to actions that appear bizarre. Problems in dealing with uncertainty can lead the PFC to instruct lower brain regions to respond with outputs that are not appropriate for the task. For example, the PFC may receive erroneous information that all of a person's shoes are missing. The response may be accusations that family members or unknown intruders stole the shoes. In reality, the person has impaired memory and forgot that she hid her shoes under the bed. The output has a delusional quality but likely results from the fact that the PFC received only part of the data necessary to come to a correct conclusion. Similarly, the PFC may direct stereotyped behavioral responses (e.g., outbursts of temper) to deal with uncertain and stress-provoking situations. Individuals who are "stressed" tend to use habitual (implicitly learned) responses in preference to higher-order goal-directed behaviors when confronted with new challenges. This is an energy-saving strategy in that habitual responses require little forethought or planning; nonetheless, these responses can be inappropriate in many settings. This may be a particular problem in individuals who have certain types of personality disorders, where over-learned and stereotyped responses seem to rule the day, particularly when the individual is stressed.

One of the major problems in detecting defects in PFC function is that current clinical tests of its higher-order processing are relatively crude compared with assessments of motor, sensory, or language function. Clinical tests as well as more sophisticated neuropsychological tests are better at monitoring defects in working memory and attention than at determining how patients respond to and make decisions in real-world and ambiguous situations. We will return to these issues later in our discussions about psychiatric disorders.

Perception Is Cognitively Complex

In any discussion of human cognition, it is important to consider how the brain actually perceives input. The brain has sophisticated systems that process unimodal types of input (e.g., input from individual primary senses), but higher-level processing involves a complex interplay between unimodal inputs to primary thalamocortical regions and cortical regions processing multimodal associations (association cortices and PFC). The structure of small-world networks is important in this regard, with regions like the PFC and parietal cortex being among the most highly connected areas in brain circuitry. This complex connectivity between primary inputs and working memory largely guarantees that most of what we consider as a conscious "perception" is highly processed information. Some cognitive scientists conclude that there is really very little primary perception in our brains and that most of what enters conscious awareness is highly filtered and interpreted—but not necessarily correct from a factual standpoint. Michael Gazzaniga described this well by referring to the brain as a "self-concerned interpreter." What we believe is happening around us and to us is actually an amalgam of sensory inputs, memories, context, and internal state (emotions and motivations) interpreted by the PFC with abstracting techniques to pigeonhole and simplify incoming data. Examples of the latter include the use of abstract categories (e.g., "plants," "animals," or "sports"), metaphors, and analogies that help to channel and organize thoughts about a new experience. In fact, as a result of the costly energy demands of higher-order processing, the brain, particularly the PFC, must take shortcuts and use its memories to make predictions about what it is experiencing. The brain rarely takes in a complete picture at one time, but rather focuses on part of a scene and makes "guesses" about the rest. As noted by Gregory Berns, these shortcuts represent a way for the brain to avoid overload. Using this type of processing, the brain changes a perception only when it realizes it has made a mistake. Recognizing mistakes and generating "error signals" are very important parts of the process of perception, and to the extent that error correction is defective, misperceptions can dominate conscious experience (e.g., bad moods, delusions). Internal error correction is a form of cognitive "reality check" and is fundamental for dealing with complex situations.

Lateralized Brain Function and Cognition

The brain uses different modes of processing to make predictive interpretations about the world, and the two cerebral hemispheres seem to process information in complementary but distinct ways. This concept is important when considering how different functions are lateralized in cortex. It is clearest with regard to language functions, which are processed in the left (dominant) hemisphere. In contrast, spatial information is processed preferentially in the right (nondominant) hemisphere.

Emotions also appear to be differentially processed in neocortex, with the right hemisphere playing the major role in interpreting and generating emotional responses. Strokes involving the right hemisphere can be associated with defects in emotional experience resulting in several types of aprosodias, which are clinical syndromes that involve expressive and/or receptive problems in emotional signaling. Examples of defects include inability to express specific emotions (e.g., appearing bland or blunted rather than sad) or difficulties in interpreting the emotions of others (mistaking anger for another emotional state or failing to even recognize that an emotion is being expressed). Both types of problems can lead to major defects in social communication and interpersonal interactions.

Studies of patients with "split brains" have been highly instructive for understanding lateralized processing in the cerebral hemispheres. Typically, these individuals have had intractable epilepsy and have had their corpora callosa severed surgically in order to prevent seizures from spreading from one hemisphere to the other. The corpus callosum is a large fiber bundle in the middle of the brain that connects the two cerebral hemispheres. Studies of split-brain individuals have yielded unique insights into how the hemispheres operate in isolation. The left hemisphere appears to seek logic and cohesiveness in its responses. It does not appear to be concerned with being factual or correct, but only with giving a coherent story. It generally doesn't admit that it doesn't know something, and it will "make up" an answer if needed. For example, in the hemineglect disconnection syndrome resulting from damage to the right hemisphere, the undamaged left hemisphere generates the story that the paralyzed hand belongs to someone else. In contrast, the right hemisphere seems concerned with accurate details and has difficulties dealing with inconsistencies. Unfortunately, this hemisphere does not have a direct language module, so it tends to express itself through emotions and feelings. These differences between the two hemispheres may contribute to the observation that strokes involving the anterior left hemisphere are more commonly associated with depression than lesions of the right hemisphere. When the left side is damaged, the right hemisphere recognizes there is a problem and becomes "worried," expressing its concerns through negative emotions. In the presence of similarly placed anterior lesions of the right hemisphere, the left hemisphere typically has no problem going about its business, but it is not held in check by the emotional control imposed by the right hemisphere. This may result in the development of manic-like (or impulsive) behaviors in some cases.

Why these differences in hemispheric function evolved, particularly with regard to logic and emotion, is not clear, but it may reflect, in part, the way information from the autonomic nervous system is processed in the brain. Input from the sympathetic nervous system conveying data about arousal and survival is preferentially processed in the right forebrain, while input from the parasympathetic nervous system involving relaxation and affiliation is processed on the left. Interestingly, these different inputs and modes of processing appear to have different energy requirements, with left (holistic) processing being more energy-sparing and right (detail-oriented) processing being more energy-intensive.

Intelligence and Cognitive Flexibility

Before leaving this initial discussion about cognition, we would like to make a few comments about human intelligence and its potential relevance to psychiatric disorders. "Intelligence" is a difficult and politically charged concept to define precisely. It reflects the contributions of a variety of brain regions and ICNs and is something of an emergent property of the brain. Although debated, it also appears that there may be different types of intelligence and that individuals can vary significantly across these domains. These include abilities involving language, mathematics and logic, music, movement/athletics, spatial relationships, and social function. Social intelligence reflects the ability to understand one's own mind and the minds of others. Emotional understanding and empathy might constitute a separate form of intelligence, although this may be a subset of general social intelligence. These various forms of intelligence can be difficult to measure, and many clinically used instruments based on verbal and nonverbal intelligence quotients (IQ) are subject to cultural biases and leave a lot to be desired. Nonetheless, defects in IQ performance can be important for identifying areas of functional impairment that can impede educational, social, and occupational activities. Also, while high performance on IQ tests is not protective against neuropsychiatric disorders, low intellectual performance is associated with increased risk for several major disorders, including depression, substance abuse, and psychosis. Similarly, intellectual capacity may be important for predicting persons at greatest risk for dementing illnesses as well as the course of dementia. An example of this comes from the Nun Study, a longitudinal study that examined the long-term outcomes of women living in a cloistered religious order. In early adulthood, those entering the convent were asked to write autobiographies. Women whose writings demonstrated more advanced and complex writing styles fared better as they aged in terms of cognitive performance and risk of dementia. The reasons for the differences are not certain but are consistent with a "cognitive reserve" hypothesis in which greater intellectual capacity may help to buffer illness. Top-down processing and emotional control also appear to benefit from greater intellectual capacity. Nonetheless, being "smart" in one domain does not necessarily predict intelligence in the other spheres, and it is unclear whether different forms of intelligence result in different abilities to top-down process and control emotions and motivation. It is also clear that the brain circuits underlying "intelligence" involve multiple cognitive processes and that these functions often involve computations in frontal, parietal, and temporal cortices and the interconnections among these regions. In particular, high intelligence may reflect the benefits of small-world network processing outlined earlier.

Humans are inherently social animals, and our ability to relate to others has a lot to do with life satisfaction. Defects in a person's social network and support system can have significant impact on the outcome of mental disorders as well. Thus, the area of social intelligence is important in psychiatry. In particular, the ability of an individual to recognize that others have their own minds (experiences and agency) and to draw inferences about the mental states of others based on facial expressions, speech, verbal tone, and nonverbal cues is important in connecting socially with others and in developing satisfying interpersonal relationships. Understanding this ability has led to the concept of "theory of mind" (TOM); that is, we develop a "theory" about what others are actually thinking and meaning. TOM implies that humans are often (if not always) trying to "read" the minds of others. This is an interesting concept when one considers how bothersome such thoughts can be to individuals with psychosis, who often struggle with the notion that people are reading their minds or putting thoughts into their heads. Reading each other's mind is a basic tenet of how we relate and develop understanding of the intentions, actions, emotions, and words of others. Activity in the medial and inferior PFC and superior temporal sulcus, likely including the face area in the fusiform gyrus, appears to contribute significantly to TOM processing. Interestingly, some parts of the PFC have neurons (called "mirror neurons") that seem particularly adept at TOM-type processing. These neurons fire in response to perceived actions of others and initiate actions that mimic what is perceived in the other person's behavior, including his or her movements. Defects in TOM have been observed in multiple psychiatric disorders, but they may be most prominent in autism, where major defects in social attachment and reciprocity are cardinal features. Individuals with autism-spectrum disorders appear to have diminished capacity to perceive agency (planning, intention and self-control) in others. Similarly, misattributions about mental states may represent a type of cognitive defect in other disorders. For example, attribution of agency to inanimate objects is observed in schizotypal thinking (called "magical" thinking).

EMOTIONS: COMPUTING VALUES AND MEANING

What Values, What Meaning?

Emotional processing, the second component of the mind in LeDoux's scheme, allows humans (and other animals) to attach value to the things they encounter. The brain systems involved in emotion are evolutionarily old compared to the PFC; even rodents have emotional-processing systems that are organized in a fashion similar to the networks found in primates and humans. There is little doubt that these systems play an important role in survival: emotions allow us to assess a situation rapidly and unconsciously, and determine whether it is safe or a threat. These are the computations that allow us to make "gut" decisions. Emotional systems are also designed to take control of brain function and drive behavior when activated. For example, we have all had the experience of becoming startled upon hearing a sudden noise, taking defensive postures before we ever become consciously aware of what is happening. The initial sensory input (vision or sound) is processed subcortically and activates key survival systems. Cortex is involved secondarily and can then put conscious constraints on motor behavior (called "response inhibition" in cognitive terms). For example, we may move away from a snake before we consciously realize that we are even doing so. After moving away from the snake, we then understand the danger and consciously decide to move to even safer ground.

There is some agreement that humans have six "primary" emotions: happiness, sadness, fear, anger, surprise, and disgust. Contempt is also included in some schemes. These are considered primary emotions for two reasons: they appear to occur in all human populations and they are expressed in a similar fashion (using similar facial expressions) by people of different cultures. Human emotional life is much richer than the primary emotions, however, and we also have many secondary emotions that relate to social interactions. These include guilt, shame, embarrassment, jealousy, pride, and love, among others. Although these secondary emotions have major impacts on our lives, it is not clear that they are processed in the same way as the primary emotions or how they may derive from the primary emotions.

Given that primitive brain systems underlie emotional processing, it is also useful to think about emotions from the perspective of other animals. Jaak Panksepp has described the existence of seven major emotional systems in animals. These include networks for lust (sexual approach), care (maternal nurturing), joy (play), fear (danger), rage (anger), panic (separation distress), and seeking (exploration). Similar to emotions in humans, Panksepp views these systems as rapidly encoding information about whether an encounter is life-sustaining or life-threatening and driving adaptive and instinctual responses to appropriate action. Panksepp has further argued that these primary systems in animals extend to humans and could serve as potential "endophenotypes" for describing the underpinnings of psychiatric disorders. Endophenotypes are observable (and usually quantifiable) traits that are likely tied much closer to genes and neural systems than complex illness phenotypes (such as disorders and syndromes).

How Are Emotions Processed?

All emotions represent brain computations that include an analysis of incoming information and a subsequent output based on that analysis. In this model, a stimulus is initially perceived either consciously (in the cortex) or unconsciously (in subcortical structures). Specific brain systems process this perception and generate a bodily response. This response is often a change in the output of the autonomic nervous system, the system regulating basic body physiology (e.g., heart rate, blood pressure, respiration, and temperature). These bodily changes are also detected by the brain and can be incorporated into the computational mix. For example, becoming afraid increases heart rate. This in turn can be perceived by the brain, leading to further increases in heart rate in a positive feedback loop. At the point when bodily sensations and context are recognized consciously in working memory, we experience what Antonio Damasio calls a "feeling," the conscious representation of an emotional state. At several places along this processing path, we can take behavioral action in response to the emotion. This might occur once we become consciously aware of the "feeling." At that point, the PFC can drive voluntary behavior. Alternatively, and perhaps more interestingly, a behavioral response can occur before or simultaneous with changes in heart rate and respiration, before neocortex has become involved and before we are conscious of what is going on. This is one of the major principles of emotional systems: they do not need cortex to do their computations and to effect behavioral change. This makes them both powerful and potentially problematic.

How does this happen? It appears that there are several subcortical and cortical networks that contribute to emotional processing. As a result of work by LeDoux, Michael Davis, Michael Fanselow, and numerous others, the system that is understood in most detail is the one involved in processing fear, a primary emotion experienced as clearly in rodents as it is in humans. In fear processing, the amygdala, a complex walnut-shaped brain structure with multiple sub-nuclei deep within the temporal lobe, is a principal player. When a fear-generating stimulus is encountered, information is routed initially through the thalamus, a subcortical way-station for processing sensory and other inputs. The thalamus connects directly to the amygdala for rapid assessment of inputs and also sends input to sensory neocortex for more detailed assessment and interpretation. This simple routing allows the amygdala to drive defensive action via its own direct connections to stress and alerting systems in the hypothalamus and brain stem as well as to the striatum and motor system before cortex ever gets involved. The nature of synaptic contacts and synaptic delays ensures that the amygdala gets the information before the cortex, given that more synapses are required to get the data to cortex and distributed within cortex to working memory. Adding to this, recent studies indicate that the amygdala also has direct chemo-sensing properties of its own and uses acid-sensing ion channels (ASICs) to detect changes in brain carbon dioxide levels or acid–base balance. Thus, the amygdala can do its own direct sensory processing; in turn, this can generate rapid emotional responses, including fear. This may be one of the reasons why changes in respiration (hyperventilation) are so closely intertwined with emotions. Figure 4-4 highlights neural circuitry involved in fear processing (and anxiety) and the central role of the amygdala.

The direct input from the thalamus (or cortex) flows to the lateral nucleus of the amygdala for initial processing. The lateral nucleus connects directly to the central and basolateral amygdaloid nuclei, which regulate emotional processing and generate output to regions controlling alertness, defensive behaviors, and hormonal responses, with the central nucleus playing the key role as a driver of outputs to other brain regions. These output regions include brain-stem nuclei governing arousal and motivation (e.g., the norepinephrine, serotonin, and dopamine transmitter systems) as well as systems regulating neuroendocrine hormonal responses in the hypothalamus and systems mediating freezing responses (behavioral inhibition) in periaqueductal gray. The amygdala is an important activator of stress hormones like cortisol via its connections with the paraventricular nucleus (PVN) of the hypothalamus, resulting in the release of corticotrophin-releasing factor (CRF), which in turn stimulates the pituitary to release ACTH (adrenocorticotrophic hormone). ACTH acts on the adrenal glands to promote secretion of cortisol. Cortisol does many things to mediate stress responses, including acting on the brain in a feedback fashion. Interestingly, changes in the regulation of cortisol secretion (altered diurnal

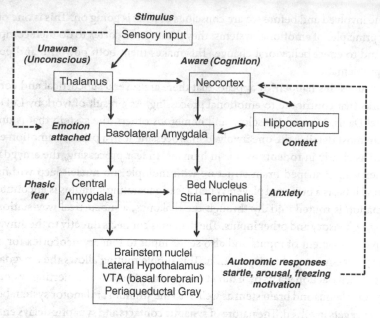

Figure 4-4. Fear and anxiety. The diagram depicts neural circuitry involved in processing fear and anxiety and highlights the central role of the amygdala. While much of this circuitry is shared between fear and anxiety, it is currently thought that the circuitry involved in anxiety engages the extended amygdala, including the bed nucleus of the stria terminalis. See the Appendix for location of key structures.

variation and diminished suppression with dexamethasone) are among the most replicated biological findings in major depression and stress-related disorders.

The amygdala is also capable of synaptic plasticity, and thus it can "learn" to be afraid. Repeated exposure to a fearful stimulus can result in a type of conditioning that leads to an otherwise innocuous stimulus becoming associated with a fear-producing stimulus. This is the basis for Pavlovian conditioning, and similar implicit effects in humans may play a role in certain mood and anxiety disorders. The amygdala also has strong bidirectional connections with the hippocampus, a brain region that is critical for declarative memory formation and that helps to process novelty and context. These connections can lead to even more complex forms of emotional learning that can have adverse effects on behavior. For example, a person can become conditioned to be afraid of paired stimuli via the amygdala (e.g., becoming afraid of a bell that is paired with a shock); one can also become conditioned to be afraid of the place where a bad thing happened (e.g., being stressed in a classroom). When "context" is added to the conditioning, the hippocampus likely plays a role in the learning. This is called "contextual fear conditioning" and can result in excessive and inappropriate responses when one re-enters the conditioned place—for example, generalizing a bad classroom experience to all classrooms. The importance of the interplay between amygdala and hippocampus in emotional processing has been highlighted in a recent study demonstrating the contributions of these regions to anxious temperament as a predisposing risk for mood and anxiety disorders. In primates, hippocampal metabolic activity contributing to anxious temperament is heritable whereas amygdala activity is not. This suggests different roles for genes and environment affecting different brain regions in this behavioral phenotype.

The important point to remember is that there are different components to fear-generated memories, and these different components have implications for how the memories can be controlled or eradicated. Interestingly, studies in rodents indicate that animals can also be conditioned to recognize safety signals and environments where bad things will not happen (e.g., being conditioned to a place where a shock will never occur). This type of learning could contribute to the effects of certain forms of psychotherapy in humans and may help to form the basis of desensitization (deconditioning) therapies as well as extinction learning and conditioned inhibition. Importantly, such learning is not necessarily "unlearning," but more likely is an alternative type of learning that involves amygdala, striatum, and possibly hippocampus.

The amygdala also has connections to the PFC, with strong ties to the ventral (orbital) PFC and the medial (midline) PFC. It is interesting to note that the amygdala does not have strong connections to regions involved in working memory in the dorsolateral PFC, again highlighting the idea that conscious thinking is not really critical for amygdala function. In fact, when the amygdala is in control, working memory is temporarily suspended. Think how difficult it is to perform well on an examination when anxiety levels are running high; things that we ordinarily know well sometimes cannot be consciously recalled when anxiety is in control. Lateral PFC and working memory, however, can override the amygdala (i.e., you can think your way out of being afraid). The relationship of working memory to amygdala processing and the ability of the amygdala and its connections to serve as learning devices have major implications for psychiatry and are the basis for psychotherapies used to treat mood and anxiety disorders.

Other Emotions and Other Brain Regions

The amygdala is only one part of the "limbic system," a distributed subcortical brain system that is thought to play the conductor's role in emotional processing. The concept of the limbic system is sometimes debated—not because subcortical systems aren't involved in emotions, but because defining what constitutes a "limbic" structure can be difficult based on complex connectivity. While the amygdala is a key player in emotional processing, it is not the only structure involved. It is also clear that the amygdala participates in processing more than fear. For example, the amygdala plays a substantial role in rage (the "fight" part of the "fight-or-flight" response) and may also trigger positive emotions, including sexual behaviors. Different nuclei of the amygdala may be involved in different primary emotions. The medial and posterior nuclei are thought to be involved in processing sexually oriented emotions and behaviors, while, as noted previously, the lateral and central nuclei are involved in processing fear. There is also evidence that the amygdala, particularly its medial portion, is part of a basic "threat" system that appears to regulate aggressive behaviors.

Importantly, the amygdala itself is only one component of an extended system that includes the bed nucleus of the stria terminalis (BNST), the striatum (particularly the ventral striatum), hypothalamic nuclei that regulate hormone output via the pituitary, and brain-stem nuclei that regulate the output of monoamine neurotransmitters. Examples of these brain-stem nuclei include the locus coeruleus (site of norepinephrine synthesis), the dorsal raphe nucleus (serotonin), and the ventral tegmental area (dopamine). The connections and involvement of these structures in distributed emotion-processing networks provide a framework for understanding how catecholamines, indoleamines, peptide transmitters, and hormones are involved in psychiatric disorders. Interestingly, studies in rodents and humans suggest that anxiety, a more persistent state of unease with less well-defined triggers than fear, differs from primitive acute fear responses in engaging an extended amygdala network, including the BNST (see Fig. 4-4). Also, involvement of the nucleus accumbens and dopamine in emotional processing provides a link for understanding how emotions relate to motivation. We will discuss this in greater detail later.

Work on the fear-processing network has been greatly aided by the fact that there are well-characterized rodent models of fear conditioning. This has allowed anatomical pathways and synaptic mechanisms to be mapped in considerable detail. Similar models for other emotions are less well developed. Nonetheless, growing evidence indicates that specific regions in cortex are involved in emotional processing and in the generation of conscious awareness of feelings. These cortical regions include the anterior insular cortex (AIC), the rostral anterior cingulate cortex (ACC), and somatosensory cortex. AIC and ACC are deeper cortical structures that receive multimodal inputs from emotional systems and work in concert with the emotional systems. They appear to be critical for conscious awareness of several emotions, including disgust, affective components of pain, and motivation. Disgust is a particularly interesting example. This primary emotion reflects a visceral (gut-level) response to a perception and may have evolved as a mechanism to assess whether something in the environment is edible or noxious. This "gut feeling" eventually may have taken on other meanings of social importance, such as determining "right and wrong" (our moral standards). In other words, the level at which we experience a twinge of disgust may be the level beyond which we will not proceed with an act. Human neuroimaging studies of moral decision making strongly suggest that our initial assessment in these decisions involves our emotional networks, including brain regions involved in disgust. The AIC plays a key role in these experiences and is adept at pulling together information about homeostatic state (state of the autonomic nervous system, hormonal levels, and arousal), emotional state, hedonic conditions, and social situations. The concept that moral standards are closely related to emotional processing demonstrates the amazing integration of cognitive and emotional systems. Figure 4-5 shows the location of the AIC in the human brain.

In concluding this discussion of emotional processing we also want to highlight the key role of the hypothalamus, a part of the diencephalon located below the thalamus (hence the name; see the Appendix for location). This region, like the amygdala, is a collection of multiple small nuclei that, in effect, connect the brain and endocrine systems

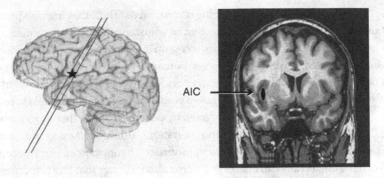

Figure 4-5 Insular cortex. The figure depicts the location of insular cortex. This region plays a role in higher-level processing of several emotions. Abbreviation: AIC (anterior insular cortex). (Adapted from Damasio, 2005, with permission.)

via the pituitary gland. The various hypothalamic nuclei regulate many behavioral and homeostatic processes, including food intake, metabolism, sexual behaviors, circadian rhythms, stress responses, and the autonomic nervous system (blood pressure, respiration, temperature). Even more complex behaviors such as maternal and social affiliation appear to have strong ties to hormones regulated by the hypothalamus (e.g., oxytocin). The details of hypothalamic function and its regulation are complex, with more than 15 subnuclei involved. The importance of the hypothalamus is highlighted by the notion that some neuroscientists liken its actions to those of a thermostat, adjusting bodily function to meet demands. Other scientists go a step further and suggest that most of the higher brain is designed to keep the hypothalamus under control. The importance of the hypothalamus to behavior and psychiatric disorders cannot be overemphasized. In recent years, some illnesses have been directly linked to hypothalamic dysfunction. A clear example is the finding that narcolepsy, a disorder characterized by sleep attacks and cataplexy (loss of muscle tone), involves the loss of specific hypothalamic neurons that release the peptide orexin (also known as hypocretin). It is possible that similar findings will be discovered in other neuropsychiatric disorders in the future.

What Triggers Emotional Responses in the Brain?

Emotions are incredibly dynamic and powerful aspects of our mental lives. They are capable of taking control to help us survive. Thus, it would seem that the stimuli that trigger these responses are critical for us to recognize quickly. While there is still much to be learned about what triggers emotions in humans, there is evolving evidence that effective triggers seem to involve "error" detection in our brains—rapid (and not necessarily conscious or correct) assessments of whether a stimulus (or an action) meets expectations or not. When there is a mismatch between expectation and perceived (or experienced) outcome, emotional systems can be activated to make rapid adjustments. As you might guess, the most intense emotions are triggered by negative assessments. Furthermore, the computations that activate emotions can be quite crude, reflecting perhaps not much more than educated guesses (predictions) about what is going on around us. Thus, they are also prone to error and require their own error correction to adjust inappropriate responses.

In his book *Iconoclast*, Gregory Berns, a cognitive neuroscientist and psychiatrist, discusses categories of things that trigger human anxiety. Berns describes several types of human fears, and his assessment provides interesting food for thought that may also be relevant to how other negative emotions (e.g., anger, sadness) are activated. At its most base level, fear is triggered by perceived harm: threats to our well-being. These are fairly straightforward interpretations, although learning and memory can generalize these responses to less appropriate circumstances (e.g., becoming afraid of things that really can't harm us). Berns also indicates that fear responses can be triggered by perceptions of loss or failure, which in many cases can be accompanied by a fear of personal humiliation. This might lead to a fear of rejection or of being isolated and ostracized from a social network. Humans are highly social animals and loss of contact with our "herd" is bad for our well-being. The final trigger for fear responses described by Berns may be the most interesting and the one that provides deepest insight into how our brains process abstract information: this is the fear of the unknown. We have already emphasized the concept that our brains don't tolerate uncertainty very well. This is particularly true of our left hemispheres, which tend to make up answers if things don't seem coherent. Similarly, dealing with ambiguity and the fact that most decisions don't have clear-cut right or wrong answers is a major challenge for the PFC. In the absence of certainty, emotional systems can be used to provide more definitive responses—though not necessarily correct or useful responses. Some cognitive scientists believe that difficulties in dealing with ambiguity may be one of the earliest manifestations of serious dysfunction involving higher brain centers. Again, this doesn't necessarily mean that there is pathology in those centers, only that they are struggling with the data they are confronting.

From a neuroscience perspective, it is not clear why different emotions are triggered under different circumstances or why different emotions are triggered in the same individual when confronted by relatively similar circumstances. It is also not known why some individuals are prone to anxiety and others to anger or sadness when confronted with similar situations. At one level of analysis, the computation that a perceived (or real) outcome does not meet expectation might trigger anxiety if the perception is one of harm, sadness if the perception is one of loss or defeat, or anger if the perception is one of unfairness. The factors that bias individuals toward one or another of these determinations may have a lot to do with how our motivational system works and how our expectations are determined by our brains.

MOTIVATION: THE IMPORTANCE OF HAVING GOALS
How Does Motivation Work?

Motivation is the third component of LeDoux's mental trilogy. It involves the computations that determine how we set and achieve goals. Motivation is closely coupled to our concepts of reward and the factors that dictate our expectations. The motivational (and reward) system, like the emotional systems, is old from an evolutionary perspective, and it is closely entwined with the subcortical emotional systems. For example, in Jaak Panksepp's scheme, the emotion called "seeking" may reflect some of what is considered motivation since it involves the computations that drive animals to explore their environment. Also, the way that certain incentives pique our interest may involve activation of emotions. These incentives can be innate or learned. Some seem to be basic drives (e.g., food, sex, survival) while others are more complex and are derived from our learning and environment. Interestingly, humans have a unique ability to use their own abstract thinking as an incentive (or at least as a motivator). As noted by Read Montague, humans are probably the only animals that are willing to die for abstract beliefs—religious or political ideas, for example. He sums this up well by saying "sharks don't go on hunger strikes." As we will discuss in more detail later, almost all abused drugs modulate and usurp the activity of our motivational system via effects on the neurotransmitter dopamine.

Our motivational system involves a subcortical network that includes the nucleus accumbens, the ventral pallidum, and the midbrain ventral tegmental area (VTA) (Fig. 4-6). This system interacts strongly with thalamocortical systems, including the PFC, and appears capable of computing both motivation and reward, although these are not necessarily the same thing from a processing perspective. The VTA is a region that synthesizes dopamine, and the dopamine released by projections from the VTA is a key modulator in the nucleus accumbens. Dopamine's influence also

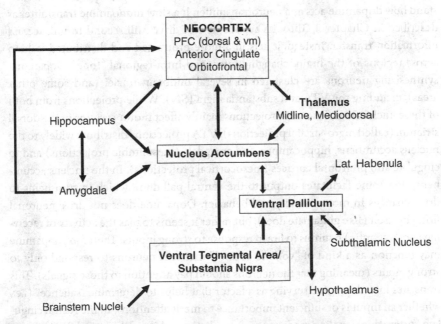

Figure 4-6 Reward circuit. The diagram depicts key structures and connections within the motivational system, highlighting the central role of the ventral tegmental area, nucleus accumbens, and regions of neocortex. See the Appendix for location of key structures.

spreads beyond the nucleus accumbens to connected areas in the rostral cingulate cortex that are important for error detection and areas in the PFC that regulate working memory. Based on imaging studies, it appears that anticipation of a reward activates the nucleus accumbens and VTA, while experiencing a reward seems also to involve the medial caudate nucleus, putamen, and eventually dorsal caudate and supplemental motor cortex. Dopamine helps to drive initial responses and to recruit the more distributed circuit involved in behavioral outcomes.

How does the motivation system work? It appears that the nucleus accumbens is a key region that integrates input about goals, emotions, and memories, and then generates signals that act via the ventral pallidum to help drive motor output and behavior. In this system, dopamine seems to play a major role as an error-detection signal. Some have considered dopamine to be a reward signal, but current thinking suggests it plays a different role. Dopamine seems to help determine whether a perception meets expectations, and it helps other regions in the network direct their attention to important (salient) activities. What this means in practical terms is that the firing of dopamine neurons in the VTA reflects a computational comparison of observations and expectations. When outcomes are better than expected, dopamine neurons in the VTA fire action potentials at increased rates, resulting in more dopamine being released in the nucleus accumbens, cingulate cortex, and PFC. When outcomes fail to meet expectations, firing diminishes and dopamine levels drop. Thus, it is the firing of these specific neurons and the release of dopamine that serves as a "critic signal," in the words of Montague.

What makes dopamine "motivating?" To answer this, it is important to understand how dopamine acts as a neurotransmitter. It a slow monoamine transmitter as described in Chapter 3. Thus, its actions do not drive millisecond-to-millisecond information transfer. Instead, it acts in a more protracted and distributed fashion across regions of the brain, changing inter- and intra-regional "tone." Dopamine-synthesizing neurons are clustered in several midbrain nuclei (and some other areas), including the VTA and substantia nigra (SN). While projections from both of these nuclei are diffuse, SN projections mainly affect motor systems in the dorsal striatum (called nigro-striatal projections). VTA projections distribute widely to the nucleus accumbens, hippocampus, and amygdala (mesolimbic projections) and to cingulate and prefrontal cortices (mesocortical projections). In the nucleus accumbens, dopamine facilitates output to the ventral pallidum, which in turn helps to drive changes in motor activity and behavior. Dopamine does not drive neuronal firing by itself (like glutamate does), but rather it seems to bias the activity of receiving (postsynaptic) neurons to fire in response to strong inputs. Therefore, dopamine may function as a kind of "volume control" that tells neurons to respond only to strong inputs (meaning that the neurons should pay attention to those signals). This translates into dopamine serving as a factor that helps to determine "salience" (i.e., whether an input is of sufficient importance to merit attention). In the rostral cingulate cortex, this signaling mediates error prediction, while in the lateral PFC it helps to focus attention and working memory. In the PFC, this can also be viewed as a type of "filtering" function. Under pathological conditions, where there is too much or too little dopamine, the brain can have trouble determining whether a stimulus is important or irrelevant. This may be a big problem for patients with schizophrenia, where changes in dopamine transmission are thought to contribute to defects in working memory and cognition.

Dopamine transmission in the motivational system also appears to be critical for reinforcement (incentive-based) learning, a type of experience-dependent processing that helps us update and select goals. According to Terry Sejnowski and colleagues, reinforcement learning is the mechanism that allows us to use an ancient prediction system (dopamine) to engage with the modern world and to learn from that world what works and what doesn't work. Montague describes this process as a series of computational steps. First, a perception (either internal or external) generates an immediate signal that is compared to a stored value function in longer-term memory. This comparison results in a "critic signal" (dopamine cell firing) as described earlier. The product of the critic signal (dopamine) is then used to guide choices and to select the next goal by biasing the responses of receiving neurons. This so-called "reward prediction error signal" not only biases subsequent decision making but also influences what is learned from the experience and is used to set future expectations. The learning part of this experience likely reflects the involvement of the hippocampus, where dopamine inputs play a modulating role and seem to be important for the generation of certain long-term memories. Recent imaging studies in humans have focused on understanding how the brain distinguishes between error detection and reward processing. It appears that errors strongly activate the posterior medial PFC (including pre-supplemental motor areas and the rostral cingulate zone) regardless of whether the perceived error is being made by us or by others. The latter is an example of how we learn from the behaviors of others. In contrast, activity in the striatum (particularly ventral striatum) is engaged by reward regardless of error status.

What Determines Our Expectations?

Comparisons of expectations to outcomes play a major role in reinforcement learning—but what sets our expectations? Clearly, they are not static and are often context-dependent. Thus, they are subject to modifications from our emotions and our memories. Nonetheless, our expectations often reflect core and longstanding aspects of our selves, aspects that likely fall under the broad heading of "personality." Personality refers to enduring patterns of how we think about ourselves and the world. It can be described in a number of ways, but one that we find helpful from a brain systems perspective has been championed by C. Robert Cloninger. According to Cloninger, there are two major dimensions to personality: temperament and character. Temperament reflects basic habits and skills that influence how we interact with and respond to the world. Cloninger defines four aspects of temperament: novelty seeking, harm avoidance, reward dependence, and persistence. Character traits determine how we participate in the world and include cooperativeness, self-directedness, and self-transcendence.

Genetics plays a large role in determining a person's temperament and character traits, although both are also modified by experience. Temperament traits appear to be particularly important in determining things that catch our attention and that are important to us. Thus, it appears that these traits also help to determine salience and to set our internal expectation barometer. Are we happiest when things are static or changing? Do we prefer safety over riskier undertakings? How much does the approval of others mean to us? Neuroimaging studies are helping to elucidate the neural systems that contribute to and help to drive these traits. For example, novelty seeking appears to involve a network that includes the hippocampus, amygdala, and nucleus accumbens, while reward dependence appears to engage regions of the PFC and striatum. Persistence involves lateral orbital and medial prefrontal cortices as well as the nucleus accumbens. The role of the nucleus accumbens in these traits is intriguing in light of its apparent role in motivation, error detection, and reinforcement learning. Also, studies of novelty seeking indicate that persons with high exploratory tendencies have diminished expression of a specific class of dopamine receptors (D2 receptors) in ventral midbrain dopamine neurons. These individuals also have enhanced dopamine responses to novel stimuli compared to individuals with low novelty seeking.

These observations are important for thinking about the role of personality in psychiatric disorders as well as potential strategies to help individuals with personality disorders deal with difficulties arising from their temperament and character. According to Cloninger, defects in character traits are the features that indicate the likely presence of a personality disorder, while differences in temperament traits determine the form the disorder takes. For example, uncooperative behavior and lack of self-directedness is observed in many personality disorders. However, the presence of high novelty seeking and low harm avoidance in the face of these character problems correlates with exhibiting antisocial behaviors (lying, poor school and job performance, sexual promiscuity, and fighting). Similar analyses can be applied to other personality disorders.

We want to end this discussion by emphasizing further the important role that motivation plays in brain function and how motivations, cognition, and emotions are intimately intertwined. Karl Friston has hypothesized that all of us have an internal representation of the world against which we compare things to determine whether they meet or don't meet expectations. He argues that motivation based on this stored "model of the world" helps the brain quickly overcome disorder (and the second law of thermodynamics). It forms the basis for biased attention and competition among inputs, allowing values assigned by ascending modulators (emotions) to regulate how inputs are handled and outputs are generated. This goes a long way toward sharpening executive function and minimizing "surprises" to the brain (a bane for higher-order cognitive function), but this also ensures that what is sampled and how it is sampled is biased, as are the strategies used for processing. An example of the latter is the finding that highly reward-dependent individuals exhibit greater improvement in working memory performance when in an environment where they are rewarded for performance, but, interestingly, the improvement in working memory typically occurs during tasks that are not directly rewarded. They improve their performance by adopting a proactive cognitive control strategy (see earlier sections of this chapter) that enhances the likelihood of reward. This again highlights how motivation and cognition are intertwined.

Appetitive (approach) aspects of motivation are largely driven by ventral striatal circuits. Motivation can also be considered to have avoidance aspects, driven in large part by amygdala-based circuits, and regulatory components mediated by PFC networks, again highlighting how the three components of mind are intertwined.

SUMMARY: A SIMPLIFIED OVERVIEW OF BRAIN SYSTEMS AND MIND

We believe that conceptualizing the mind as a trilogy comprising interrelated brain networks is heuristically valuable for thinking about psychiatric symptoms and disorders. At the risk of oversimplifying these points, we will conclude this discussion by providing a more basic summary of what we have described in this chapter. Admittedly, the descriptions below are unsophisticated from scientific and brain processing perspectives, but we think such simplification can help clinicians think practically about how brain systems contribute to psychiatric problems and how to approach those problems therapeutically.

The brain networks underlying thinking, emotions, and motivation interact strongly, and defects across these spheres occur in all major psychiatric disorders. Conscious thinking is the purview of the neocortex, and the PFC is central to this process. It is the moderator, decision maker, and interpreter of everything that happens in the conscious brain. While the PFC may not be able to solve all problems by itself, it has the best handle on where in the brain problems can be solved. Just like the way other small-world networks self-organize and operate, the PFC contains very highly connected nodes and has long-range connections to influence many other brain regions. It is also subject to dysfunction and error generation when it gets defective information from other systems.

The amygdala is critical for emotional processing. It might be considered a bit like a "watchdog" that detects challenges and then works with the hypothalamus and other homeostatic systems to alert the individual and rapidly correct things when deemed appropriate. The dopamine-nucleus accumbens system along with key parts of the PFC is important in motivation and can be viewed a bit like a behavioral "thermostat." When mismatches between expectation and outcome occur, this system helps the brain adjust and reset its compass. We will deal with the hippocampus in future chapters, but for now it is important to understand its key role in handling convergent inputs. It functions a bit like an "integrator" and binds a lot of things together, including our memories and emotions, resulting in even richer associations and memories based on experience. Almost all processed information eventually finds its way to the hippocampus and it, in turn, is capable of sharing its own processing with multiple brain systems. The hippocampus is also critical for novelty detection, so things that are considered "new" end up in this system. Finally, the anterior insula and rostral cingulate cortex serve important roles as "interpreters" helping to bring interoceptive (internal) representations and subjective experiences to awareness and thus to influence behavior. These two areas help to interpret the activity of the ancient evolutionary systems for the more recently evolved PFC. While we have singled out a few key regions, it is also important to keep the general ICN concept in mind: these regions do not function in isolation and are all parts of distributed brain circuits that interact and guide mental processing. Furthermore, our understanding of the complexities of interactions within and across brain systems remains in its infancy and as new information is gained systems neuroscience advances. For example, the cerebellum contains more than 50% of all brain neurons and has largely been thought to regulate motor function. Some evidence suggests that this is overly simplistic and this region may also participate in networks underlying language, mood, and executive control.

It is also important to realize that these brain systems do not result in anything akin to a computer or camera. They make mistakes by taking energy-saving shortcuts, but in healthy brains, they do an amazing job of correcting those mistakes, leading to coherent thinking, feeling, and behavior. This is even more amazing when we take into account the fact that our brains combine ancient systems (amygdala and nucleus accumbens) with intermediate (hippocampus) and relatively modern (neocortex) additions. In his book *The Accidental Mind*, David Linden refers to such an arrangement as a "kludge," a term that loosely means a bunch of things piecemealed together that somehow seem to get the job done. From an engineering perspective, it is not clear that this is the optimal way to design a great computational device, yet this system does more than even the most sophisticated computers in terms of pattern recognition, abstraction, and concept generation. It is amazing how well it works . . . most of the time.

Points to Remember

Psychiatric disorders are brain disorders and reflect dysfunction across all aspects of mind—cognition, emotion, and motivation.

Certain symptoms may predominate in certain illnesses (e.g., emotional problems in mood or anxiety disorders), but problems with cognition, emotion, and motivation are almost always comorbid. The way the brain is wired as a global network almost ensures comorbid symptoms across these three domains when things go wrong.

While the brain is a complex organ, mental processing can be effectively described and understood in terms of systems neuroscience and ICNs. As we will discuss further in subsequent chapters, defects in specific ICNs can predict psychiatric symptoms and can serve as targets for rehabilitative efforts and psychotherapies. Defects in molecular mechanisms are more likely to be amenable to specific pharmacological interventions.

SUGGESTED READINGS

Buckner, R. L., Andrews-Hanna, J. R., & Schacter, D. L. (2008). The brain's default network: Anatomy, function and relevance to disease. *Annals of the New York Academy of Science, 1124,* 1–38.

LeDoux, J. (2002). *Synaptic self: How our brains become who we are.* New York: Viking Press.

Montague, R. (2006). *Why choose this book? How we make decisions.* New York: Dutton Press.

OTHER REFERENCES

Berns, G. (2008). *Iconoclast: A neuroscientist reveals how to think differently.* Boston: Harvard Business Press.

Bisley, J. W. (2011). The neural basis of visual attention. *Journal of Physiology (London), 589,* 49–57.

Blair, R. J. R. (2010). Neuroimaging of psychopathy and antisocial behavior: A targeted review. *Current Psychiatry Reports, 12,* 76–82.

Bledowski, C., Rahm, B., & Rowe, J. B. (2009). What "works" in working memory? Separate systems for selection and updating of critical information. *Journal of Neuroscience, 29,* 735–741.

Braver, T. S., Paxton, J. L., Locke, H. S., & Barch, D. M. (2009). Flexible neural mechanisms of cognitive control within human prefrontal cortex. *Proceedings of the National Academy of Sciences (USA), 106,* 7351–7356.

Casey, B. J., Duhoux, S., & Cohen, M. M. (2010). Adolescence: What do transmission, transition and translation have to do with it? *Neuron, 67,* 749–760.

Cloninger, C. R. (2004). *Feeling good: The science of well-being.* New York: Oxford University Press.

Cohen, M. X., Schoene-Bake, J.-C., Elger, C. E., & Weber, B. (2009). Connectivity-based segregation of the human striatum predicts personality characteristics. *Nature Neuroscience, 12,* 32–34.

Conway, A. R. A., Kane, M. J., & Engle, R. W. (2003). Working memory capacity and its relation to general intelligence. *Trends in Cognitive Sciences, 7,* 547–552.

Corbetta, M., Patel, G., & Shulman, G. L. (2008). The reorienting system of the human brain: From environment to theory of mind. *Neuron, 58,* 306–324.

Damasio, A. (1999). *The feeling of what happens: Body and emotion in the making of consciousness.* San Diego, CA: Harcourt.

Davis, M., Walker, D. L., Miles, L., & Grillon, C. (2010). Phasic vs. sustained fear in rats and humans: Role of the extended amygdala in fear vs. anxiety. *Neuropsychopharmacology Reviews, 35,* 105–135.

de Bruijn, E. R. A., de Lange, F. P., von Cramon, D. Y., & Ullsperger, M. (2009). When errors are rewarding. *Journal of Neuroscience, 29,* 183–186.

Dosenbach, N. U. F., Fair, D. A., Cohen, A. L., Schlaggar, B. L., & Petersen, S. E. (2008). A dual-networks architecture of top-down control. *Trends in Cognitive Sciences, 12,* 99–105.

Friston, K. (2010). The free-energy principle: A unified brain function? *Nature Reviews Neuroscience, 11,* 127–138.

Gazzaniga, M. S. (2008). *Human: The science behind what makes us unique.* New York: HarperCollins.

Goldberg, E. (2001). *The executive brain: Frontal lobes and the civilized mind.* New York: Oxford University Press.

Gray, K., Jenkins, A.C., Heberlein, A.S., & Wegner, D.M. (2011). Distortions of mind perception in psychopathology. *Proceedings of the National Academy of Sciences (USA), 108,* 477–479.

Greene, J. D., Nystrom, L. E., Engell, A. D., Darley, J. M. & Cohen, J. D. (2004). The neural basis of cognitive conflict and control in moral judgment. *Neuron, 44,* 389–400.

Gusnard, D. A., Ollinger, J. M., Shulman, G. L., Cloninger C. R., Price, J. L. Van Essen, D. C., et al. (2003). Persistence and brain circuitry. *Proceedings of the National Academy of Sciences (USA), 100,* 3479–3484.

Haber, S. N., & Knutson, B. (2010). The reward circuit: Linking primate anatomy and human imaging. *Neuropsychopharmacology Reviews, 35,* 4–26.

Hawkins, J. (with Blakeslee, S.). (2004). *On intelligence.* New York: Times Books.

He, J. J., Shulman, G. L., Snyder, A. Z., & Corbetta, M. (2007). The role of impaired neuronal communication in neurological disorders. *Current Opinion in Neurology, 20,* 655–660.

Javanovic, T., & Ressler, K. J. (2010). How the neurocircuitry and genetics of fear inhibition may inform our understanding of PTSD. *American Journal of Psychiatry, 167,* 648–662.

Jimura, K., Locke, H. S., & Braver, T. S. (2010). Prefrontal cortex mediation of cognitive enhancement in rewarding motivational contexts. *Proceedings of the National Academy of Sciences (USA), 107,* 8871–8876.

Khalsa, S. S., Rudrauf, D., Feinstein, J. S., & Tranel, D. (2009). The pathways of interoceptive awareness. *Nature Neuroscience, 12,* 1494–1496.

Kouneiher F., Charron, S., & Koechlin, E. (2009). Motivation and cognitive control in the human prefrontal cortex. *Nature Neuroscience, 12,* 939–945.

Laird, A. R., Eickhoff, S. B., Li, K., Robin, D. A., Glahn, D. C., & Fox, P. T. (2009). Investigating the functional heterogeneity of the default mode network using coordinate-based meta-analytic modeling. *Journal of Neuroscience, 29,* 496–505.

Lakoff, G., & Nunez, R. (2000). *Where mathematics comes from: How the embodied mind brings mathematics into being.* New York: Basic Books.

Linden, D. E. J. (2007). The working memory networks of the human brain. *Neuroscientist, 13,* 257–267.

Linden, D. J. (2007). *The accidental mind: How brain evolution has given us love, memory, dreams, and God.* Cambridge, MA: Belknap Press.

Liu, H., Stufflebeam, S. M., Sepulcre, J., Hedden, T., & Buckner, R. L. (2009). Evidence from intrinsic activity that asymmetry of the human brain is controlled by multiple factors. *Proceedings of the National Academy of Sciences (USA), 106,* 499–503.

Newberg, A., D'Aquili, E., & Rause, V. (2001). *Why God won't go away. Brain science & the biology of belief.* New York: Ballantine Books.

Nomura, E. M., Gratton, C., Visser, R. M., Kayser, A., Perez, F., & D'Esposito, M. (2010). Double dissociation of two cognitive control networks in patients with focal brain lesions. *Proceedings of the National Academy of Sciences (USA), 107,* 17–22.

Oler, J. A., Fox, A. S., Shelton, S. E., Rogers, J., Dyer, T. D., Davidson, R. J., et al. (2010). Amygdalar and hippocampal substrates of anxious temperament differ in their heritability. *Nature, 466,* 864–868.

Panksepp, J. (2004). *Affective neuroscience: The foundations of human and animal emotions.* New York: Oxford University Press.

Panksepp, J. (2006). Emotional endophenotypes in evolutionary psychiatry. *Progress in Neuro-Psychopharmacology and Biological Psychiatry, 30*, 774–784.

Quartz, S. R., & Sejnowski, T. J. (2002). *Liars, lovers and heroes: What the new brain science reveals about how we become who we are.* New York: William Morrow.

Raichle, M. E., & Snyder, A. Z. (2007). A default mode of brain function: A brief history of an evolving idea. *Neuroimage, 37*, 1083–1090.

Riley, K. P., Snowden, D. A., Desrosiers, M. F. & Markesbery, W. R. (2005). Early life linguistic ability, late life cognitive function, and neuropathology: Findings from the Nun Study. *Neurobiology of Aging, 26*, 341–347.

Shin, L. M., & Liberzon, I. (2010). The neurocircuitry of fear, stress and anxiety disorders. *Neuropsychopharmacology Reviews, 35*, 169–191.

Vann, S. D., Aggleton, J. P., & Maguire, E. A. (2009). What does the retrosplenial cortex do? *Nature Reviews Neuroscience, 10*, 792–802.

Zald, D. H., Cowan, R. L., Riccardi, P., Baldwin, R. M., Ansari, M. S., Li, R., et al. (2008). Midbrain dopamine receptor availability is inversely associated with novelty-seeking traits in humans. *Journal of Neuroscience, 28*, 14372–14378.

Ziemann, A. E., Allen, J. E., Dahdaleh, N. S., Drebot, I. I., Coryell, M. W., Wunsch, A. M., et al. (2009). The amygdala is a chemosensor that detects carbon dioxide and acidosis to elicit fear behavior. *Cell, 139*, 1012–1021.

5

Psychiatric Disorders and Brain Networks

Understanding how psychiatric syndromes arise and how best to treat them requires understanding how the brain processes information and how dysfunctional brain networks result in symptoms. Psychiatric illnesses likely involve primary dysfunction in one or a few specific intrinsic connectivity networks (ICNs). This dysfunction results in compensatory changes in other ICNs; some of these changes may improve function and some may compound the primary deficits. Importantly, we would argue that, over time, all major psychiatric disorders involve dysfunction across the three spheres of the mind. Thus, symptoms reflecting cognitive, emotional, and motivational deficits are the rule and not the exception, particularly in full-blown illnesses. This cross-modality dysfunction mirrors how the brain is organized, how ICNs interact to generate thinking and behavior, and how synaptic interactions and brain plasticity across neural systems can work both to the benefit of and to the detriment of the individual. We believe that these concepts can help psychiatrists understand the nature of mental disorders more rigorously. In addition, we believe that understanding how malfunction in specific brain systems generates particular symptoms will ultimately help to simplify and correct some of the current problems in psychiatric diagnosis, including the overdiagnosis of numerous comorbid disorders in the same individual based on symptoms that share the neural networks making up the mind. It is possible that a better understanding of psychotic disorders, for example, will result from understanding which ICNs are primarily malfunctioning and which ICNs are involved in compensating for missing or inappropriate input. In this chapter, we provide an overview of brain networks and their relationship to psychiatric disorders. This approach of relating psychiatric syndromes to brain systems is in its infancy, so the concepts discussed here are not statements of absolute fact, but rather represent ideas percolating in the field as well as our own interpretation and speculation.

PSYCHIATRIC DISORDERS AND DEFECTS IN MENTAL ERROR CORRECTION

To start this discussion, we again emphasize that psychiatric disorders may ultimately reflect problems in neural homeostasis and in how the brain corrects the errors that it generates. We have referred to this problem earlier in the book and will now consider the idea in greater detail. The human brain is a complex computing device that processes and keeps track of tremendous amounts of information about our external and internal worlds. To do this in an efficient way, the brain must use shortcuts to save energy and shorten processing time. Unconscious emotions and motivations are examples of brain shortcuts; the brain uses shortcuts in higher-order thinking as well. For example, we routinely draw inferences and conclusions about ambiguous situations on the basis of limited information. Once drawn, these conclusions can be difficult to reverse, even in the face of contradictory evidence. Our "perceptions" almost always reflect a combination of new sensory inputs and past experiences. Because the brain takes shortcuts connecting the old with the new, the resulting computations are not necessarily factual or based in the reality experienced by a neutral observer. This contributes to the fact that the brain is prone to making "errors"—mistakes that are minor in most cases (e.g., simple misperceptions, faulty recollections, misunderstandings) but sometimes can be profound (major emotional overreactions, psychotic ideas, for example).

Damage to the brain exaggerates error generation as a result of defective ICNs ineffectively processing information or sending misinformation to normally functioning ICNs that either compensate for the defect or don't realize that the information is defective. Our brains ultimately create all of our "realities," and in some cases what is perceived as reality is simply wrong from the standpoint of others. Importantly, healthy brains are good at correcting errors. Error correction involves updating information processing based on new inputs and outcomes, and typically involves brain plasticity and our ability to learn and remember new information, including utilizing reiterative, reinforcement-based forms of learning. Our brains constantly compare the information we receive to what we expect to receive (i.e., our reality). If there is disagreement, the brain tries to correct the magnitude of this disagreement. Brain plasticity provides the substrate for updating internal and external realities—updating that usually, but not always, leads to congruence between the two worlds.

We would argue that humans, including those without psychiatric disorders, often get odd ideas about the world, develop bad moods, and experience periods of aberrant motivation. We previously noted that about one-fourth of adults report significant obsessions and/or compulsions that include magical ideas (e.g., superstitions and peculiar beliefs), counting or numbering rituals, and hoarding behaviors. About one-third of adults report some type of persecutory ideas—for example, the belief that they have been purposefully wronged by others, been held back in their lives by others, or been the target of derision by others. Most of these individuals are not psychiatrically ill, or at least they have not come to clinical attention for having obsessive-compulsive disorder (OCD) or a psychotic illness. They are able to keep their peculiar thinking and behaviors under sufficient control to function in their lives. For unclear reasons, people whose behavior reaches the threshold of psychiatric disorder fail to correct or adjust to errors in thinking, mood, and motivation. These errors, particularly those that are emotionally charged, compound over time and lead to persistent, unusual behaviors that become uncomfortable for the individuals and for those around them.

Cognitive neuroscientists Paul Fletcher and Chris Frith have discussed problems in error correction from a psychiatric perspective. They postulate that an inability to distinguish between relevant and irrelevant inputs is a major problem for persons with psychiatric disorders. Thus, individuals with illness have a propensity to act on irrelevant information and appear to have defects in self-monitoring. For example, in schizophrenia, the problem does not appear to be a defect in logical reasoning per se, but rather a defect in *probabilistic reasoning*—a tendency to discount strong evidence against a belief while overvaluing weak information in favor of the belief. By working with incorrectly weighted information, people with schizophrenia come to inaccurate conclusions about themselves and the world, and are unable to update their beliefs on the basis of new input—a type of learning or plasticity defect. Interestingly, schizophrenia is often thought to involve defects in the dopamine transmitter system, and one of dopamine's principal functions is to generate error-prediction signals. Thus, problems in error correction in people with schizophrenia may reflect defects in neural circuits using dopamine-mediated transmission. These defects may in turn influence working memory and explicit learning, and lead to difficulties in using new information as a corrective device.

Persons with other psychiatric illnesses also demonstrate defects in error correction, although the characteristics of the defects appear to differ from those seen in schizophrenia. Based on cognitive testing studies, Farshad Mansouri and colleagues report that individuals with major depression are capable of error detection and error correction; however, they require increased time and neuronal effort to process and correct their mental errors. During this temporal delay, the yet-to-be corrected errors have more time to become incorporated into new learning, hence perpetuating and compounding the defect. The problem is not that the depressed person always inaccurately evaluates information. Rather, the correction system works too slowly and the error becomes ingrained in thinking and perception. Depressed individuals are also known to assess situations inaccurately because of negative emotional bias, and this compounds problems with error generation and correction: the negatively charged events take precedence over positive experiences, reflecting, again, an emotion-based bias in probabilistic reasoning.

OCD offers a third example of problems encountered with error processing. Individuals with this disorder can accurately evaluate relevant information and can process the information fast enough. However, they seem to have difficulty preventing irrelevant inputs from interfering with relevant ideas—a type of attentional and cognitive inflexibility problem. In effect, relevant and irrelevant thoughts and perceptions become intertwined and carry a high emotional (anxiety and dysphoria) component. In some ways, the problems observed in OCD seem more akin to the error correction problems noted in schizophrenia, including having magical beliefs about things (for example, the power of their own thinking or actions to result in a bad outcome). This is consistent with clinical observations indicating that it can sometimes be difficult to distinguish delusional ideas from severe obsessional thinking.

When the brain is unable to correct its mental errors, various symptoms can develop. Persons with schizophrenia may develop persecutory delusions because of an inability to weigh the relevance of information accurately. Depressed patients may have misperceptions about their self-worth, and when they are unable to correct these thoughts in a timely manner, the thoughts become ingrained in their thinking, leading to thoughts of guilt and death. Persons with OCD may have extraneous inputs interfere with error correction, and they may keep trying to return to the relevant information, developing habitual obsessions or compulsive actions in the process. Over time, erroneous ideas become incorporated into routine thinking and become more persistent and habitual. This situation is compounded by psychosocial stress; with increasing stress, humans and other species become more habitual (implicit) in their responses as a way the brain uses to conserve energy.

WHY DO INDIVIDUALS WITH PSYCHIATRIC DISORDERS FAIL TO CORRECT MENTAL ERRORS?

Error correction and its role in psychiatric disorders are complex topics and not yet understood in great detail. We believe that error correction reflects an important set of mechanisms that the brain uses to work efficiently, and when these mechanisms aren't working correctly, problems develop. In this section, we speculate about factors that may contribute to faulty error correction. These are highlighted in Table 5-1.

Error correction often requires the ability of higher brain systems to override mistakes in emotions, motivation, and perception, more primitive modes of neural processing. Thus, one likely contributor to faulty error correction and homeostasis is a failure of top-down control. This could arise in multiple ways. For example, impaired intellectual development could limit the ability of the brain to handle the complex array of information that bombards it regularly. Cognitive inflexibility and cognitive control defects associated with impaired intellectual development likely contribute to the observation that individuals with lower general intelligence (as measured by standard IQ testing) are at increased risk of several major psychiatric disorders, including schizophrenia, substance abuse, and major depression. Similarly, developmental problems arising from severe early life stress (e.g., malnourishment, abuse, and neglect) could interfere with higher cortical function as a result of neural injury and aberrant learning. Problems in cortically driven top-down control could also arise at other times in life from specific brain lesions (for example, traumatic brain injury or stroke) or neurodegenerative disorders that lead to dysfunction and disconnections among ICNs involved in cognition, attention, emotion, and motivation.

Table 5-1 Why Failure to Self-Correct?

Altered top-down control
    Neurodevelopmental problem (IQ/early stress)
    Lesions/neurodegeneration (cell loss, cortical thinning)
    Disconnections between emotions/motivation/cognition (synaptic/connectivity problem)
Primary overriding defect in emotional, motivational, or cognitive systems
Faulty learning (plasticity problem)
Usurped motivation (drugs/drives/ideas)

In addition to failures of top-down processing, some individuals may have primary pervasive problems in emotional and motivational systems that make it difficult for higher centers to correct erroneous information. For example, early childhood abuse and neglect are associated with hyperreactive stress responses in which relatively innocuous events can trigger inappropriate emotional and bodily responses. It is possible, perhaps even likely, that stressful events early in childhood, particularly when coupled with certain genetic predispositions, interfere with emotional development and result in stress and emotional systems that override cortical control. This could combine with early stress-mediated changes in cortical development to cause significant difficulties in emotional regulation. Similar considerations could affect motivational and reward systems. For example, individuals who abuse certain drugs have changes in their motivation-salience systems that make it difficult for these systems to self-correct. All abused drugs profoundly influence the brain's motivation and reward systems and lead to long-term, persistent effects on the structure and function of these systems, effects that often persist well beyond the period of drug use. Normally, neocortex exerts control over drives generated by the motivation system. Drugs of abuse can cause a rebalancing of functional connectivity among these systems, diminishing the effectiveness of cortical connections and allowing poorly regulated emotionally driven actions to substitute for healthier pathways to reward and stress reduction. This functional and physical rewiring of the motivational system likely contributes to the fact that substance-abuse syndromes are often difficult to treat and are subject to repeated relapses.

Interestingly, drugs of abuse are not the only way in which motivation can be usurped and made difficult to regulate. As humans evolved the capacity for abstract thinking, we also developed the ability to use our abstract thoughts as motivators. Thus, in addition to more physiological drives (food, sex, survival), humans can use abstract concepts to drive actions (for example, striving to win a game or fighting for a political cause). When taken to extremes, abstract beliefs can so override logic that humans will sometimes destroy themselves for their beliefs, as witnessed by political or religious suicides. In effect, we are probably the only species that can be so "seduced" by our own thinking. The point here is that certain thoughts can become so ingrained in our brain's processing that, like drugs of abuse, they override rational control.

RETHINKING PSYCHIATRIC CLASSIFICATION AND ENDOPHENOTYPES

As we have stated before, we view major psychiatric disorders as involving dysfunction across the three spheres of the mind: thinking, emotion, and motivation. This does not imply, however, that the primary pathology driving dysfunction in any given illness equally affects the ICNs that make up these computational systems. For example, cortical centers involved in executive function are prone to dysfunction when abnormalities arise in other brain systems. In Alzheimer's disease, individuals typically develop problems with executive function (planning and decision making), but the initial pathology attacks and percolates within memory systems; higher-order dysfunction represents a secondary manifestation. It is also important to consider how brain plasticity can work against an individual in the context of illness. Mental errors generated within one system can propagate as illness persists and progresses. Erroneous processing can become more crystallized and pervasive, involving expanding degrees of brain circuitry over time. Substance-abuse disorders may represent an instructive example of this concept in which an expanding neural circuitry comes to play a role as illness progresses over time and repeated drug use. We will discuss this in greater detail later in this chapter. For now, we want to consider whether it is useful to think about psychiatric classification according to the tripartite constructs of the mind—that is, is it useful to conceptualize psychiatric disorders as reflecting *primary* dysfunction in cognition, emotion, or motivation? Such a classification would attempt to define a primary locus of dysfunction within one of these major constructs of mind, and might help in defining the earliest manifestations of illness and in understanding how the illness progresses over time to affect all three components of the mind. If illnesses can be staged according to such a scheme, it might be possible to design rational therapeutic and rehabilitative strategies that are targeted toward stage of illness, including individuals at high risk who have not yet developed full-blown dysfunction. Such a scheme might also help us to understand why it is more difficult to treat major depression in the context of a personality disorder (or substance abuse disorder) than "primary" depression in an individual without other psychiatric disorders, and why it may be inappropriate to use similar treatment strategies in these two scenarios.

Table 5-2 presents a simple example of how such a classification scheme might be constructed. In this example, dementing illnesses, mental retardation syndromes, and delirium are viewed as primary disorders of *cognitive* function resulting from

Table 5-2 Mental Disorders and Mind: Primary Defects and Disabilities?

Primary cognitive disorders?

  Working memory/attention/executive function (PFC-parietal networks)

- Dementia, mental retardation, delirium
- Psychotic disorders
- Obsessional disorders?

Primary emotional disorders?

  Negative emotions (mPFC-pgACC-extended amygdala network)

- Mood disorders
- Anxiety disorders

Primary motivational disorders?

  VTA-nucleus accumbens-PFC network

- Substance abuse/alcoholism
- Eating disorders
- Paraphilias
- Personality disorders

major defects in higher-level processing; all of these disorders exhibit significant problems with learning, memory, and reasoning. We are less certain about including deliria in this group because these are complex syndromes that strongly involve arousal and more primitive brain dysfunction. Similarly, we wonder whether psychotic disorders and perhaps obsessional disorders might also be viewed as involving major, but different, defects in cognition that are present early in the illness process. The aligning of psychotic disorders with dementias and developmental cognitive disorders would be consistent with the frequent association of the latter disorders with psychotic symptoms. Furthermore, there is evidence that varying degrees of neuropsychological dysfunction accompany all psychotic disorders and these defects are often present at the onset of the first episode. We would also note that in such a scheme the designation of an illness as "psychotic" would take on *primary* importance in classification, reflecting the more aggressive course and cognitive dysfunction associated with psychosis regardless of how we currently classify the disorder (e.g., schizophrenia, bipolar disorder, or psychotic major depression). This would also mean that the presence of psychosis would result in certain mood disorders being aligned more closely with schizophrenia than with non-psychotic mood disorders. This might be more consistent with shared genetics across psychotic disorders and may result in the development of strategies for rehabilitative efforts targeting the defects in cognition that lead to or are associated with the generation of psychotic thinking. This classification would also be consistent with the importance of cognitive defects in psychotic disorders as prime drivers of work-related disability.

A problem with this approach might lie in determining the presence of psychotic symptoms in individual patients or even in determining what constitutes a psychotic symptom (Chapter 1). However, we don't see this as a major issue in clinical settings, where disorders with psychotic features are typically viewed and treated as being distinct from non-psychotic illnesses. What is less clear, in the case of mood disorders, is whether each episode of depression or mania in a given patient is also associated with psychosis. Some persons with a mood disorder may exhibit periods of illness with or without psychotic symptoms, and this complicates the proposed conceptualization. We would argue, however, that once an individual has developed unequivocal psychosis, almost regardless of cause, he or she has a more complex illness than the non-psychotic versions of the disorder.

Other disorders, specifically non-psychotic mood disorders and anxiety disorders, might be viewed as reflecting primary defects in *emotional* systems, involving genetic and acquired changes in the function of the extended amygdala, reward system, and associated ICNs. Consistent with this, depressed individuals exhibit major difficulties in sustaining positive emotions, and this correlates with a failure to maintain activity in a circuit involving frontal cortex and nucleus accumbens when processing pleasant experiences. Shared brain circuitry could account for the large degree of comorbidity among mood and anxiety syndromes. Again, as these illnesses progress, they might secondarily involve cognitive and motivational systems, but the primary defect is likely to be found in the emotional system.

Some psychiatric disorders could also be viewed as arising from primary deficits in *motivation* pathways. The substance-abuse disorders are the clearest examples based on the known pharmacology of abused drugs and their propensity to target the ventral tegmental–nucleus accumbens network. We would also speculate whether eating disorders, paraphilias, gambling disorders, and perhaps personality disorders fit into such a scheme, since each of these groups of disorders exhibits major issues with aberrant motivation.

While it is clearly premature to reclassify psychiatric disorders along these lines, it is possible that a conceptual scheme like this could help define intermediate phenotypes that are more closely linked to brain ICNs and possibly to the genetics and biology of the disorders. As an example, we would return to recent work on the role of brain ICNs in the pathology and clinical presentation of dementia syndromes (Chapter 2). In these syndromes, clinical phenotype is driven by dysfunction within specific ICNs, while the molecular mechanisms underlying the dysfunction can be shared across phenotypes. For example, the usual clinical phenotype of Alzheimer's disease appears to involve a primary attack on the default network, but less commonly the molecular pathological hallmarks of Alzheimer's disease, plaques and tangles, can also lead to the clinical presentation of behavioral variant frontotemporal dementia. This occurs when the plaques and tangles attack a different ICN (the emotional-salience system). More often, the neurodegeneration accompanying behavioral variant frontotemporal dementia involves molecular pathology that differs from that found in Alzheimer's disease. While it is not yet clear what renders a given ICN vulnerable in a given individual, the high activity and energy requirements of default network processing seem to be important in Alzheimer's disease, and this provides one clue that could be helpful in devising future treatment and prevention strategies.

Expanding these concepts to psychiatric disorders, one might also look for endophenotypes based on primary emotions observed in animals and humans, as proposed by Jaak Panksepp. What we are tentatively calling *primary emotional disorders* (non-psychotic mood and anxiety disorders) largely reflect a strong negative emotional bias: sadness/defeat in the case of depression, fear/anxiety in the case of anxiety disorders, and perhaps anger/rage in other disorders. Manic euphoria might be viewed as an exception, but even here elation often degenerates into irritability and anger as well as mixed manic and depressed states. The neural computations leading to a particular mood state are becoming better understood and appear to involve a comparison of real or perceived outcomes to one's internal expectations (Table 5-3). When outcomes are below expectations, emotions are triggered as brain systems attempt to reset. The specific emotion that is experienced may reflect an internal bias of the individual's emotional ICNs, with perceived defeat/loss generating sadness, perceived threat triggering anxiety (flight), or perceived unfairness triggering rage (fight). The emotional triggers themselves seem to revolve around several themes, including perceived harm, failure, rejection, and ambiguity. Ambiguity (uncertainty) might be the most difficult for humans to deal with because it is the least specific. Ambiguity may also be the emotional trigger that requires the

Table 5-3 Negative Emotional Bias

Sadness (loss)	Triggers
Outcome < expectation → defeat	Harm
Anxiety (fear)	Failure
Outcome < expectation → flight	Rejection
Anger (rage)	Ambiguity
Outcome < expectation → fight	

highest degree of coordination among executive, emotional, and motivational systems because it requires more brain effort to analyze.

This discussion raises an important question about the factors that determine "expectations" in our brains. We described these concepts in Chapter 4 but will expand the theme a bit here. At the most primitive level, humans are motivated by *drives* that influence survival and reproduction (e.g., food, sex, protection). Humans are also motivated by *wants*—things that aren't necessary for survival and evolution but that are attractive and advantageous. In these cases, the brain calculus reflects a determination of whether a perceived outcome or behavior is worth the cost. This calculation can take into account concepts like social approval and even our own abstract ideas about the things that we find attractive. Inherent features of our personalities seem to be a major variable in these determinations, particularly dimensions of personality that C. Robert Cloninger and others refer to as *temperament*. Cloninger defines temperament as habits and skills that are elicited by relatively simple stimuli perceived by our senses. Temperament is described in terms of features like harm avoidance, novelty seeking, reward dependence, and persistence—traits that are heritable, developmentally stable, and not driven primarily by social learning. These traits help to determine the things that catch our attention and that have a high degree of emotional salience. Interestingly, and as described in Chapter 4, neuroimaging studies indicate that these temperament traits reflect activity in specific neural circuits that are part of the motivational ICN.

WHAT DO WE KNOW ABOUT ICNs AND PSYCHIATRIC DISORDERS?

Cognitive Disorders: Psychosis

While it is safe to say that we don't yet understand how ICNs are involved in any primary psychiatric disorders, lessons learned from behavioral neurology where specific brain lesions result in psychiatric symptoms can be helpful in pointing directions (see Chapter 1). Thus, we believe that psychosis can be examined as a primary defect involving components of our cognition systems. For example, some psychotic symptoms involve delusional misidentification of people in the environment. In Capgras syndrome, individuals develop the belief that a person close to them has been replaced by an exact double. Certain brain lesions are also associated with delusional misidentification. These lesions typically involve the nondominant hemisphere or both frontal lobes and result in defects in the abilities to monitor one's self and correct inaccurate perceptions. Clinical examples include the syndrome of reduplicative paramnesia, in which a person develops the belief that he or she is in a place that is an identical replica of the place he or she is. As noted in Chapter 1, similar brain lesions can also be associated with anosognosia-for example, a person's inability to recognize a limb as being part of his or her own body. In these cases, damage to the right hemisphere results in the primary neurological defect (e.g., left-sided hemiparesis), but the intact left hemisphere becomes overactive and provides an aberrant explanation. In these syndromes, faulty input from the lesioned region combines with overgeneralization from the left hemisphere to generate symptoms. While mechanisms underlying Capgras syndrome are less certain, defects in cognitive processing could interact with emotional changes to produce symptoms. V. S. Ramachandran has suggested that Capgras syndrome may involve altered connectivity between perception (seeing and hearing a family member) and emotion (lack of positive valance), with a failure to experience the expected emotion leading to a delusional explanation. When the perceived loved one evokes little or no emotion (or even negative emotion), the left hemisphere generates the explanation that the person can't be the loved one, but instead must be an imposter. In this case, the primary cause of the syndrome is a disconnection between the emotional and cognitive systems, but the cognitive system, in an effort to make sense of the defective input, develops the mistaken belief that the loved one was replaced by an exact double. As noted, a major defect in probabilistic reasoning may lie at the heart of the delusion. Perhaps related to this, some evidence suggests that individuals with schizophrenia have difficulties differentiating new and old information, and that defects in right hemispheric processing contribute to problems with recognition memory. The left hemisphere then appears to supply a delusional conclusion for the misperceived information. Other evidence suggests that impairments in threat responses in conjunction with diminished recognition memory contribute to worsening of psychotic symptoms.

A number of studies have examined mental factors that contribute to persecutory ideas in people with and without psychiatric disorders. Across human populations, persecutory ideas and suspiciousness represent the most common forms of delusion, and these types of ideas are relatively common among individuals with no clear psychiatric disorder, although in the latter individuals they don't become as unshakable or bizarre as they are in persons with true delusions. Factors contributing to persecutory ideation seem to include a combination of emotional and cognitive processing problems leading to persistently defective thinking. Individuals with persecutory ideas and delusions typically exhibit a negative emotional bias (i.e., a tendency toward pessimism, dysphoria, and low self-esteem) along with defects in executive function and decision making (e.g., a tendency to jump to conclusions and to misinterpret the mental states of others). Problems with problem solving and probabilistic reasoning contribute as well and may be major factors in the transition from odd "ideas" to "delusions." The influence of negative emotional bias coupled with defects in executive function results in cognitive biases in how attention is focused, how situations are assessed, and how attributions are made. The important point is that delusional thinking has a cognitive basis but is not simply a thought problem: it reflects a combination of cognitive defects and emotional bias. Multiple ICNs contribute to symptoms, but cognitive misinterpretation plays the lead role in how the symptoms are manifest and likely in determining how fixed the aberrant ideas become.

The involvement of multiple ICNs in psychosis is highlighted further when one considers illnesses like schizophrenia. This psychotic disorder is characterized by positive symptoms (delusions, hallucinations, and thought disorder), negative symptoms (blunted affect, asociality, alogia, anergia, and amotivation [the so-called "5 A's"]), cognitive defects (problems in selective attention, recognition memory, and working memory, among others), and, at times, motor symptoms. Interestingly, the cognitive defects appear to be longstanding problems in many individuals; they are often present at the onset of illness and remain relatively stable over time. They also play a major role in determining the long-term course of the illness and the level of disability, serving as a principal reason that individuals with schizophrenia have difficulty completing school or holding gainful employment (the "dementia" of Kraepelin's dementia praecox). Cognitive deficits are also likely contributors to the aberrant thinking associated with the illness, including persecutory ideas.

What goes wrong in the brains of patients with schizophrenia to produce cognitive dysfunction and symptoms? While this is still a work in progress, some insights are being gained from studies of brain networks. Individuals with schizophrenia exhibit defects across brain regions with structural changes (shrinkage and loss of cells) in the hippocampus and multiple parts of the neocortex, including the PFC. We previously noted that brain networks have a small-world connectivity that reflects high degrees of local clustering among regions in a network (short path length) and efficient transfer of information between more distant regions mediated by a few longer-range connections. Danielle Bassett and colleagues used functional imaging to examine how healthy controls and individuals with schizophrenia compare with regard to brain network connectivity. Persons with schizophrenia exhibit abnormal multimodal network organization with reduced hierarchical structure of neocortex and diminished connectivity of frontal cortex hubs. Non-frontal cortical regions, in contrast, exhibited highly connected hubs not seen in controls. This results in a brain architecture that is less efficient in handling multimodal data, and is consistent with a type of dysconnectivity involving the frontal lobes. Figure 5-1 presents an overview of this work and highlights differences in cortical network connectivity and hierarchy in controls and individuals with schizophrenia.

Changes in small-world connectivity among cortical regions have practical consequences for information processing. Van den Heuvel and colleagues found that the *resting-state* path length of cortical networks inversely correlates with IQ measures of intelligence: a longer resting-state path length is associated with diminished processing efficiency and lower general intelligence. Thus, dysconnectivity and loss of hierarchical processing in schizophrenia, particularly involving right-sided

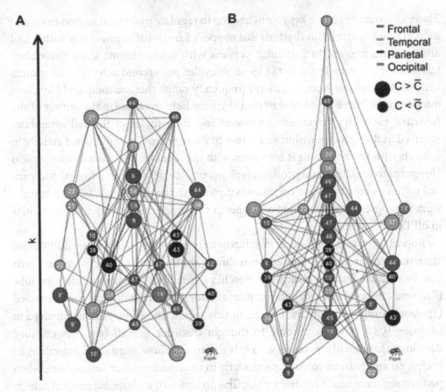

A

B

— Frontal
— Temporal
— Parietal
— Occipital

● $C > \bar{C}$
● $C < \bar{C}$

Figure 5-1 Connectivity maps: controls vs. persons with schizophrenia. The diagram depicts differences in cortical connectivity between control subjects (A) and individuals with schizophrenia (B) based on functional MRI data. The diagram shows altered local clustering in frontal cortex and longer path lengths linking cortical regions in individuals with schizophrenia. (Reproduced with permission from Bassett et al., 2008.) See color insert.

frontoparietal networks, may account for the observed difficulties in working memory, executive function, and distinguishing new and old information, the latter perhaps contributing to problems in correcting defective premises about one's self and the external world.

David Lewis and Robert Sweet have cogently discussed schizophrenia from a neurocircuitry perspective, highlighting defects in working memory and auditory processing. The working memory defects involve abnormalities in dorsolateral prefrontal cortex (dlPFC), a region critical for the ability to hold thoughts on line in focused attention. When asked to do tasks in which working memory load is low, subjects with schizophrenia are able to perform the tasks but show higher levels of activation of dlPFC compared to controls. This reflects higher cognitive demand and the need for greater energy use to do the task. When working memory demand is high, persons with schizophrenia exhibit diminished dlPFC activity and experience difficulty with task performance. In addition to these functional defects, subjects with schizophrenia have structural abnormalities in pyramidal neurons and certain types of GABAergic interneurons in dlPFC. The latter cells are a class of fast spiking inhibitory neurons that express the calcium binding protein, parvalbumin.

These interneurons play a key role in helping to regulate pyramidal neuron firing and help to synchronize brain rhythms that support functional connectivity within and among brain regions. In particular, persons with schizophrenia show diminished task-related rhythms in the beta (15 to 30 cycles per second activity) and gamma (30 to 80 cycles per second activity) frequency range that are modulated by these interneurons. These types of electrical rhythms help to organize the output of the principal excitatory (pyramidal) neurons and help to select the cell assemblies involved in doing a task within and across brain regions. The diminished activity in subjects with schizophrenia is consistent with the idea that there is a dysconnection (longer path length) among cortical regions, particularly between frontal and parietal regions, contributing to cognitive symptoms in the disorder. While this is still a work in progress, it appears that one aspect of schizophrenia involves abnormalities in dlPFC processing.

Importantly, cortical defects in schizophrenia are not restricted to dlPFC, and alterations in gamma rhythms are seen throughout neocortex. For example, Lewis and Sweet also describe changes in Heschl's gyrus in the dominant temporal lobe that result in problems in interpreting auditory input, including the expressed (spoken) emotions of others. Defects in this region and other regions involved in language ICNs likely contribute to thought disorder as well (e.g., tangentiality, derailment). Similarly, persons with schizophrenia show attenuated activation of prefrontal and parietal cortices, particularly in the nondominant hemisphere, when performing recognition memory tasks. The presence of widespread cortical defects may be a major contributor to the defects in focused attention observed in schizophrenia. A recent large-scale meta-analysis of neuroimaging data has added support for these ideas and indicates that when doing cognitive control tasks, patients with schizophrenia activate the same cortical and subcortical networks as controls, but differ in having diminished activation of regions required to maintain context and task, a type of cognitive control problem.

Other studies have found that persons with schizophrenia have an overactive default system and problems shifting out of the default mode when asked to focus attention. Defects in focused attention and working memory could be major contributors to the blurring of internal and external worlds associated with schizophrenia, leading to delusions and hallucinations when combined with higher-level cognitive defects and negative emotional biases. Consistent with this, a recent study examining a genetic risk factor for psychosis (schizophrenia and bipolar disorder) found that risk was associated with diminished connectivity between right and left dlPFC (likely reflecting problems in working memory) and enhanced connectivity between hippocampus (part of the default system) and dlPFC. Normal subjects showed little direct connectivity between hippocampus and dlPFC. Interestingly, genetic risk was also associated with greater connectivity between the amygdala, hippocampus, and PFC, perhaps reflecting the emotional bias associated with psychotic symptoms. Thus, it is possible that primary defects in cortical systems involved in cognitive processing lead to both the negative and positive symptoms of schizophrenia. Some of these cognitive defects may create unbalanced communication between cognitive, emotional, and motivational systems. Recent studies suggest that treatment with antipsychotic medications may help to modulate activity within the default ICN and that early changes in blood flow in ventral striatum and hippocampus (in the first week of treatment) are predictive of good clinical response, with changes in anterior cingulate and frontal cortex occurring later in the process (after 6 weeks of treatment). This again highlights the interdependence of neural circuits underlying the mind.

In our thinking, we include psychotic mood disorders and the complicated syndrome of schizoaffective disorder among the "cognitive" disorders. This is consistent with the cognitive impairment associated with these disorders and with their more aggressive course. We admit, however, that changes in neurocircuitry are much less well defined in these disorders. In a comprehensive 2009 review, Jonathan Savitz and Wayne Drevets concluded that subjects with bipolar disorder have diminished volume in several brain regions, including hippocampus, orbital PFC, and ventral PFC, with hypometabolism in dorsal PFC. They emphasized that subjects with bipolar disorder also share some abnormalities with individuals with major depressive disorder involving a "viscero-motor emotion regulating network" that includes medial PFC, amygdala, hippocampus, ventral striatum, hypothalamus, and brain stem. We will describe this circuitry in more detail later in this chapter.

Obsessive-Compulsive Disorder: Cognitive or Emotional Disorder?

OCD is usually considered an anxiety disorder, emphasizing the strong emotional component in this illness. While anxiety is clearly a key symptom, we will consider OCD separately from other anxiety disorders and focus on how cognitive aspects of the disorder may arise and the relationship between cognitive and emotional symptoms. OCD is a heterogeneous condition in which individuals have recurrent and intrusive thoughts (obsessions) that are often accompanied by repetitive motor behaviors (compulsions) performed to allay associated negative emotions. A large-scale meta-analysis found that symptoms of OCD cluster around four major themes: symmetry (repeating, ordering, and counting rituals), forbidden thoughts (usually with sexual, religious, or aggressive content), cleanliness (concerns about contamination), and hoarding behaviors. While most characteristic of OCD, these symptoms are observed in other psychiatric disorders and are also found in individuals without defined psychiatric illness. Even in nonclinical populations, however, these symptoms can cause distress. Often, negative emotions (anxiety and low mood) are associated with such symptoms and are a driving force behind seeking clinical care.

The brain changes associated with OCD appear to involve pathways connecting the striatum (basal ganglia) and PFC, particularly the ventral and orbital PFC, where emotional inputs are received, processed, and regulated. These circuits are important because they allow the cortex to exert inhibitory control over behaviors and drive more flexible patterns of behavior. OCD is associated with structural and functional changes in this striatocortical circuitry, especially changes involving orbitofrontal cortex.

This region is important for *reversal learning*, a form of learning that uses negative feedback to alter behaviors that are ineffective or unproductive. These observations draw attention to the cognitive aspects of OCD and raise the possibility that defects in a specific form of learning are a major contributor to clinical phenotype. Interestingly, patients with OCD and their clinically unaffected close relatives show diminished activation of lateral orbitofrontal cortex and other cortical regions during reversal learning, suggesting that defects in reversal learning may be endo-phenotypes for the disorder. How defects in reversal learning arise is not certain but could involve changes in modulatory monoamine neurotransmitters. At the mini-mum, key cognitive defects in OCD seem to include problems in reversal learning as well as difficulties shifting attention among thoughts and an overall inflexibility in thinking. Defects in executive function, including problems with decision making and planning, are also associated with the disorder.

There is some evidence that different OCD symptoms have distinct neural corre-lates with increased connectivity within fronto-striato-thalamic circuits. For example, when performing a symptom provocation task, persons with cleansing rituals have increased activation in ventromedial PFC and right caudate nucleus, whereas indi-viduals with hoarding behaviors have increased activation in left precentral gyrus and right orbitofrontal cortex. Persons with checking rituals exhibit increased connectiv-ity among putamen/globus pallidus, thalamus, and dorsal aspects of neocortex. Interestingly, individuals with OCD also show reduced functional connectivity between lateral PFC and dorsal striatum and between ventral striatum and the ventral tegmental area. The latter findings suggest reasons that conscious cognitive control can be difficult for OCD patients and error correction may be defective.

The findings in OCD again highlight key interactions between cognitive and emotional systems leading to clinical dysfunction. Furthermore, the involvement of both the dorsal and ventral striatum in OCD provides circuitry that can translate aberrant thinking into motor output, namely implicit, habit-driven behaviors appearing in the form of compulsive acts and rituals. Based on this, we suggest that OCD involves significant problems in cognitive processing and, therefore, might be more appropriately classified as a subtype of primary cognitive disorders. It is less clear, however, that individuals with OCD exhibit the working memory problems associated with other cognitive disorders, although the intrusion of unwanted thoughts into consciousness may reflect a type of filtering problem.

Anxiety Disorders as Primary Emotional Disorders

Anxiety disorders are a heterogeneous group of illnesses involving forms of exces-sive and inappropriate fear. Other negative emotional symptoms, particularly depressed mood, are often observed, and there is considerable overlap between mood and anxiety disorders, both in terms of symptoms and treatments. It is also important to consider that anxiety, while having its closest ties to the primary emo-tion of fear, differs from fear in several regards. While fear is usually a rapid response to a perceived and better-defined threat, anxiety can be much more persistent and less directly tied to specific external cues or circumstances. The fear observed in anxiety disorders can be directed toward discrete things (phobias) and/or other people (social phobias). It can be pervasive and relatively unfocused (generalized anxiety) or time-linked to various life stressors (acute or posttraumatic stress), or can occur as discrete episodes with clear or unclear triggers (panic attacks). How and why different forms of anxiety disorders arise is uncertain, but it appears that all forms engage the brain's fear circuitry. Hence, the amygdala and its distributed connections play a central role.

The neuroscience of anxiety has been significantly aided by the existence of well-characterized models of fear in rodents. We described this circuitry in some detail in Chapter 4 and highlighted the existence of two pathways for fear processing: a subcortical path that allows rapid and unconscious assessment of stimuli and a path that includes neocortex and conscious feelings. Furthermore, work in rodents has demonstrated that chronic and less-directed fear responses, resembling anxiety in humans, engage and require a more distributed extended amygdala circuit that includes the bed nucleus of the stria terminalis (BNST) and the shell (outer) region of the nucleus accumbens. How the more extended amygdala is engaged in this process is not completely understood but appears to involve release of corticotrophin-releasing factor (CRF) from output terminals of the central amygdaloid nucleus in the BNST. In these studies, the BNST takes on a key role in differentiating fear from anxiety, although circuitry is clearly shared. We would also further emphasize interactions between the extended amygdala and hippocampus in fear-based learning, particularly with regard to context. Figure 4-4 (Chapter 4) presents an overview of the neural systems involved in fear and anxiety.

What happens to brain circuitry in human anxiety disorders? A complete answer to this question is not known, but it appears that there are several types of information processing that likely contribute to the spectrum of anxiety disorders. As described by Daniel Pine and colleagues, there is an attentional component to anxiety that allows individuals to orient to a perceived threat. This process is followed by an appraisal of the threat and includes social and physiological responses. There are also strong components of learning and memory in anxiety disorders (akin to fear conditioning in rodents). In many ways, these processing components resemble components observed in animals and likely reflect analogous brain circuitry. Thus, the amygdala, and to a lesser extent the hippocampus, are thought to play a major role in determining initial threat assessment and orienting responses. Just as in rodents, there is evidence for the involvement of the ventral and medial PFC, and this involvement may be particularly important for the appraisal component of anxiety processing and for performance monitoring and response prevention. Anxiety disorders also engage circuitry in the striatum, including the caudate-putamen and nucleus accumbens. This striatal involvement is likely important for driving motor and habitual responses, conflict monitoring, and error correction. This circuitry is excessively active in anxiety states, although the changes observed in social phobias appear to differ from those observed in specific phobias or OCD.

Parts of this fear/anxiety network also show structural changes in certain anxiety disorders. For example, there is evidence for shrinkage of the hippocampus and perhaps the amygdala in posttraumatic stress disorder (PTSD). Structural changes in the hippocampus may distinguish PTSD from other anxiety disorders. We will deal with the role of stress in psychiatric disorders in subsequent chapters, but for now we question whether PTSD should be classified with other anxiety disorders given the types of symptoms encountered (e.g., emotional numbness, intrusive re-experiencing of events). Further work on the neurocircuitry of these disorders should help to clarify this issue.

Recent studies in generalized anxiety disorder (GAD) highlight potentially important changes in functional connectivity within anxiety/fear circuits, including possible compensatory changes associated with illness. Amit Etkin and colleagues found that there is little connectivity between executive control networks in cortex (dlPFC and posterior parietal cortex) and amygdala in healthy controls. Subjects with GAD, in contrast, exhibit enhanced connectivity between amygdala and executive control regions, but diminished connectivity to a salience network involving insula and cingulate cortex. These authors speculate that the enhanced engagement of a cortical control network is a compensatory adaptation that helps to maintain control over emotional outputs, while the altered connectivity to the salience system may result in problems regulating autonomic nervous system outputs (e.g., heart rate, sweating).

Emotional Disorders: Primary Major Depression

Depressive disorders, like the anxiety disorders, are a heterogeneous group of illnesses. We emphasized this in Chapter 2 but highlight this again as we now consider how brain networks may be involved in major depression. Our focus in the following discussion is on "primary" non-psychotic mood disorders that exist either in the absence of other psychiatric illnesses or that clearly antedate the onset of other disorders, with particular attention paid to highly familial forms of major depression. We will also consider depression occurring in the context of bipolar (type I) disorder, but we believe this may be a different form of illness, given its propensity to manifest psychotic symptoms during both depression and mania. We believe these considerations are important because lumping all depressions together, including the so-called "minor" depressions, is likely to result in confusing data with regard to brain networks.

Studies by Wayne Drevets, Helen Mayberg, and others have played a major role in describing the involvement of cognitive, emotional, and motivational systems in major depressive disorder (MDD) and the way functional connectivity changes contribute to symptoms and recovery. These studies have also helped to define circuitry in emotional systems that may be the drivers of the dysfunction in major depression. Using well-characterized subjects with highly familial forms of MDD and bipolar disorder, Drevets and colleagues found increases in blood flow and metabolism in circuits involving orbital frontal cortex, ventrolateral prefrontal cortex

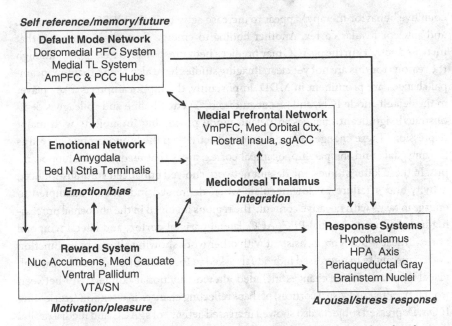

Figure 5-2 Depression circuitry. The diagram depicts key regions and connections thought to be involved in primary major depression. This circuitry highlights the role of emotional, cognitive, and motivational systems in this complex set of disorders. (Adapted from descriptions provided by Wayne Drevets and Joel Price.) For locations of anatomic structures, please refer to the Appendix. Abbreviations: TL (temporal lobe), PCC (posterior cingulate cortex), sgACC (subgenual anterior cingulate cortex).

(vlPFC), and the subgenual and pregenual anterior cingulate cortices (sgACC and pgACC). The critical circuit also includes the amygdala, ventral striatum, and medial thalamus. Other studies have highlighted the importance of abnormalities in the PFC, sgACC, hippocampus, and amygdala. The cortical changes associated with MDD are thought to contribute to higher-level emotional experiences and cognitive dysfunction, while the subcortical changes are thought to contribute to changes in emotional processing, emotional memory, memory retrieval, and motivation, particularly motivation to perform goal-oriented tasks. Figure 5-2 presents an overview of neural circuitry involved in major depression.

In imaging studies, the sgACC has emerged as a key node, with increased activity in the sgACC and amygdala correlating with the severity of active depressive symptoms. In contrast, changes in vlPFC and lateral orbital cortex correlate negatively with depression severity. Interactions among these sites and within this network are thought to be important in symptom production, with diminished activity in medial PFC resulting in disinhibition of the amygdala and changes in endocrine, autonomic, reward, and attentional systems in MDD. Interestingly, different treatments for depression seem to affect the core network in different ways, perhaps reflecting the basic underlying mechanisms of the treatments. Antidepressant medications and deep brain stimulation targeted to sgACC appear to diminish overactivity in sgACC and amygdala, while psychotherapeutic interventions (interpersonal therapy and cognitive behavior therapy) appear to increase activity in the vlPFC, orbital cortex, and anterior insular cortex. Another finding to emerge from these studies is that increased activity in the pgACC may predict a better response to treatment, although the reasons for this are not yet clear. Imaging studies have also found that hippocampal changes are prominent in MDD. Importantly, the hippocampus is a key player in the default-mode ICN, and recent studies by Yvette Sheline and colleagues demonstrated significant changes in default-mode processing in subjects with major depression. These changes include increased activity in the hippocampus, as well as the amygdala and the parahippocampal cortex, areas that feed into the hippocampus. In these latter studies, the default network showed enhanced stimulus-induced activity and a failure to downregulate when depressed individuals attempted to engage in tasks with negative content. The regions involved in the abnormal processing included ventromedial PFC, ACC, lateral parietal cortex, and lateral temporal cortex. These studies are consistent with other work showing altered brain function and connectivity in depressed individuals asked to focus attention on tasks with high visual demand. These changes included altered functional connectivity between frontal, parietal, and visual cortices, perhaps reflecting changes in attention/reorienting ICNs. Depressed subjects also showed increased activity of sgACC and medial orbital cortex that was modulated by the attentional demand required for task performance. A recent meta-analysis of 19 studies highlights the importance of increased rostral ACC activity as a predictor of treatment response and speculates that low activity in this region may contribute to difficulties in deactivating the default network and bringing task-activated networks on line.

A number of regions involved in the functional circuitry of major depression also exhibit structural changes. We will discuss this in greater detail in the next chapter. For now, it is important to note that there is evidence indicating structural changes in the hippocampus, amygdala, and sgACC as well as other regions of the PFC and lateral aspects of the cerebral cortex. How these changes arise is not clear, but some individuals with depression show changes early in the disorder, possibly antedating the onset of illness, while others have changes that appear to correlate with illness duration. Structural changes have also been linked to changes in specific cell populations in various regions. For example, the sgACC and the amygdala exhibit a loss of glial cells, particularly a loss of oligodendrocytes in the amygdala. Oligodendrocytes help to form the myelin insulation for axons that carry information from one neuron to another; they also help form white matter tracts that link brain regions. In the sgACC, Dost Öngür and colleagues reported more than 20% reduction in glial cells in subjects with MDD, whereas subjects with bipolar disorder showed about 40% reduction. Other studies indicate loss of glial and neuronal cells in other regions of cortex. Changes have also been found in interneurons in some regions such as hippocampus, particularly in bipolar disorder. Francine Benes and colleagues reported about 40% reduction in non-pyramidal neurons in the CA2 region with a trend toward diminished cell number in area CA3 of subjects with bipolar disorder. Psychosocial stress is known to affect synapse development and maintenance and results in shrinkage of the dendritic arborization of neurons. Dendrites are sites at which neurons typically receive inputs from other neurons. These changes are likely to conspire with cell loss to produce the decrease in regional brain volume observed in subjects with major mood disorders. Although changes in specific regions are important and likely contribute to processing defects in those regions, it is important to consider that changes in specific regions do not occur in isolation and affect overall network performance. It is network dysfunction that lies at the heart of psychiatric symptoms and disorders.

Finally, it is also important to consider that emotional processing, like a number of other forms of brain computation, shows hemispheric lateralization. This is most clearly observed in people who suffer strokes affecting frontal cortex. Here, damage to the left frontal region is typically associated with depressed mood, while right frontal strokes are associated with either no change in mood or manic-like symptoms in some subjects. This observation may reflect the fact that information from the sympathetic nervous system, a part of the autonomic nervous system that monitors arousal and survival, is preferentially processed in the right hemisphere, whereas input from the parasympathetic nervous system dealing with relaxation and affiliation is handled by the left hemisphere. The anterior insular cortex and the associated rostral ACC are also important participants in autonomic processing and in the generation of associated subjective feelings associated with mood states. Following a left-sided stroke, the right hemisphere can become overactive, and this may be a driver of the negative mood state.

The studies outlined here indicate that major depressive disorders are complex in terms of categorizing them as primary defects in emotion, cognition, or motivation. Although emotional ICNs appear to be at the heart of these disorders, they also involve prominent cognitive, attentional, and motivational defects. The cognitive changes associated with depression may be particularly important in causing disability. Luke Clark and colleagues have highlighted problems with executive function, memory, emotional processing, and feedback sensitivity in individuals with depression resulting from dysfunction within the PFC-subcortical circuitry described above. Thus, major depressive disorders might represent disorders of systems required to integrate all three aspects of mind. A major question concerns how altered connectivity and function across multiple brain networks occurs. While answers are incomplete, it appears that highly connected and highly plastic neural hubs may play a critical role. For example, Sheline and colleagues recently observed that emotional, cognitive-control, and default-mode neural networks show increased resting-state connectivity to the same areas of bilateral dorsal medial PFC in depressed subjects. They refer to this region of dorsal medial PFC as a "dorsal nexus." This dorsal nexus seems to serve as a nidus for linking the networks together in illness, and the degree of connectivity of the three networks with the dorsal nexus correlates with illness severity. Other recent work suggests that regions such as the lateral habenula that link key forebrain and midbrain areas play a key role in regulating a number of behaviors associated with depression, including changes in motivated behaviors, movement, sleep, and reward-based decision making. Thus, it is possible that multiple nodes are involved in pulling together the circuitry underlying depression. These nodes could become key regions for targeted therapeutic interventions.

Motivational Disorders: Substance Abuse

Because almost every (if not every) addictive drug attacks the same neural system, more might be known about the neurocircuitry and cellular mechanisms of substance-abuse disorders than any other group of psychiatric illnesses. The primary network involved in these disorders is organized similarly in rodents and humans. This similarity has allowed the development of well-characterized animal models and the use of sophisticated physiological and molecular tools to work out the details of changes at cellular, synaptic, and system levels. A host of scientists, including Eric Nestler, Steve Hyman, George Koob, Rob Malenka, Peter Kalivas, Nora Volkow, Read Montague, and others, have played significant roles in this work, and the results have provided a model for understanding how to think about the biology of other psychiatric conditions.

As we have noted, addictive drugs modulate the actions of the neurotransmitter dopamine in a network that includes the midbrain ventral tegmental area (VTA), the origin of the mesolimbic and mesocortical dopamine systems (Fig. 5-3). Neurons in the VTA project to the nucleus accumbens, hippocampus, PFC, and other areas. The VTA–accumbens–PFC network is the principal circuit involved in the acute effects of drugs of abuse, and it is also the circuitry thought to underlie our

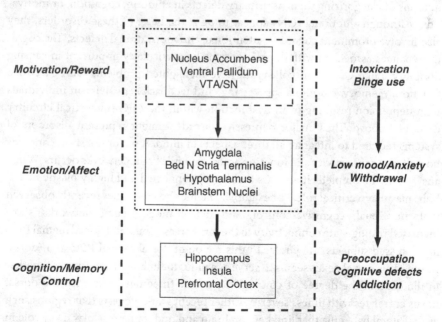

Figure 5-3 Brain circuitry and addiction. The diagram depicts neural circuitry involved in the effects of addictive drugs and how the circuitry becomes increasingly complex as addiction progresses. (Adapted from descriptions provided by George Koob and Nora Volkow.) For locations of anatomic structures, please refer to the Appendix.

motivation and reward systems. In this network, the firing of dopamine neuro.
seems to serve as a reward-prediction signal that indicates whether an experience is
better or worse than expectations. Experiences that exceed expectations enhance
firing of these neurons, while those below expectations diminish firing. Dopamine
neurons continuously send information to the nucleus accumbens and PFC, and
changes in their firing rate result in increases or decreases in dopamine levels in the
postsynaptic structures, allowing dopamine to serve as a "valuation" signal, in the
words of Read Montague.

Dopamine is a classic slow transmitter (see Chapter 3) that helps to organize and
coordinate activity within and across brain regions; it also is involved in regulating
the inputs and outputs of those regions. In the nucleus accumbens, dopamine signaling influences value judgments and helps to determine whether something
should be approached or avoided. Different circuitry within the nucleus accumbens
may play a role in approach and avoidance decisions. The output of the nucleus
accumbens via the ventral pallidum and the dorsal striatal-pallidal systems helps to
coordinate motor responses. In PFC, dopamine helps to determine which signals
neurons pay attention to, in effect performing a type of gating function that helps to
determine the "salience" of inputs.

The VTA–nucleus accumbens–PFC loop represents the most simplified circuitry
involved in substance abuse. Other regions also contribute, including the amygdala
(and its connections) and the hippocampus (and its affiliated ICNs). These connections and the influence of dopamine on these regions and networks provide a conduit for the involvement of emotional systems as well as learning and memory in
substance-abuse disorders. Studies of the circuitry involved in the actions of abused
drugs highlight the distributed anatomy and connectivity of the amygdala, including
the amygdala proper, the shell (outer) region of the nucleus accumbens, and the
BNST. Most abused drugs directly affect one or more of these regions. Several
regions within the PFC are also involved in this extended network. Cortical regions
include ventromedial PFC, involved in goal-directed decision making and perhaps
in interpreting value signals, and dlPFC, critical for working memory, emotional
regulation, and cognitive control. The ACC is also involved, and this region is hypo-
active in individuals with substance-abuse disorders, leading to problems with performance monitoring and cognitive control. The involvement of higher brain centers
in substance-abuse disorders has prompted Nora Volkow and colleagues to refer to
these disorders as problems of "neurocognition" and not simply defects in impulse
control or motivation. This is a profound statement and one that we would emphasize runs through all of psychiatry: all full-blown major psychiatric disorders are
"neurocognitive" disorders.

In popular terminology, most addictive drugs "hijack" the brain's motivation
circuitry, in effect substituting for natural rewards. These drugs accomplish this feat
by enhancing the release of dopamine from VTA terminals using several mechanisms. Cocaine and amphetamines alter the function of dopamine transporters in
the nucleus accumbens and other regions, either by blocking dopamine uptake
(cocaine) or by enhancing dopamine release via heteroexchange (amphetamines).

The latter point means that amphetamines are taken up by dopamine transporters in exchange for dopamine being released. Other drugs (e.g., opiates) increase dopamine levels by altering the firing of dopamine neurons in VTA.

Because of the profound effect of addictive drugs on dopamine, there has been interest in determining whether other "addictive" behaviors influence the dopamine system. For example, changes in the dopamine system may occur in certain human "impulse control disorders," such as pathological gambling, compulsive shopping, and perhaps compulsive sex and overeating. Similarly, neuroimaging studies suggest that playing certain video games is associated with enhanced dopamine release, contributing to the belief that these games might be "addicting." Therapeutic drugs that influence the dopamine system, including some used to treat Parkinson's disease, a disorder resulting from the loss of dopamine neurons in substantia nigra, can also lead to addictive behaviors, including some of the impulse-control disorders mentioned above. These findings have contributed to our evolving understanding of the complexities of Parkinson's disease and the role of dopamine in modulating numerous motivated behaviors. Importantly, abused drugs are particularly good at increasing dopamine levels, and thus they are much more effective, and thus more addicting, than other behaviors.

The effects of addictive drugs on dopamine release happen quickly, as soon as the drugs reach their targets in the brain. Substance-abuse disorders, however, are chronic problems that require repeated drug exposures to become manifest in their most severe form. This has prompted studies examining the long-term adaptations in the VTA-accumbens system induced by these drugs, including effects on second messengers, gene expression, and protein synthesis. In the nucleus accumbens, dopamine binds to D1-type receptors and activates adenylate cyclase via a GTP-binding protein (G-protein); this leads to synthesis of cyclic AMP, a second messenger. In turn, cyclic AMP activates protein kinase A, an enzyme that phosphorylates various proteins, including CREB (cyclic AMP response element binding protein). CREB is a transcription factor that allows dopamine to alter gene expression. CREB promotes the activation of immediate early genes (e.g., c-fos, fos-B) that are also transcription factors driving expression of other genes. This cascade of events results in long-term effects on neuronal function and structure, and these changes are likely to be critical for driving the long-term effects of abused drugs on individual neurons and networks.

Addictive drugs have major effects on the function of synapses in the VTA and its connected regions, using synaptic plasticity mechanisms that we will discuss in Chapter 6. Dopamine neurons in the VTA receive excitatory glutamate inputs from the PFC, hypothalamus, and tegmental nucleus. Compelling evidence indicates that these excitatory synapses exhibit long-term potentiation (LTP) following exposure to abused drugs. VTA LTP is important for the early behavioral responses to the drugs, leading to increased output of the dopamine neurons, and is observed in live animals following administration of a variety of drugs, including cocaine, amphetamine, nicotine, and ethanol. This persistent synaptic enhancement, like LTP in the hippocampus (Chapter 6), involves activation of N-methyl-D-aspartate (NMDA)–type glutamate receptors. Interestingly, some drugs (cocaine and ethanol, for example) produce LTP in the VTA of rodents after just a *single in vivo* exposure, indicating that only one drug exposure is sufficient to set long-lived processes in motion. Other drugs (e.g., antidepressants) do not have this effect. Early LTP in the VTA is believed to play a role in attaching motivational significance to the drug experience and results in a form of learning that helps to drive even longer-term changes in function within this system.

Synaptic changes also occur in the nucleus accumbens, a primary target of VTA dopamine neurons. The nucleus accumbens has two main parts, a "core" region that is an extension of the dorsal striatum (caudate-putamen) and a "shell" region that is part of the extended amygdala. In addition to LTP, there is another form of long-term synaptic plasticity, long-term synaptic depression (LTD), that results in a persistent decrement in synaptic transmission. Importantly, drug exposure produces LTD of glutamate synapses in the shell region of nucleus accumbens, but not in the core region. This LTD appears to correlate with behavioral sensitization to the abused drug. Over time, non-addicted animals recover from acute LTD in the nucleus accumbens, while animals that exhibit persistent "addiction-like" behaviors (meaning a propensity to self-administer drugs) have lasting synaptic changes. Drugs of abuse are also associated with long-term changes in the extracellular levels of glutamate in the nucleus accumbens, and these changes appear to be mediated by effects on a type of glutamate transporter (called the cystine-glutamate transporter) in glial cells.

Sophisticated cellular and molecular studies in rodents in combination with functional imaging studies in humans have led to insights into how addictive disorders can be conceptualized from a "neurocognitive" perspective. In a model described by George Koob and Nora Volkow, drug addiction is seen to progress through three stages (Table 5-4). Initially, there is a phase of repeated binge drug use and intoxication that strongly engages the VTA-accumbens circuitry already discussed. With continued drug use, individuals enter a phase in which repeated bouts of drug intoxication and withdrawal result in associated negative moods and anxiety. This phase expands the circuitry outside of VTA-accumbens to engage the extended amygdala and its role in emotional modulation.

With more protracted drug use, individuals enter a phase of drug preoccupation and enhanced anticipation of drug use, involving an even more distributed neural network that includes circuits underlying cognition and higher-level control. Key structures in

Table 5-4 Three Stages of Addiction

Binge use and intoxication
  VTA-nucleus accumbens "reward" circuit involved
Repeated withdrawal and negative affect
  Extended amygdala (including the bed nucleus of the stria terminalis) also becomes
    involved
Preoccupation, habit, and executive dysfunction
  Hippocampus, orbitofrontal cortex, PFC, anterior insula, and dorsal striatum also
    become involved

---

this third phase include the orbitofrontal cortex, dorsal striatum, PFC, hippocampus, and insula, an expanded network that seems to be involved in drug craving and in the contextual aspects of drug abuse, as well as memory dysfunction. Context plays an important role in drug use, and it is one of the reasons that effective treatments require restructuring the lives of addicted persons. Other areas involved in the third stage of drug abuse include the ACC, inferior frontal cortex, and dlPFC, a circuit that is important for inhibitory control, attention, and working memory.

Importantly, the synaptic plasticity associated with the repetitive cycle of drug use and withdrawal is key to the expansion of this circuitry over time, and it leads to an interconnected dysfunctional network that has a negative impact on all aspects of the mind. It is not a great extrapolation to consider that analogous expansion in dysfunctional circuitry over time and with repeated bouts of illness could contribute to the pathogenesis and complexities of other psychiatric disorders. The advantage of studying the circuitry of substance abuse is that the disorder starts in specific circuitry that can be defined and studied in detail. Progression of illness then layers in expanding and more complicated neural networks. Figure 5-3 presents an overview of neural circuitry thought to be involved in the stages of drug addiction.

While many aspects of this story remain uncertain, the important point is that much is now known about how the motivational system works and how drugs of abuse attack the system to produce their acute and long-term effects. This information has inspired various ideas for the development of novel treatment strategies for drug-abuse syndromes. For example, there is interest in determining whether the cystine-glutamate transporter described above can serve as a target for therapeutic pharmacology by altering extracellular levels of glutamate and whether transporter-mediated changes in extracellular glutamate levels affect the actions of glutamate on specific subtypes of glutamate receptors (particularly metabotropic receptors). These receptors could then become targets for therapeutic intervention.

The effects of addictive drugs on the motivational system are long-lived at cellular and synaptic levels. Thus, it is not surprising that substance-abuse syndromes often involve chronic and relapsing dysfunction. The involvement of the amygdala and hippocampus adds emotional and learning components to these syndromes, compounding the chronic effects of the drugs. Work in the area of addiction also has implications for understanding how motivational, emotional, and cognitive systems are intertwined and how these neural systems become engaged in increasingly complex circuitry as illness progresses.

Other Abused Drugs: Hallucinogens

The studies outlined above involve addictive drugs that primarily attack the dopamine system. Another group of abused drugs have different mechanisms of action and are referred to as "hallucinogens," reflecting their ability to modify perception and cognition. These drugs are interesting because their predominant effects seem to influence sensory processing, perhaps providing insights into mechanisms involved in higher-order perceptual processing. We will briefly discuss two classes of hallucinogens: a group containing LSD (lysergic acid diethylamide) and psilocybin ("mushrooms"), and a class represented by MDMA (3,4-methylenedioxymethamphetamine, aka "Ecstasy"). Although these drugs are abused, they are not addictive in the traditional sense of the term. Because the body develops very rapid tolerance to these hallucinogens, they are prone to occasional use and do not usually lead to the cycle of craving, obsessive drug seeking, and painful withdrawal seen with addictive drugs. Interestingly, hallucinogens do not primarily influence central motivational systems, although they do have deleterious effects on mental function.

LSD and psilocybin can produce time distortion, visual sensory images (including illusions), and, occasionally, synesthesias. Synesthesia refers to a phenomenon in which senses become interwoven (e.g., one might hear colors or see sounds). Users indicate that some of these experiences lead to profound self-transcendence, mystical insight, and knowledge, although this is more anecdotal than fact, given the severe adverse effects these drugs can have. David Nichols and colleagues have shown that LSD-type hallucinogens act as agonists on serotonin 5HT2A receptors that are coupled to intracellular signaling pathways via a specific subtype of G protein. Javier González-Maeso and colleagues extended these findings by demonstrating that the hallucinogens, but not non-hallucinogenic 5HT2A agonists, may act by directly influencing specific cortical neurons via a 5HT2A receptor subtype with unique signaling characteristics. These findings suggest that even when a drug influences a distributed transmitter system such as serotonin, highly specific effects can be achieved via molecular subtypes of receptors and signaling cascades. This opens doors to understanding how manipulation of specific cortical neurons and regions can influence network properties and result in altered sensory experiences.

MDMA (Ecstasy) has been reported to increase alertness and feelings of empathy, caring, and intimacy together with decreased aggressiveness. This agent has effects on the serotonergic and adrenergic systems as well as the hormone/transmitter oxytocin. The oxytocin system appears to play a role in mating and social bonding behaviors, and investigations of this drug may provide insight into brain systems involved in social interactions. Psilocybin and MDMA have been studied as possible treatments for anxiety in patients with late-stage cancer. Such clinical use is complicated by the possibility that chronic exposure to MDMA may have toxic effects on the serotonin system.

SUMMARY: RECURRING THEMES

Functional neuroimaging studies have convincingly demonstrated overlap among brain regions involved in various psychiatric disorders. What is becoming clearer is how specific brain regions contribute to specific processing tasks and how dysfunction in a given region can have profound effects on the function of remaining nodes in an ICN or even in other ICNs. Understanding what a network does—how it handles its inputs, how it processes information locally, and how it uses that information to communicate with other regions—is critical for understanding psychiatric symptoms and disorders. Some brain regions, by virtue of their high connectivity, participate in multiple circuits; thus it is not unexpected to find functional changes in these regions across multiple illnesses. The hippocampus, amygdala, nucleus accumbens, and PFC are clear examples of such regions. It is not always clear how illness specificity arises within these shared circuits underlying cognition, emotion, and motivation, but we speculate that the primary nodes or networks involved early in a given disorder may play a big role in defining the nature of that clinical disorder. For example, addictive drugs clearly attack the motivation/reward system early, and thus, defects in this type of processing are primary issues in these disorders. We would also argue that because there is so much overlap among these circuits and the different illnesses, it is not surprising that there is substantial "comorbidity" of disorders, particularly given the potential for illness-driven plasticity across networks as illnesses persist and progress. Again, all three aspects of the mind are involved in all disorders. This fact guarantees comorbidities. The key to sorting this out seems to lie in understanding which processing defects are most prominent in a given illness and ultimately what makes those ICNs vulnerable at synaptic, cellular, and molecular levels. It is also important to know which brain changes occur earliest in the course of an illness and which changes are secondary, tertiary, or compensatory. Compensatory changes, however, are not necessarily beneficial and ultimately can contribute to illness phenotype. As we have mentioned previously, cellular and synaptic changes are potential targets for pharmacological interventions, while functional changes at the ICN/system level are potential targets for psychotherapeutic and rehabilitative strategies. Both types of intervention are likely to be required for optimal clinical results in most patients.

At the risk of being overly simplistic, we will end this discussion by describing what various brain regions outlined in this chapter are likely to contribute to information processing and psychiatric dysfunction. This discussion is based on a recent paper on the "neurobiology of wisdom" by Thomas Meeks and Dilip Jeste. Neocortex, particularly the PFC, provides the highest-level processing and the highest level of abstraction in the brain. Lateral and dlPFC are critical for working memory and for cognitive aspects of conscious top-down control over emotions and impulses. These regions also play a significant role in dealing with ambiguity, one of the recurring challenges our brains face. Medial and ventromedial PFC are important for self-reflection and affective components of decision making, while orbitofrontal cortex plays a role in controlling impulsivity via response inhibition and in attaching affective value to stimuli and rewards. Parts of parietal cortex, particularly parietal-frontal connections, are important for focusing attention, reorienting responses, and a number of higher-order cognitive processes underlying intellect, whereas regions of the superior temporal sulcus seem to be critical for differentiating between ourselves and others and for determining social relevance. Subcortical structures are involved in emotions and motivation. The amygdala plays a key role in almost all emotional processing and in determining how we react to things. Its broad connectivity to cortex and subcortex likely is the basis for its important roles in modulating multiple functions, handling ambiguity, and determining salience and significance. The nucleus accumbens/striatal system is critical for goal selection and motivation, helping to determine reward valence and reinforcement. Somewhere between subcortical and higher centers in PFC and parietal cortex, regions such as the anterior cingulate cortex seem to detect conflicts and activate circuitry to deal with conflicts. Posterior cingulate cortex helps to determine self-relevant (interoceptive) stimuli and along with insular cortex may be important in providing a sense of moral judgment, perhaps via the emotion of disgust. Importantly, none of these regions functions in isolation, and the computations provided by each region contribute to the intra- and inter-network processing that is critical for healthy functioning of the brain. Illnesses can arise via defects in specific key regions, particularly a combination of regions, or perhaps through altered connectivity within these networks. Ultimately, the goal of much brain function may well be to keep primitive centers (amygdala, VTA-accumbens, and hypothalamus/brain stem) under wraps.

Points to Remember

Psychiatric disorders are complex problems involving the structure and function of brain networks. While changes in transmitter systems contribute to the disorders, the illnesses are not simply the result of "chemical imbalances."

Work on the role of specific ICNs is still in the early stages. Nonetheless, this level of analysis has tremendous potential for defining the symptoms and phenotypes of psychiatric disorders and may lead to more valid approaches to diagnosis. ICN-level analyses also have potential for contributing to the development of better psychotherapeutic and rehabilitative strategies.

Because well-characterized animal models of fear and substance abuse exist, we are further along in understanding how cellular and synaptic changes conspire to produce changes in network function in these conditions, and in turn, how changes in network function result in behavioral changes. Findings in animal studies are leading to new ideas about how to treat anxiety and substance-abuse disorders at pharmacological and psychotherapeutic levels.

SUGGESTED READINGS

Bassett, D. S., Bullmore, E., Verchinski, B. A., Mattay, V. S., Weinberger, D. R., & Meyer-Lindenberg, A. (2008). Hierarchical organization of human cortical networks in health and schizophrenia. *Journal of Neuroscience, 28,* 9239–9248.

Davis, M., Walker, D. L., Miles, L., & Grillon, C. (2010). Phasic vs. sustained fear in rats and humans: Role of the extended amygdala in fear vs. anxiety. *Neuropsychopharmacology Reviews, 35,* 105–135.

Drevets, W. C., Price, J. L., & Furey, M. L. (2008). Brain structural and functional abnormalities in mood disorders: Implications for neurocircuitry of depression. *Brain Structure and Function, 213,* 93–118.

Koob, G. F., & Volkow, N. D. (2010). Neurocircuitry of addiction. *Neuropsychopharmacology Reviews, 35,* 217–238.

LeDoux, J. (2002). *Synaptic self: How our brains become who we are*. New York: Viking Press.

Lewis, D. A., & Sweet, R. A. (2009). Schizophrenia from a neural circuitry perspective: Advancing toward rational pharmacological therapies. *Journal of Clinical Investigation, 119,* 706–716.

Nutt, D., King, L. A., Saulsbury, W., & Blakemore, C. (2007). Development of a rational scale to assess the harm of drugs of potential misuse. *Lancet, 369,* 1047–1053.

OTHER REFERENCES

Benes, F. M. (2007). Searching for unique endophenotypes for schizophrenia and bipolar disorder within neural circuits and their molecular regulatory mechanisms. *Schizophrenia Bulletin, 33,* 932–936.

Bentall, R. P., Rowse, G., Shryane, N., Kinderman, P., Howard, R., Blackwood, N., et al. (2009). The cognitive and affective structure of paranoid delusions. *Archives of General Psychiatry, 66,* 236–247.

Bloch, M. H., Landeros-Weisenberger, A., Rosario, M. C., Pittenger, C., & Leckman, J. F. (2008). Meta-analysis of the symptom structure of obsessive-compulsive disorder. *American Journal of Psychiatry, 165,* 1532–1542.

Buckner, R. L., Andrews-Hanna, J. R., & Schacter, D. L. (2008). The brain's default network: Anatomy, function and relevance to disease. *Annals of the New York Academy of Science, 1124,* 1–38.

Bullmore, E., & Sporns, O. (2009). Complex brain networks: Graph theoretical analysis of structural and functional systems. *Nature Reviews Neuroscience, 10,* 186–198.

Cavedini, P., Zorzi, C., Piccinni, M., Cavallini, M. C., & Bellodi, L. (2010). Executive dysfunctions in obsessive-compulsive patients and unaffected relatives: Searching for a new intermediate phenotype. *Biological Psychiatry, 67,* 1178–1184.

Chamberlain, S. R., Menzies, L., Hampshire, A., Suckling, J., Fineberg, N. A., del Campo, N., et al. (2008). Orbitofrontal dysfunction in patients with obsessive-compulsive disorder and their unaffected relatives. *Science, 321,* 421–422.

Clark, L., Chamberlain, S. R., & Sahakian, B. J. (2009). Neurocognitive mechanisms in depression: Implications for treatment. *Annual Review of Neuroscience, 32,* 57–74.

Cloninger, C. R. (2004). *Feeling good: The science of well-being*. New York: Oxford University Press.

Dagher, A., & Robbins, T. W. (2009). Personality, addiction, dopamine: Insights from Parkinson's disease. *Neuron, 61,* 502–510.

Desseilles, M., Balteau, E., Sterpenich, V., Dang-Vu, T. T., Darsaud, A., Vandewalle, G., et al. (2009). Abnormal neural filtering of irrelevant visual information in depression. *Journal of Neuroscience, 29,* 1395–1403.

Devinsky, O. (2009). Delusional misidentifications and duplications. Right brain lesions, left brain delusions. *Neurology, 72,* 80–87.

Eisenberg, D. P., & Berman, K. F. (2010). Executive function, neural circuitry and genetic mechanisms in schizophrenia. *Neuropsychopharmacology Reviews, 35,* 258–277.

Etkin, A., Prater, K. E., Schatzberg, A. F., Menon, V., & Greicius, M. D. (2009). Disrupted amygdalar subregion functional connectivity and evidence of a compensatory network in generalized anxiety disorder. *Archives of General Psychiatry, 66,* 1361–1372.

Fineberg, N. A., Potenza, M. N., Chamberlain, S. R., Berlin, H. A., Menzies, L., Bechara, A., et al. (2010). Probing compulsive and impulsive behaviors, from animal models to endophenotypes: A narrative review. *Neuropsychopharmacology, 35*, 591–604.

Fletcher, P. C., & Frith, C. D. (2009). Perceiving is believing: A Bayesian approach to explaining the positive symptoms of schizophrenia. *Nature Reviews Neuroscience, 10*, 48–58.

Giacobbe, P., Mayberg, H. S., & Lozano, A. M. (2009). Treatment resistant depression as a failure of brain homeostatic mechanisms: Implications for deep brain stimulation. *Experimental Neurology, 219*, 44–52.

González-Maeso, J., Weisstaub, N. V., Zhou, M., Chan, P., Ivic, L., Ang, R., et al. (2007). Hallucinogens recruit specific cortical 5-HT_{2A} receptor-mediated signaling pathways to affect behavior. *Neuron, 53*, 439–452.

Hare, T. A., Camerer, C. F., & Rangel, A. (2009). Self-control in decision making involves modulation of the vmPFC valuation system. *Science, 324*, 646–648.

Harrison, B. J., Soriano-Mas, C., Pujol, J., Ortiz, H., Lopez, M., Hernandez-Ribas, R., et al. (2009). Altered corticostriatal functional connectivity in obsessive-compulsive disorder. *Archives of General Psychiatry, 66*, 1189–1200.

Heller, A. S., Johnstone, T., Schackman, A. J., Light, S. N., Peterson, M. J., Kolden, G. G., et al. (2010). Reduced capacity to sustain positive emotion in major depression reflects diminished maintenance of fronto-striatal brain activation. *Proceedings of the National Academy of Sciences (USA), 106*, 22445–22350.

Hikosaka, C. (2010). The habenula: From stress evasion to value-based decision-making. *Nature Reviews Neuroscience, 11*, 503–513.

Hyman, S. E., & Malenka, R. C. (2001). Addiction and the brain: the neurobiology of compulsion and its persistence. *Nature Reviews Neuroscience, 2*, 695–703.

Kalivas, P. W. (2009). The glutamate homeostasis hypothesis of addiction. *Nature Reviews Neuroscience, 10*, 561–572.

Kapur, S. (2003). Psychosis as a state of aberrant salience: A framework linking biology, phenomenology and pharmacology in schizophrenia. *American Journal of Psychiatry, 160*, 13–23.

Kasanetz, F., Deroche-Gamonet, V., Berson, N., Balado, E., Lafourcade, M., Manzoni, O., et al. (2010). Transition to addiction is associated with a persistent impairment in synaptic plasticity. *Science, 328*, 1709–1712.

Kauer, J. A., & Malenka, R. C. (2007). Synaptic plasticity and addiction. *Nature Reviews Neuroscience, 8*, 844–858.

Kaye, W. H., Fudge, J. L., & Paulus, M. (2009). New insights into symptoms and neurocircuit function of anorexia nervosa. *Nature Reviews Neuroscience, 10*, 573–584.

Lahti, A. C., Weiler, M. A., Holcomb, H. H., Tamminga, C. A., & Cropsey, K. L. (2009). Modulation of limbic circuitry predicts treatment response to antipsychotic medications: A functional imaging study in schizophrenia. *Neuropsychopharmacology, 34*, 2675–2690.

Lesh, T. A., Niendam, T. A., Minzenberg, M. J., & Carter, C. S. (2011). Cognitive control deficits in schizophrenia: Mechanisms and meaning. *Neuropsychopharmacology Reviews, 36*, 316–338.

Lisman, J. E., Coyle, J. T., Green, R. W., Javitt, D. C., Benes, F. M., Heckers, S., et al. (2008). Circuit-based framework for understanding neurotransmitter and risk gene interactions in schizophrenia. *Trends in Neuroscience, 31*, 234–242.

Mansouri, F. A., Tanaka, K., & Buckley, M. J. (2009). Conflict-induced behavioral adjustment: A clue to the executive function of the prefrontal cortex. *Nature Reviews Neuroscience, 10*, 141–152.

Mataix-Cols, D., Wooderson, S., Lawrence, N., Brammer, M. J., Speckens, A., & Phillips, M. L. (2004). Distinct neural correlates of washing, checking, and hoarding symptom dimensions in obsessive-compulsive disorder. *Archives of General Psychiatry, 61*, 564–576.

Meeks, T. W., & Jeste, D. V. (2009). Neurobiology of wisdom: A literature overview. *Archives of General Psychiatry, 66*, 355–365.

Mirzenberg, M. J., Laird, A. R., Thelen, S., Carter, C. S., & Glahn, D. C. (2009). Meta-analysis of 41 functional neuroimaging studies of executive function in schizophrenia. *Archives of General Psychiatry, 66*, 811–822.

Montague, R. (2006). *Why choose this book? How we make decisions.* New York: Dutton Press.

Nemeroff, C. B. (2004). Neurobiological consequences of childhood trauma. *Journal of Clinical Psychiatry, 65*(Suppl. 1), 18–28.

Nestler, E. J. (2005). Is there a common molecular pathway for addiction? *Nature Neuroscience, 8*, 1445–1449.

Nichols, D. E. (2004). Hallucinogens. *Pharmacology & Therapeutics, 101*, 131–181.

Ongur, D., Drevets, W. C., & Price, J. L. (1998). Glial reduction in the subgenual prefrontal cortex in mood disorders. *Proceedings of the National Academy of Sciences (USA), 95*, 13290–13295.

Panksepp, J. (2006). Emotional endophenotypes in evolutionary psychiatry. *Progress in Neuro-Psychopharmacology and Biological Psychiatry, 30*, 774–784.

Pessoa, L., & Adolphs, R. (2010). Emotion processing and the amygdala: From a "low road" to "many roads" of evaluating biological significance. *Nature Reviews Neuroscience, 11*, 773–782.

Pine, D. S., Helfinstein, S. M., Bar-Haim, Y., Nelson, E., & Fox, N. A. (2009). Challenges in developing novel treatments for childhood anxiety disorders: Lessons from research on anxiety disorders. *Neuropsychopharmacology, 34*, 213–228.

Pizzagalli, D. A. (2011). Frontocingulate dysfunction in depression: Toward biomarkers of treatment response. *Neuropsychopharmacology Reviews, 36*, 183–206.

Price, J. L., & Drevets, W. C. (2010). Neurocircuitry of mood disorders. *Neuropsychopharmacology Reviews, 35*, 192–216.

Ragland, J. D., Laird, A. R., Ranganath, C., Blumenfeld, R. S., Gonzales, S. M., & Glahn, D. C. (2009). Prefrontal activation defects during episodic memory in schizophrenia. *American Journal of Psychiatry, 166*, 863–874.

Ramachandran, V. S., & Blakeslee, S. (1998). *Phantoms in the brain: Probing the mysteries of the human mind.* New York: William Morrow.

Ressler, K. J., & Mayberg, H. S. (2007). Targeting abnormal neural circuits in mood and anxiety disorders: From the laboratory to the clinic. *Nature Neuroscience, 10*, 1116–1124.

Rotge, J. Y., Aouizerate, B., Tignol, J., Bioulac, B., Burbaud, P., & Guehl, D. (2010). The glutamate-based genetic immune hypothesis in obsessive-compulsive disorder. An integrative approach from genes to symptoms. *Neuroscience, 165*, 408–417.

Sambataro, F., Blasi, G., Fazio, L., Caforio, G., Taurisano, P., Romano, R., et al. (2010). Treatment with olanzepine is associated with modulation of the default mode network in patients with schizophrenia. *Neuropsychopharmacology, 35*, 904–912.

Satterthwaite, T. D., Wolf, D. H., Loughead, J., Ruparel, K., Valdez, J. N., Siegel, S. J., et al. (2010). Association of enhanced limbic response to threat with decreased cortical facial recognition memory response in schizophrenia. *American Journal of Psychiatry, 167*, 418–426.

Savitz, J., & Drevets, W. C. (2009). Bipolar and major depressive disorder: Neuroimaging the developmental-degenerative divide. *Neuroscience and Biobehavioral Reviews, 33*, 699–771.

Schwabe, L., & Wolf, O. T. (2009). Stress prompts habit behavior in humans. *Journal of Neuroscience, 29,* 7191–7198.

Seeley, W. W., Crawford, R. K., Zhou, J., Miller, B. L, & Greicius, M. D. (2009). Neurodegenerative diseases target large-scale human brain networks. *Neuron, 62,* 42–52.

Seeley, W. W., Menon, V., Schatzberg, A. F., Keller, J., Glover, G. H., Kenna, H., et al. (2007). Dissociable intrinsic connectivity networks for salience processing and executive control. *Journal of Neuroscience, 27,* 2349–2356.

Seminowicz, D. A., Mayberg, H. S., McIntosh, A. R., Goldapple, K., Kennedy, S., Segal, Z., et al. (2004). Limbic-frontal circuitry in major depression: A path modeling metanalysis. *Neuroimage, 22,* 409–418.

Sheline, Y. I., Barch, D. M., Price, J. L., Rundle, M. M., Vaishnavi, S. N., Snyder, A. Z., et al. (2009). The default mode network and self-referential processes in depression. *Proceedings of the National Academy of Sciences (USA), 106,* 1942–1947.

Sheline, Y. I., Price, J. L., Yan, Z., & Mintun, M. A. (2010). Resting-state functional MRI in depression unmasks increased connectivity between networks via the dorsal nexus. *Proceedings of the National Academy of Sciences (USA), 107,* 11020–11025.

Shin, L. M., & Liberzon, I. (2010). The neurocircuitry of fear, stress and anxiety disorders. *Neuropsychopharmacology Reviews, 35,* 169–191.

Van den Heuvel, M. P., Stam, C. J., Kahn, R. S., & Hulshoff Pol, H. E. (2009). Efficiency of functional brain networks and intellectual performance. *Journal of Neuroscience, 29,* 7619–7624.

Weiss, A. P., Ellis, C. B., Roffman, J. L., Stufflebeam, S., Hamalainen, M. S., Duff, M., et al. (2009). Aberrent frontoparietal function during recognition memory in schizophrenia: A multimodal neuroimaging investigation. *Journal of Neuroscience, 29,* 11347–11359.

Whitfield-Gabrieli, S., Thermenos, H. W., Milanovic, S., Tsuang, M. T., Faraone, S. V., McCarley, R. W., et al. (2009). Hyperactivity and hyperconnectivity of the default network in schizophrenia and in first-degree relatives of persons with schizophrenia. *Proceedings of the National Academy of Sciences (USA), 106,* 1279–1284.

Zanelli, J., Reichenberg, A., Morgan, K., Fearon, P., Kravariti, E., Dazzan, P., et al. (2010). Specific and generalized neuropsychological deficits: A comparison of patients with various first-episode psychosis presentations. *American Journal of Psychiatry, 167,* 78–85.

6

The Hippocampus
Synapses, Circuits, and Networks

In prior chapters, we highlighted the important role that the hippocampus plays in brain function. It is one of the brain's most highly connected hubs, and it is a participant in several major intrinsic connectivity networks (ICNs), including the default system. In addition, it is a part of the traditional "limbic system," a largely subcortical brain network that contributes significantly to emotional processing. The concept of the limbic system has evolved over the years in response to increasing information about the complex interactions of brain networks, and the hippocampus is now viewed as a key structure operating at the interface of cognitive, emotional, and motivational systems. Joseph LeDoux has described highly connected regions of the brain as "convergence zones," areas where multimodal inputs are processed and concepts are generated. In his terminology, the hippocampus holds an even loftier position as a "superconvergence zone," reflecting its role as a site of extremely high connectivity. It is becoming increasingly clear that the hippocampus is involved in multiple major psychiatric disorders; abnormalities of hippocampal structure or function have been associated with Alzheimer's disease and other dementias, amnestic disorders, major depression, bipolar disorder, schizophrenia, and posttraumatic stress disorder, among others. Because the hippocampus has been a favored site for studies of synaptic function and synaptic plasticity, its connectivity and internal operations are better understood than many other brain regions. Thus, we will describe its function in some detail, attempting to synthesize how cellular and synaptic processing relates to the function of neural systems and the generation of clinical symptoms. While studied in greatest detail in the hippocampus, these cellular and synaptic mechanisms are also relevant to the function of other brain regions and networks. Thus, the principles outlined in this chapter have general importance for understanding the physiology of brain systems. The following discussion requires some basic knowledge of neurophysiology, including information outlined in Chapter 3. We would also refer readers to Eric Kandel's neuroscience textbook or to the review by Zorumski and colleagues in the current edition of *Kaplan and Sadock's Comprehensive Textbook of Psychiatry* for background information.

WHY IS THE HIPPOCAMPUS IMPORTANT?

The hippocampus is pivotal in the formation of new memories. Memories are critical components of our lives and influence all aspects of mental function, including our ability to recognize novelty, envision the future, and make decisions. As noted in Chapter 1, there are several types of memory that are processed in different regions of the brain. For example, emotional memories are largely encoded in the amygdala, while procedural memories (like how to ride a bicycle) utilize motor pathways, including the dorsal striatum, motor cortex, and cerebellum. The hippocampus is involved in the generation of "declarative memories," a type of learning that includes the ability to recall life experiences ("episodic memories") and facts about the world ("semantic memories"). Declarative memory is sometimes referred to as "explicit memory" to distinguish it from procedural, conditioned, and emotional memories ("implicit memories"). The hippocampus is not required for implicit memories.

Although declarative memories involve multiple brain regions, the hippocampus plays an important and time-limited role in their formation and in the transfer of the initial memory traces to longer-term storage in neocortex. When the hippocampus is damaged bilaterally, the effects on memory are devastating. Individuals lose the ability to form new declarative memories. They can behave in an appropriate fashion and interact socially, but they have no recollection of new experiences. Similar, but less persistent, amnestic states are observed under the influence of certain drugs (e.g., alcohol and benzodiazepines). Here, individuals have distinct periods of time (called "blackouts") during which they are alert and interactive but cannot form new memories. These blackouts are temporary and result from the effects of the drugs on the distributed hippocampal memory network.

By examining how the hippocampus works, we can begin to understand many of the mechanisms the brain uses to process and integrate information. A conceptual understanding of such processes is important because therapies for psychiatric disorders have direct influence on various components of these processes. In this chapter, we will integrate concepts that involve anatomical and neuronal structure, electrical processing of information, chemical signaling, and gene expression. In a subsequent chapter, we will review basic principles of transmitters and receptors that are pertinent to psychiatry.

WHAT IS THE HIPPOCAMPUS?

The hippocampus is a brain region located bilaterally in the medial temporal lobe. It is described by anatomists as "archicortex," meaning a phylogenetically older part of cortex that has three distinct layers instead of the six layers typically found in neocortex, such as in prefrontal cortex (PFC). The name "hippocampus" was coined by early histologists because the dissected structure bears a resemblance to a seahorse (*hippocampus* in Latin). Other anatomists thought it resembled a ram's horn and referred to the structure as "cornu Ammonis" (Ammon's horn) after Ammon, an Egyptian god who had the body of a human and the horns of a ram. The cornu

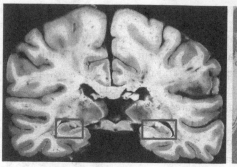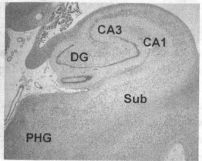

Figure 6-1 Human hippocampus. The photographs depict the location and structure of the human hippocampus. The hippocampus is an infolded region deep within the medial temporal lobe (left panel). The right panel shows the microscopic anatomy of the human hippocampus and highlights the location of the dentate gyrus (DG), areas CA3 and CA1, the subiculum (Sub), and parahippocampal gyrus (PHG). (Figures are courtesy of Nigel Cairns, Washington University in St. Louis.)

Ammonis (CA) designation is still used today to describe subregions of the hippocampus (areas CA1, CA2, CA3, and CA4; note that area CA4 is a transition zone from dentate gyrus to CA3 and is rarely considered separately).

Within the hippocampus there are several major structural subdivisions (Fig. 6-1). One of these is the *dentate gyrus*, a sideways-V–shaped structure that serves as the port of hippocampal entry for excitatory neuronal inputs from a nearby brain region called the entorhinal cortex. These neuronal inputs release the neurotransmitter glutamate. Glutamate, a classical fast excitatory transmitter, stimulates dentate *granule cells*, the principal (excitatory) neurons in the dentate, by depolarizing the membrane of these cells. In fact, glutamate excites granule cells in a variety of ways by taking advantage of several different glutamate-specific receptors, including both ionotropic (ion channel) and metabotropic (G-protein coupled) receptors. These different types of receptors become important for understanding how information is processed and will be discussed later in this chapter. The incoming connections (called "afferents") enter the dentate gyrus via nerve fibers called the *perforant path* and synapse onto the dendrites of granule cells. In turn, the granule cells send excitatory (glutamate) inputs to pyramidal (excitatory) neurons in area CA3 via the *mossy fibers*, a pathway that uses large and very potent synapses to drive firing of CA3 neurons. Area CA3 then sends its excitatory axons to pyramidal neurons in area CA1 via an axonal system called the *Schaffer collateral pathway*.

The perforant path, mossy fibers, and Schaffer collaterals are referred to collectively as the "trisynaptic pathway" to indicate that they often function as a three-synapse unit. This system represents an effective feed-forward hippocampal-centric excitatory network that uses glutamate as its principal neurotransmitter for information processing (Fig. 6-2). As we will describe later, the trisynaptic pathway does the primary work of initial declarative memory formation. There are additional excitatory inputs to hippocampal neurons from the contralateral hippocampus (providing input from the other cerebral hemisphere), the amygdala (adding emotional content), and

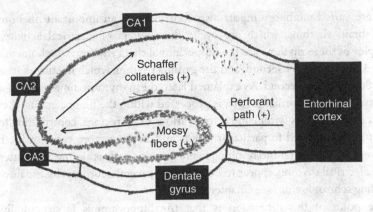

Figure 6-2 Hippocampal slices and the trisynaptic pathway. The diagram depicts a transverse slice of the hippocampus, highlighting the internal structure of the hippocampus and the pathways for information flow from entorhinal cortex via the trisynaptic pathway. The (+) sign indicates excitatory input. Hippocampal slices can be prepared from rodent brains and kept viable for hours while maintaining the synaptic pathways. These slices have been a favored preparation for studying hippocampal synaptic physiology. (The drawing is courtesy of Yukitoshi Izumi, Washington University in St. Louis.)

midline thalamic nuclei (providing a conduit for input from medial PFC). The entorhinal cortex also sends direct excitatory inputs to pyramidal neurons in areas CA1 and CA3 in addition to its input via the dentate gyrus. Finally, pyramidal neurons in the various CA regions (particularly in area CA3) recurrently innervate each other, adding to the excitatory power of the local network. These various connections provide ways for the cortex and other structures to communicate directly with various hippocampal regions and influence the way they process information. The trisynaptic pathway, however, is the backbone of information processing within the hippocampus; other inputs largely modify and complement this core mode of processing.

Before examining how the trisynaptic pathway is involved in memory formation, it is important to understand that there must be some mechanism in place to regulate all of the excitatory (glutamatergic) loops just described. In fact, the strong excitatory drive within the hippocampus makes it vulnerable to damage by over-excitation via a process that John Olney has called "excitotoxicity." Excessive hippocampal excitability can result in seizure initiation in temporal lobe epilepsy, serving as a nidus for partial complex seizures. To help control its excitability, the hippocampus has an array of interneurons that use GABA as a fast inhibitory neurotransmitter. These interneurons regulate excitatory inputs to various hippocampal regions and help to control the output of granule cells and pyramidal neurons. Current studies indicate that there are about 21 different types of inhibitory interneurons in the CA1 region alone, demonstrating how diverse, complex, and important this inhibitory control is. Different inhibitory interneurons synapse at various places along the dendrites, cell bodies, and axons of principal neurons and help to regulate how rapidly and rhythmically these neurons fire action potentials, as well as the effectiveness of excitatory inputs from other regions.

These varied inhibitory inputs also contribute to an important phenomenon called brain rhythms, which are cyclic fluctuations of electrical activity. Two examples of these rhythms are the hippocampal theta rhythm, which fluctuates at about 4 to 8 cycles per second, and the gamma rhythm, which fluctuates at rates of 30 to 80 cycles per second. As explained later, these rhythms appear to add a time dimension to the information that is processed within the hippocampus; they also appear to link activity within and across various brain regions, contributing to how neurons are entrained to particular inputs and develop more complex inter- and intra-regional computations resulting in phenomena such as alertness and attention. These electrical rhythms appear to be altered in several neuropsychiatric disorders, including schizophrenia (see Chapter 5).

The point of this discussion is that the hippocampus is structurally well designed to process excitatory inputs from the cortex. As is true for all regions of the brain, however, runaway excitation can be devastating, so checks and balances exist to keep regional activity under control. In addition to fast glutamatergic and GABAergic inputs, the hippocampus receives a variety of important inputs from neuromodulatory transmitter systems, including dopamine, serotonin, norepineph-rine, and acetylcholine. These slower transmitters help to set tone in the region, influencing neuronal firing and the effectiveness of glutamate synapses. These modulatory inputs are also likely to be important in helping to focus the "attention" of the hippocampus on specific inputs and processing tasks, just as they do in the PFC and other regions of the cortex.

HOW DOES INFORMATION FLOW WITHIN THE HIPPOCAMPAL SYSTEM?

For the hippocampus to form complex memories with multiple components, it must have the ability to link several different types of data: sensory information (visual, auditory, tactile, olfactory, and gustatory); emotional information; information dealing with the importance of an event (i.e., salience); and information related to the "meaning" of an event (including abstract interpretations involving PFC). Such varied types of data are initially processed via specific ICNs and then funneled to a cortical region called the rhinal cortex. This is a region in the temporal lobe that further processes the input before sending it to the entorhinal cortex, the main direct cortical connection to the hippocampus. The rhinal cortex includes the parahip-pocampal cortex, which, among other things, appears to gather information from pathways determining "where" things are located, and the perirhinal cortex, which gathers details determining "what" something is. The parahippocampal cortex and the perirhinal cortex send input to the lateral (outer) and medial (inner) subpor-tions of the entorhinal cortex, respectively. The entorhinal cortex, a region of typical six-layered cortex, sends its excitatory output from layer II neurons to the dentate gyrus via the perforant pathway. Thus, up to this point in the circuit, information has been gathered from distant parts of the brain, processed, and sent to the ento-rhinal cortex. This partially processed information then enters the machinery of the

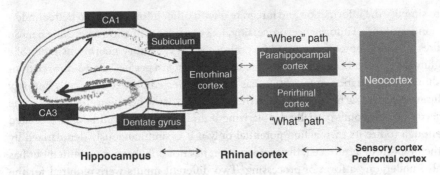

Figure 6-3 Hippocampal information flow. The diagram depicts how information flows from neocortex via the rhinal cortex and entorhinal cortex into the hippocampal trisynaptic pathway and back to cortex via the subiculum.

hippocampus, where it is bound together in a manner that eventually forms a declarative memory.

Once information gets to granule cells in the dentate gyrus via the perforant pathway, it is available for processing via the trisynaptic pathway in areas CA3 and CA1. Output from the trisynaptic pathway exits CA1 and flows to the subiculum and eventually to the neocortex as well as back to the entorhinal cortex; output to the entorhinal cortex is the predominant path. Figure 6-3 presents an overview of how information flows to and from the hippocampus.

Information returning to the entorhinal cortex from the hippocampus is further integrated with new information from the rhinal cortex and other regions before re-entering the hippocampus for another round of informational integration. This process provides a powerful mechanism by which the hippocampus can feed the results of its computations back to the cortex, allowing for modulation of informational integration in other brain regions, including modulation of subsequent inputs to the hippocampus via entorhinal cortex. This loop seems to provide an important tool for enriching the associations formed within the hippocampus. As mentioned previously, there are additional direct connections to the CA areas from various regions such as the midline thalamus and amygdala; these connections further influence the processing that occurs in the trisynaptic pathway. This notion of data looping within neural networks is not unique to the hippocampus and is found in other systems, such as the cortico-thalamic-striatal system.

WHAT DO HIPPOCAMPAL SUBREGIONS DO?

Once information moves from various brain regions into the trisynaptic pathway, what do the neurons within the hippocampus actually do to help solidify this information into something we call memories? Utilizing the structural relationships between the various components of the trisynaptic pathway, hippocampal neurons use an elaborate system of informational "fine tuning" to process the inputs they receive. Fine tuning involves taking a large amount of information and deciding how to simplify the information and integrate it with other information. To better understand this kind of information processing, let's consider a situation where one neuron fires an action potential, causing (via release of an excitatory neurotransmitter like glutamate) a receiving cell to fire an action potential in a perfect one-to-one relationship. In this situation, information has been transferred between the cells but only limited processing has occurred. On the other hand, if the first neuron influences the second cell by only partially depolarizing it and this second cell becomes excited enough to fire its own action potential only if it is simultaneously depolarized by the input from a third cell, then information has not only been transmitted but has also undergone a form of processing. Two different inputs were required for the receiving cell to send a message further downstream. This process of several cells working together to influence another cell is called *convergence*. Similarly, each of the two cells that converged on the third cell might also influence other, different cells. This process is called *divergence*. Each type of neuron in the trisynaptic pathway has remarkably different properties in terms of how much converging input is required for that cell to fire an action potential. Each cell type also differs in terms of how divergently its output is spread.

To perform its computations, the hippocampus takes advantage of these principles of convergence and divergence. Many of the specific details have been worked out in great detail within the rodent hippocampus, and we will use this model to discuss how the hippocampus functions as an information-processing machine. As noted, inputs to the trisynaptic pathway originate in layer II of entorhinal cortex and synapse upon granule cells in the dentate gyrus. In the rat, there are about 1.2 million dentate granule cells, and each of these neurons receives about 5,000 excitatory inputs. Of these 5,000 converging inputs, about 200 to 400 must simultaneously depolarize the granule cell in order for that cell to fire an action potential. Therefore, each excitatory synapse from entorhinal cortex to a particular granule cell has a relatively weak influence. Because it takes a lot of input to trigger a granule cell, the dentate gyrus is sometimes thought to act as a "gatekeeper" within the hippocampus. It allows information to flow into the rest of the hippocampus *if and only if* the message is strong—that is, input is arriving from many entorhinal neurons simultaneously. This may help protect the hippocampus from excessive excitatory bombardment from cortex during pathological conditions like seizures. Figure 6-4 presents an overview of how information flows within the hippocampus.

Convergence and divergence also occur in subsequent stages of the trisynaptic pathway. There are about 250,000 pyramidal neurons in the rat CA3 region. Each dentate granule cell contacts about 10 to 15 CA3 pyramidal neurons (divergence). Each CA3 pyramidal neuron fires an action potential when simultaneously stimulated by only 3 to 5 granule cells (convergence). Thus, individual granule cells can have a strong influence on a CA3 neuron since a single granule cell provides up to one-third of the depolarization needed to trigger the CA3 cell. Since each CA3 neuron receives input from about 50 to 80 different granule cells, about 5% (3 to 5 of the 50 to 80 granule cells) of an individual CA3 neuron's inputs must fire simultaneously in order to excite it. Further down the trisynaptic pathway, a CA1 pyramidal

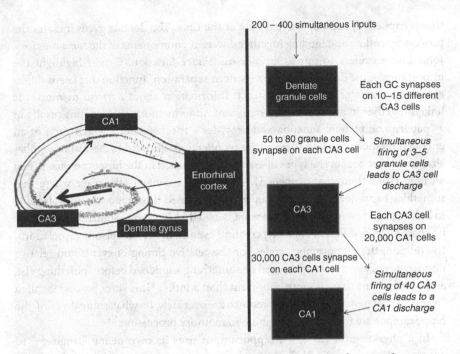

200 – 400 simultaneous inputs

Dentate granule cells

Each GC synapses on 10–15 different CA3 cells

50 to 80 granule cells synapse on each CA3 cell

Simultaneous firing of 3–5 granule cells leads to CA3 cell discharge

CA3

Each CA3 cell synapses on 20,000 CA1 cells

30,000 CA3 cells synapse on each CA1 cell

Simultaneous firing of 40 CA3 cells leads to a CA1 discharge

CA1

CA1

Entorhinal cortex

CA3

Dentate gyrus

Figure 6-4 Information flow within the hippocampus. The diagram depicts information flow within the hippocampus, highlighting the principles of convergence and divergence and how they contribute to hippocampal computations.

neuron fires an action potential when about 40 CA3 neurons stimulate it simultaneously. Each CA1 neuron receives about 30,000 inputs, so it can be triggered by a relatively small number of the CA3 neurons that connect to it. Thus, each CA1 cell serves to integrate information from a large number of inputs. In terms of divergence, each CA3 neuron can influence about 20,000 CA1 cells, allowing each CA3 cell to have far-reaching influence on many CA1 cells. CA1 pyramidal neurons send their axons (output) into the subiculum and to entorhinal cortex as well as to the PFC and other subcortical structures. From this discussion, it should be apparent that it takes a lot to get information into the trisynaptic pathway, but once it is accepted, the system processes the information very effectively and rapidly.

The above discussion is largely based on the anatomy and physiology of the rodent hippocampus. The human hippocampus is larger and more complex, but the overall architecture and the principles underlying its function appear to be very similar. For example, the human dentate gyrus has about 18 million granule cells, compared to 1.2 million in the rat. The transition between areas CA3 and CA1 is another place where increased complexity in the human hippocampus is apparent: humans have about 5 times more neurons in area CA1 than CA3 (14 million vs. 2.8 million), while rats have only about 1.5 times more neurons in CA1. This difference gives humans the potential for even greater divergence of information in the CA1 region.

The hippocampus is a master of declarative memory formation, binding together information about context and novelty; the what, where, who, and when things happened; and our internal state at the time. The dentate gyrus initiates the process by coding and binding together different components of the *same* memory. John Lisman refers to this as an *auto-associative* function. Others highlight the importance of the dentate gyrus in a "pattern separation" function that keeps different components of a memory distinct. Information about *different* memories is linked together in area CA3 in a *hetero-associative* memory process; this results in a "pattern completion" function and provides a mechanism by which parts of an encoded memory can lead to an entire recollection. Howard Eichenbaum emphasizes that there are several types of associations formed in the hippocampus. When an item (something that happened) is linked to a context (the place where that something happened), memory for an "event" is created. The hippocampus is also able to link chains of events together into what is called an "episode." Similarly, events may be shared across different episodes, creating even richer cross-episode associations. In addition, the hippocampus codes for the relative timing of events and relative importance of events—that is, whether something happened before something else and whether one thing is more important than another. This latter process is called "transitive inference." Table 6-1 presents an overview of what subregions of the hippocampus are thought to contribute to memory processing.

In a physiological sense, the hippocampus uses its own neural "language" to process information. For hippocampal processing to be useful for other brain regions, it must be converted to a form that can be understood by other networks, particularly higher centers in neocortex. The CA1 region seems to facilitate this, converting output from CA3 to a form that is recognized by neocortex; thus, CA1 is sometimes referred to as a "decoder." CA1 also has the ability to analyze the input it receives directly from the entorhinal cortex and to compare that information to the processed information it receives from area CA3. Thus, CA1 also plays a role as a "mismatch detector," helping to maintain checks and balances on processing performed in the dentate gyrus and CA3 relative to inputs from cortex. This is a type

Table 6-1 What Do Hippocampal Subregions Do?

Dentate gyrus: "pattern separation" network
Codes *different components* of the same memory • Facts, context, novelty . . . what, where, when?
CA3: "pattern completion" network
Codes *sequences* linking one memory to another • Item + Context = Event • Event 1 + Event 2 + . . . = Episode • Links Events to different Episodes • Codes transitive associations (A > B > C > D > E)
CA1: "decoder" and "mismatch detector"
Converts hippocampal representation to a cortical form

of neural error detection that we have mentioned in prior chapters. Certain aspects of memory coding, such as the ability to keep track of place and certain aspects of incremental learning, may also benefit from this ability of CA1 to use both direct inputs from entorhinal cortex and processed inputs from CA3.

As an aside, it is interesting to consider how the hippocampus (and brain) keeps track of time, since timing is an important part of memory context. This area is under active study, but two factors seem to be important. Earlier, we mentioned that the hippocampus demonstrates rhythmic electrical activity (e.g., the theta rhythm). Such rhythmic activity sets a temporal background for interpreting new inputs. Put another way, data are processed within the hippocampus at various points in a theta cycle, and this provides a potential temporal organizing principle. Another way the hippocampus tracks time involves gradual changes in network activity that occur over time, changes that may progress in waves over the entire expanse of the structure, creating what some scientists refer to as "time zones" within the hippocampus. Thus, the representation of context can change over time. Some scientists have likened this concept to the notion that "inputs never step into the same hippocampus twice." The major point to remember is that the processing of information that leads to memory involves several biological mechanisms, including convergence and divergence of connections, comparisons of information that directly or indirectly arrives at a hippocampal location, and rhythmic changes that occur over time in the electric functioning of this magnificent brain structure.

We have emphasized the role of the hippocampus in declarative (explicit) memory and the way subregions within the structure process information, highlighting how even within a relatively simple structure there is a great deal of complexity. The trisynaptic pathway is based on the transverse anatomy of the hippocampus and the way inputs enter and exit the structure. It is also important to point out that the hippocampus has a differential organization along its dorsal–ventral (top to bottom) axis. The dorsal hippocampus (the part closest to the septal nuclei) appears to specialize in handling cognitive data (such as spatial memory, orientation, navigation, and exploration), while the ventral hippocampus (the part closest to the temporal cortex) has strong connections to the amygdala, nucleus accumbens, and infralimbic insular cortex and plays a role in processing emotional memories, particularly the context in which the emotions were experienced. The ventral hippocampus also helps to regulate motivated behaviors, autonomic functions, and neuroendocrine status, particularly release of stress hormones. Thus, the hippocampus is not simply a cognitive device; it appears to be important for integrating all aspects of mind. We should point out that the dorsal–ventral distinction pertains to the rodent hippocampus; humans appear to have similar functions distributed along the anterior–posterior (front to back) aspects of the structure, reflecting the different positioning of the hippocampus within the human brain. In humans, the posterior hippocampus corresponds to the dorsal region in rodents, while the anterior hippocampus corresponds to the ventral region. Despite having different functions, the dorsal and ventral hippocampal regions seem to use a common set of calculations to compare multiple goals and initiate corrective actions in behavior.

SYNAPTIC PLASTICITY: HOW THE
HIPPOCAMPUS LEARNS

Memories can be long-lasting; indeed, some last a lifetime. As we have discussed, information from various regions of the brain must be linked together in order to form memories. For instance, if one recalls a disturbing conversation from the previous night's dinner, activity of brain regions involving recognition of words, faces, and emotions has been tied together. This information processing involves changes in brain electrical activity. For long-lived learning and memory to take place, lasting changes in brain function must occur. We will now discuss how chemical and electrical changes encode and drive cellular and structural changes that result in longer-term memories.

The hippocampus processes the early stages of declarative memory formation using the circuitry already described. At the neuronal level, the key to developing long-term memories lies in the ability of synapses to change their longer-term responsiveness to inputs as a result of a process called "synaptic plasticity." When excitatory glutamatergic inputs are activated repeatedly by certain patterns of neuronal input, they have the ability to change how they respond to these inputs subsequently (increasing or decreasing their response). These changes regulate how the neurons pass information on to other neurons in the network via their own synaptic connections. Such changes in synaptic function can last for prolonged periods (hours to days or longer), indicating a long-term alteration of function. Because the changes persist, they are viewed as a form of synaptic memory; that is, the synapses "remember" that they have experienced a certain pattern of activation. Thus, a given input that produced a specific level of synaptic response at one point in time gives either an increased or decreased response to that same amount of input at a later point in time.

The persistence of these changes is the basis for the "synaptic plasticity and memory hypothesis," which in its simplest form states that activity-dependent, long-term synaptic plasticity induced during memory formation is both necessary *and* sufficient for information storage. This is an attractive model and has guided a lot of research on the hippocampus. As discussed cogently by Richard Morris and colleagues, considerable data support the notion that synaptic plasticity is *necessary* for learning and memory, but there is much less evidence that it is *sufficient*. Thus, it appears that while synaptic change is important for learning and memory, memory is not strictly a synaptic phenomenon; it is more likely an emergent network property involving multiple brain regions. This network property acts to coordinate the function of brain regions related to sensory, motor, and emotional mechanisms. Despite limitations in our current understanding, the synaptic plasticity-memory hypothesis remains the standard in the field, and long-term plasticity is the best model available for describing the neural machinery underlying learning.

There are several forms of long-term synaptic plasticity that are thought to contribute to memory processing. Two that have received the greatest attention are long-term potentiation (LTP) and long-term depression (LTD). Hippocampal LTP was originally described by Timothy Bliss and Terje Lomo in the early 1970s. It has subsequently been the subject of a great deal of research examining its physiological, cellular, molecular, and genetic mechanisms, as well as its potential role in behavior and learning. While hippocampal synapses readily undergo both LTP and LTD, it is important to emphasize that these forms of plasticity are not the sole property of the hippocampus: they have been observed at excitatory synapses throughout the brain, suggesting that they are general mechanisms for use-dependent synaptic change. As an example, recall the description of synaptic changes in the ventral tegmental area and nucleus accumbens following exposure to drugs of abuse outlined in Chapter 5. There is also evidence for long-term, use-dependent changes in inhibitory transmission. LTP refers to a lasting synaptic enhancement that is usually observed following brief, high-frequency stimulation of specific glutamate-using pathways. Perforant path, mossy fiber, and Schaffer collateral synapses all exhibit LTP. While all three of these synapses are important, most studies have been conducted at CA1 Schaffer collateral synapses, so we will focus on the mechanisms responsible for LTP at these synapses. It is important to understand the molecular basis of synaptic plasticity because modifications of this process may be relevant to current and future therapies in psychiatry and neurology, and genes involved in this process are candidates for contributing to a host of illnesses.

Single electrical stimulations of the Schaffer collateral pathway cause release of glutamate from presynaptic terminals on the axons of CA3 pyramidal neurons onto the apical dendrites of postsynaptic CA1 pyramidal neurons. At these synapses, which largely occur on dendritic spines (specialized outpouchings of the dendritic membrane designed to receive synaptic inputs), glutamate activates a type of receptor known as an AMPA receptor. To avoid confusion, note that AMPA is simply a synthetic chemical that selectively activates these receptors and has been used to name the receptors. Similarly, NMDA is a synthetic chemical that selectively activates another class of glutamate receptors. AMPA receptors are ligand-gated nonselective cationic channels (see Chapter 3). This means that the binding of glutamate to the receptor rapidly and briefly opens a protein pathway across the lipid cell membrane that permits sodium ions to enter the neuron and potassium ions to exit. Sodium and potassium are positively charged "cations"; because both can flow through open AMPA channels, the channels are called "nonselective." When a neuron is at its resting membrane potential (transmembrane voltage approximately −70 mV, with the inside of the cell being negative), the opening of AMPA channels largely promotes the influx of sodium ions as a result of electrical and chemical gradients acting on the neuron. The entry of sodium ions excites (depolarizes) the receiving CA1 neuron, meaning that it is easier for the CA1 neuron to fire action potentials (the "spikes" that are the principal drivers of inter-neuronal communication). AMPA receptor-mediated synaptic currents are very brief in duration, turning on and off over a period of several milliseconds.

When these same glutamate synapses are activated by a train of high-frequency pulses (e.g., 100 pulses in 1 second) instead of a single electrical stimulation, AMPA receptors produce greater depolarization of the CA1 neuron. This reflects in part the summation of repeated and closely timed depolarizations. This enhanced depolarization allows another type of glutamate receptor, the NMDA receptor, to become functional. Like AMPA receptors, NMDA receptors are nonselective cationic channels opened by glutamate, but they have two additional important properties. First, their ion channels remain closed when neurons are at rest. NMDA receptors become functional when they bind glutamate in an environment where the neuron that houses them is depolarized. Second, NMDA ion channels are highly permeable to calcium ions. Thus, when NMDA receptors bind glutamate in a cell that is partially depolarized, their ion channels open effectively and allow calcium ions (positively charged divalent [doubly charged] cations) to flow into the CA1 neuron. The increased level of intracellular calcium then activates a host of responses in the CA1 neuron. These changes involve the activation of second messengers and protein kinases that add phosphate groups to various cellular proteins (called "phosphorylation"), thus altering the function of those proteins (called "posttranslational modifications"). These calcium-mediated biochemical events are responsible for the early phases of synaptic enhancement underlying LTP. Over time, the initial calcium signals, second messengers, and induced growth factors (including brain-derived neurotrophic factor [BDNF]) drive new protein synthesis in the CA1 neuron and turn on specific genes in the nucleus of the neuron. These later events lead to even longer-lasting changes in the efficacy and structure of the glutamate synapses, including the insertion of new AMPA receptors into the membrane and the reshaping of the neuron's dendrites to make them even more effective processing devices. There is also evidence that a certain type of protein kinase (called PKM-zeta) becomes persistently activated following LTP induction, and this also contributes to lasting changes in neuronal function. The combination of these chemical and structural events results in synaptic enhancement that can be very long-lived— hence the term LTP. Figure 6-5 presents a simplified overview of the initial signaling events associated with various forms of hippocampal synaptic plasticity.

In addition to these changes in the receiving (postsynaptic) CA1 neuron, another mechanism influencing connectivity between cells involves presynaptic changes that alter the amount of glutamate released from the terminals of CA3 neurons by an action potential. This type of presynaptic enhancement also depends on NMDA receptors in postsynaptic neurons and is thought to result from the production of a "retrograde messenger" that moves from the postsynaptic cell to the presynaptic terminal and causes changes that allow increased glutamate release. Nitric oxide (NO), a small, highly reactive, and highly diffusible "gas" produced in various cells, is an example of an agent that can play this retrograde messenger role. Similar to calcium's ability to initiate long-lasting chemical events in neurons, NO can also act via intracellular messengers to drive longer-lived changes in presynaptic function. Studies using pharmacological tools to inhibit various receptors and messengers and genetic strategies to alter the expression of key proteins have provided strong support for such cascades of events. These studies also support the notion that LTP contributes to certain forms of learning in rodents, particularly spatial maze learning and contextual aspects of fear conditioning.

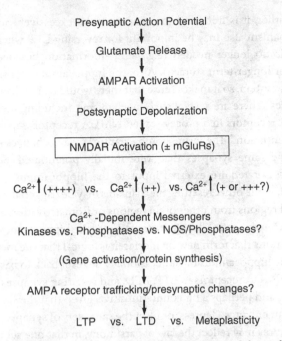

Presynaptic Action Potential

Glutamate Release

AMPAR Activation

Postsynaptic Depolarization

NMDAR Activation (± mGluRs)

$Ca^{2+}\uparrow$ (++++) vs. $Ca^{2+}\uparrow$ (++) vs. $Ca^{2+}\uparrow$ (+ or +++?)

Ca^{2+}-Dependent Messengers
Kinases vs. Phosphatases vs. NOS/Phosphatases?

(Gene activation/protein synthesis)

AMPA receptor trafficking/presynaptic changes?

LTP vs. LTD vs. Metaplasticity

Figure 6-5 Synaptic plasticity cascades. The diagram depicts synaptic and chemical events thought to underlie LTP, LTD, and metaplasticity. This is a highly simplified scheme that emphasizes the key role of NMDA receptors as molecular switches for triggering various forms of plasticity. Note that the amount of calcium entering the postsynaptic region plays a major role in determining the physiologic consequences. Abbreviations: AMPAR (AMPA receptor), NMDAR (NMDA receptor), mGluRs (metabotropic glutamate receptors), NOS (NO synthase).

Interestingly and somewhat surprisingly, many of the events described for LTP also contribute to LTD in the Schaffer collateral pathway. LTD provides a different approach to the way cells can influence connectivity. Here, activation of NMDA receptors results in calcium influx into postsynaptic neurons, activation of second messengers, and a persistent *decrease* in synaptic responses. The difference between LTP and LTD appears to involve the way synapses in CA1 are activated and the amount of calcium entering through NMDA channels. LTD is usually induced by repeated low-frequency stimulation of Schaffer collateral inputs (e.g., repeated stimulation at 1 pulse per second for periods of 10 to 15 minutes). The lower and slower calcium signals appear initially to activate protein phosphatases that remove phosphate groups from key proteins and alter the function of those proteins. This appears to be the opposite of the initial stages of LTP. However, like LTP, the long-term consequences of LTD involve new protein synthesis and gene expression with synapse remodeling and trafficking of AMPA receptors. Evidence supporting a role for LTD in learning is less compelling than with LTP, although some evidence suggests that it is important in forms of novelty learning, one-trial learning, and working memory. LTD may also be important in honing a synaptic network, working in conjunction with LTP to determine which synapses and neurons are activated by a given set of inputs and environmental conditions.

As noted earlier, it is not good for neurons to be excessively activated, so an LTD-like mechanism also may be important for reversing LTP when the synaptic enhancement is no longer needed (e.g., after information has been transferred to neocortex for longer-term storage). Also, the hippocampus is a short-term and limited capacity system, so it makes sense that there would be mechanisms to help it reset its synapses. There are several such mechanisms, including mechanisms that involve NMDA receptors in a process called NMDA receptor-dependent "homosynaptic depotentiation." The term "homosynaptic" means changes resulting from activation of the same synapses that were initially potentiated. Some resetting mechanisms do not require external input to the hippocampus (homosynaptic depotentiation), while other resetting mechanisms may be triggered by direct inputs to hippocampal regions from other brain regions or from activation of other inputs to a neuron ("heterosynaptic" depotentiation). Since the hippocampus is involved in creating connections that form new memories, it is logical that the memory-making machinery of the hippocampus must occasionally be reset back to baseline.

The role of NMDA receptors in LTP, LTD, and resetting synapses back to baseline is intriguing and perhaps a bit counterintuitive, given that the same transmitter and receptors can enhance, depress, or reset the same sets of synapses (Fig. 6-5). In a way, these features may reflect the law of parsimony, in that one set of receptors is used to drive different forms of synaptic change depending on the way the receptors are activated and the circumstances under which they are activated. Making matters even more complicated is the fact that there are types of synaptic input and receptor activation that do not result in LTP, LTD, or depotentiation but that use NMDA receptors to modulate the induction of LTP, making LTP more difficult to induce. This type of modulation is referred to as "metaplasticity" (a type of "plasticity of plasticity") and reflects changes that may result in learning being more difficult under stressful conditions (e.g., psychosocial stress or metabolic stress such as hypoglycemia or brief hypoxia). There are also other classes of glutamate receptors that contribute to synaptic plasticity and its modulation. These include a family of "metabotropic" receptors (Chapter 3) that activate second messenger systems in neurons to release calcium from intracellular stores or that alter the production of specific chemical messengers within cells. It should be evident that although much is known about synaptic plasticity, we are just starting to scratch the surface of knowledge about memory formation in humans. We would also note that our discussion has focused heavily upon synaptic plasticity in the CA1 region. Similar forms of plasticity can be observed at other glutamate synapses, but different mechanisms can be used. An example of this is found at mossy fiber synapses in area CA3 where NMDA receptors do not play a major role in LTP. Interestingly, inputs to CA3 pyramidal neurons from the contralateral hippocampus do exhibit NMDA receptor-dependent LTP, much like the LTP we described in area CA1, indicating that a single neuron can experience lasting synaptic change by different mechanisms depending on the specific synaptic input.

There are several major points in this discussion about synaptic plasticity. First, glutamate synapses are highly dynamic transducers of information and operate over a range of efficacy that is determined by how and when they are activated. Second, there are diverse types of glutamate receptors that play important roles in mediating and regulating synaptic function and have the ability to change their own activity as a result of concurrent activity in neighboring receptors. Glutamate is not unique in having multiple receptor types to accomplish its function; this is a general principle of how neurotransmitters act in the brain. Third, NMDA receptors are extremely important for synaptic plasticity. In effect, NMDA receptors are one of the brain's major "coincidence" detectors. The opening of NMDA ion channels requires the simultaneous release of glutamate from a sending cell *and* activation (depolarization) of the receiving cell. Only under these conditions does the NMDA channel allow calcium to enter a cell. This makes them ideal mediators of Hebbian-type plasticity (i.e., "neurons that fire together wire together").

NMDA receptors, however, are two-edged swords. On the one hand, they are critical for learning and memory. On the other hand, excessive activation of NMDA receptors during seizures, ischemia, or hypoglycemia can overload a neuron with calcium and other ions, leading to neuronal death ("excitotoxicity"). Thus, these receptors are subject to a great deal of regulation. For example, the reason it takes depolarization plus glutamate to activate these receptors is that extracellular magnesium ions block the ion channel when neurons are at rest. Only when the neurons are activated (depolarized) does magnesium leave the channel and allow other ions to flow. Also, glutamate binding and depolarization are not sufficient to open NMDA-receptor–associated ion channels: the receptors also must bind glycine (or a related amino acid like D-serine) as a necessary co-factor to facilitate ion channel opening. This provides yet another check on this powerful receptor system. The importance of NMDA receptors in physiological and pathological conditions is a recurring theme in modern neuroscience. These channels are also targets for a number of psychoactive drugs, including phencyclidine (PCP), memantine, and ethanol, drugs that have important effects on neuronal function, memory, and behavior.

THE HIPPOCAMPUS DOES NOT ACT ALONE

As important and elegant as the hippocampus is, it does not operate in isolation: it is part of distributed brain networks that underlie mental processing and declarative memory formation. For example, the entorhinal cortex holds a critical position in these networks, serving as both a source of direct input to the hippocampus (via the perforant pathway to dentate gyrus and via direct connections to the distal dendrites of areas CA3 and CA1) and as a target for hippocampal output. Thus, the entorhinal cortex is a critical way station, and some evidence indicates that damage to this region of cortex is even more disruptive to memory than damage to the hippocampus alone. Importantly, the entorhinal cortex is well positioned to monitor what the hippocampus does and to regulate hippocampal input and output—much like a neural traffic cop.

The hippocampus also has direct or indirect connections to other brain regions, including the prefrontal cortex, septal nuclei, amygdala, nucleus accumbens, parts of thalamus (input from nucleus reuniens and output to the medial dorsal nucleus), hypothalamus, mammillary bodies, and the contralateral hippocampus. Inputs from midbrain dopamine neurons as well as brain-stem noradrenergic and serotonergic neurons provide an influence of the motivational and arousal systems on hippocampal function. These diverse connections provide ways for the hippocampus to influence current thinking, emotions, and motivation, while incorporating inputs from these structures and their networks into the formation of new memories. Recent evidence based on intracranial electroencephalographic (EEG) recordings in humans highlights an interesting dynamic between the hippocampus and nucleus accumbens in encoding and remembering unexpected events. An early EEG potential is detected in hippocampus about 190 milliseconds after exposure to a novel stimulus. This is followed by a potential in nucleus accumbens (about 475 milliseconds after the stimulus) that precedes a late hippocampal potential (at about 482 milliseconds). The early hippocampal signal appears to reflect novelty detection, while the nucleus accumbens signal appears to provide input about expectancy and salience. The late hippocampal potential signals successful encoding of the event. These results highlight the importance of interactions between cognitive and motivational (salience) systems during learning.

In addition to its role in declarative memory, the hippocampus also serves as a node in other ICNs, including the default system, the system that is the most active in the brain when it is not focused on a specific task. Thus, it seems unlikely that the hippocampus ever gets a chance to "rest." Because of its high connectivity and highly plastic nature, the hippocampus is well positioned to use its "learning" to sculpt the activity of the resting brain and to influence the connectivity of other networks.

SLEEP AND THE HIPPOCAMPUS

The notion that the hippocampus never gets to rest takes on more concrete importance when considering the role of sleep in cognitive processing. Even during sleep, the hippocampus is highly active. Sleep–wake cycles and specific stages of sleep appear to be very important in the cortical-hippocampal interactions involved in memory function. During waking hours, we continuously take in information and our hippocampi are very active. Even when we aren't doing other tasks, the hippocampus (as part of the default network) is processing autobiographical memories and considering future activities. Such processing consumes lots of energy and likely involves the synaptic plasticity mechanisms already outlined. Eventually, however, the hippocampus must send its information to neocortex and reset its synapses for further processing. Sleep seems to play a role in this aspect, and there is evidence that during sleep the hippocampus replays circuits that were active during wakeful learning. This process is important for cortical memory storage, and disruption of sleep has adverse effects on recently learned information and the subsequent learning of new information. Slow-wave or deep sleep (SWS) may be particularly important in this regard. Although the details of how memories are processed during sleep are not completely certain, it appears that during SWS the hippocampus sends messages to the cortex. This communication during SWS involves "sharp-wave ripple" activity that consists of a burst of firing in CA3 neurons; these bursts produce an extracellular sharp-wave of electrical activity that is followed by ripple oscillations in CA1 neurons at very high frequency (200 cycles per second). These sharp-wave ripples may be the physiological signatures of the hippocampus using sleep to replay events learned during wakefulness. These waves, in turn, influence cortex and precede changes in activity of PFC neurons during SWS.

This sharp-wave ripple activity may be an important tool used by the hippocampus to assist in the learning of various forms of new information. Interestingly, short-wave ripples occur following periods when rats receive a reward for their behavior. This provides a further mechanism by which motivation can modulate learning, leading to enhanced recall of rewarded behaviors. Initial changes in the hippocampus during learning, particularly in area CA1, perhaps package the signals in a form that is useful for various other brain regions. The hippocampal sharp-wave ripple activity may be one mechanism of launching this information to more distal sites in the brain and making sure that the messages are replayed frequently enough to be learned by other brain regions.

In addition to being involved with hippocampus-to-cortex informational transfer, SWS may also be important for synaptic homeostasis. How this occurs is not certain, but cortex-to-hippocampus communication during SWS could be a way for higher centers to instruct hippocampal subregions to reset their synapses for future cycles of learning, perhaps via depotentiation. Also, SWS may contribute to synaptic refreshment by restoring energy supplies that have been depleted by intense synaptic processing during wakefulness. This process may involve the synthesis of glycogen in glial cells. Glycogen is a fuel that can be broken down for use as glucose when needed by neurons. It is in very limited supply in the brain, and only certain glia called astrocytes actually store it. Glycogen levels are depleted during wakefulness; during SWS, astrocytic glycogen levels are restored.

The role of rapid eye movement (REM) sleep in memory is less understood. During REM sleep, the cortex appears to reorganize messages from the hippocampus, and there is a general disconnection in activity between hippocampus and cortex (or at least the activity is much less coordinated between the structures). This disconnect may be a reason that dreams, which are largely REM sleep phenomena, are often not remembered: the hippocampus is largely out of the loop and can't help form the memories.

These findings are clinically important because many psychiatric disorders disrupt sleep–wake cycles. This disruption may contribute to cognitive impairment and perhaps other symptoms in the disorders, including difficulties dealing with recurring thoughts and memories. For example, there is evidence that SWS, particularly the deepest levels (stages III and IV of non-REM sleep), is disrupted in major depression. This is largely responsible for the finding that depressed patients have a shortened REM latency. Thus, defective SWS could lead to problems with synaptic energy supply, synaptic resetting, and memory consolidation. Compounding this, many psychotropic medications depress REM sleep and also have adverse effects on stage IV sleep.

With the exception of bupropion, mirtazapine, and nefazodone, most antidepressants diminish REM sleep. Mirtazapine and bupropion are among the antidepressants with the most favorable effects on sleep architecture (both REM and SWS).

NEUROGENESIS (NEW NEURONS) AND THE HIPPOCAMPUS

One of the most amazing and hopeful stories in recent neuroscience is the finding that new neurons are generated in adult brains. This raises the possibility of new avenues for brain plasticity. Data demonstrating the birth of new neurons in adult birds were described over 30 years ago, but conventional wisdom suggested that it probably did not occur in higher species. Over the past decade, considerable evidence has accumulated indicating that neurogenesis also occurs in mammals, ranging from rodents to humans. Two brain regions clearly exhibit neurogenesis in mammals: the subventricular zone of the lateral ventricles in the olfactory system and the subgranular zone of the hippocampal dentate gyrus (Fig. 6-6). In the dentate gyrus, it is estimated that about 1 new neuron is born each day for every 2,000 or so existing neurons; thus, in rodents about 1,000 to 3,000 new neurons are born each day. Over a period of several weeks, these new neurons can develop the properties of functioning adult neurons (for example, the ability to fire action potentials and to send and receive synaptic signals). As they develop, the new neurons intercalate into the circuitry of the dentate gyrus and contribute to synaptic transmission and synaptic plasticity.

The development and function of these new neurons is the subject of considerable research. Current evidence suggests that the new neurons may provide substrates that help the hippocampus deal with novelty. In effect, these neurons have no prior "history" and are thus largely blank slates from a processing standpoint. They also may be a mechanism for dealing with greater complexity of incoming

- **Learning**
  - ➤ Psychotherapy
- **Therapeutic lifestyle changes**
  - ➤ Exercise, diet, sleep, no alcohol or drug abuse
- **Environmental enrichment**
  - ➤ Stress reduction/social network
- **Antidepressant medications**
  - ➤ Almost every class
- **Brain stimulation methods**
  - ➤ ECT, rTMS, VNS, DBS?

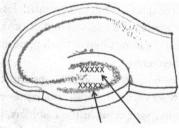

Dentate subgranular layers

Figure 6-6 Neurogenesis and psychiatry. Numerous factors, including a variety of treatments for depression, influence neurogenesis in the dentate gyrus. The diagram highlights the location of the subgranular region of the dentate gyrus, where new neurons are born in the hippocampus. Abbreviations: ECT (electroconvulsive therapy), rTMS (repetitive transcranial magnetic stimulation), VNS (vagus nerve stimulation), DBS (deep brain stimulation).

information by supplying additional computing power. Interestingly, the new neurons also provide a time stamp to the processing of new information in that they come into existence at specific times in the life of an animal. Factors that enhance or inhibit the generation and development of the new neurons demonstrate the potential importance neurogenesis may hold for psychiatry. For example, age, stress, glucocorticoid hormones (cortisol), and many drugs of abuse impair neurogenesis, whereas exercise, caloric restriction, and learning increase neurogenesis and/or survival of new neurons. Interestingly, many (if not all) classes of antidepressant medications and electroconvulsive seizures (similar to those induced with electroconvulsive therapy [ECT]) also increase dentate neurogenesis, providing a possible common substrate for the beneficial effects of these treatments. The neurogenesis effects of antidepressants are not mimicked by antipsychotics, sedatives, or opiates, suggesting some degree of specificity. We will return to this topic in a subsequent chapter when we discuss hippocampal dysfunction in psychiatric disorders. Figure 6-6 presents an overview of factors that affect neurogenesis in the dentate gyrus.

INFORMATION FLOW: A REPRISE

To end this part of the discussion, we will briefly overview information flow in the brain, borrowing the fairly simple but useful descriptions provided by Gary Lynch and Richard Granger in their book *Big Brain*. When we encounter a stimulus, input from our senses enters the thalamus, a region that plays a key role as a subcortical way station for data flow and is critical for generating the cortical electrical rhythms that underlie wakefulness and sleep. From the thalamus, information is sent to primary sensory cortex for initial processing by higher centers (as well as to the amygdala, as described in Chapters 4 and 5). These are fairly straightforward circuits that rapidly transmit "point to point" data and are geared more for data gathering than data interpretation. In addition, information, either directly from the thalamus or from primary cortex, is transmitted in parallel to at least four key processing systems. (1) The amygdala and emotional systems are activated to help determine the initial meaning and value of the incoming information (whether what we are experiencing is safe or whether it will harm us). This process can occur with or without cortical involvement. (2) The dorsal striatum is activated and provides access to the motor system for initiating movement, if necessary. This also includes initiation of habit-driven behaviors. (3) A loop between PFC, thalamus, and striatum is activated that allows higher-order processing, including conscious awareness, interpretation, and the generation of a plan for actions. (4) The hippocampus is activated and provides a way to detect novelty, context, and contingencies; it also initiates declarative memory formation. The hippocampus participates in the other systems as well, leading to even richer associations.

Importantly, these systems provide considerable, but not necessarily fully integrated, parallel processing. Some of the processing occurs simultaneously, while some occurs with varying degrees of delay, depending on how many synapses are needed in the loop and how a network deals with the information. Basal levels of arousal, emotion, and motivation can also influence how the information is processed. There is also a great deal of interconnectivity between these systems. Lynch and Granger refer to the higher-ordering processing systems (beyond thalamus and primary cortex) as "random access" circuits in computer terminology. In such circuits, parts of an input may be sufficient to denote all of the output; for example, a small piece of information may be sufficient to trigger an entire memory. While this can be highly efficient, this type of processing can be subject to mistakes, such as those leading to false memories or inaccurate recall of what actually happened during an event. As discussed previously, the need for error correction becomes an important part of the mix. In fact, the ability to recognize and correct errors at the input and output stages of processing may help determine a person's ability to exhibit good judgment and have resilience to certain illnesses (see Chapter 5).

Points to Remember

The hippocampus is critical for memory formation and is part of a declarative memory network. The hippocampus is also a contributor to other major ICNs, including the default system.

Glutamate synapses are highly plastic, and this plasticity is a key contributor to learning and memory. NMDA receptors are the linchpins of synaptic plasticity and are increasingly recognized as being important in psychiatry. While critical for learning, they can also be the harbingers of neuronal death. Thus, their regulation is a matter of fundamental importance to the brain.

Changes in hippocampal structure and function are observed in several major psychiatric disorders, including mood disorders, schizophrenia, dementing illnesses, and stress-related disorders. This may be a reason that major psychiatric disorders affect all aspects of mind; the connectivity of the hippocampus almost ensures it.

Sleep, particularly SWS, is very important in psychiatric disorders and is a critical time for memory processing. Factors that influence sleep–wake cycles can have significant impact on all aspects of mind.

Neurogenesis and its potential importance in cognitive function and learning are areas of potentially major importance to psychiatry and the biology of mood disorders.

SUGGESTED READINGS

Anderson, P., Morris, R., Amaral, D., Bliss, T., & O'Keefe, J. (Eds.). (2007). *The hippocampus book*. New York: Oxford University Press.

Fanselow, M. S., & Dong, H.-W. (2010). Are the dorsal and ventral hippocampus functionally distinct structures? *Neuron, 65*, 7–19.

Kandel, E. R. (2006). *In search of memory: The emergence of a new science of mind*. New York: WW Norton & Company.

LeDoux, J. (2002). *Synaptic self: How our brains become who we are.* New York: Viking Press.

Lynch, G., & Granger, R. (2008). *Big brain: The origins and future of human intelligence.* New York: Palgrave-Macmillan.

Zorumski, C. F., Isenberg, K. E., & Mennerick, S. (2009). Cellular and synaptic electrophysiology. In B. J. Sadock, V. A. Sadock, & P. Ruiz (Eds.), *Kaplan and Sadock's comprehensive textbook of psychiatry* (9th ed., pp. 129–147). Baltimore, MD: Lippincott Williams and Wilkins.

OTHER REFERENCES

Amaral, D. G., & Witter, M. P. (1989). The three-dimensional organization of the hippocampal formation: A review of anatomical data. *Neuroscience, 31,* 571–591.

Axmacher, N., Cohen, M. X., Fell, J., Haupt, S., Dumpelmann, M., Elger, C. E., et al. (2010). Intracranial EEG correlates of expectancy and memory formation in the human hippocampus and nucleus accumbens. *Neuron, 65,* 541–549.

Brun, V. H., Leutgeb, S., Wu, H.-Q., Schwarcz, R., Witter, M. P., Moser, E. I., et al. (2008). Impaired spatial representation in CA1 after lesion of direct input from entorhinal cortex. *Neuron, 57,* 290–302.

Buzsaki, G., & Draguhn, A. (2004). Neuronal oscillations in cortical networks. *Science, 304,* 1926–1929.

Canals, S., Beyerlein, M., Merkle, H., & Logothetis, N. K. (2009). Functional MRI evidence for LTP-induced neural network reorganization. *Current Biology, 19,* 398–403.

Eichenbaum, H. (2000). A cortical-hippocampal system for declarative memory. *Nature Reviews Neuroscience, 1,* 41–50.

Eichenbaum, H., & Lipton, P. A. (2008). Towards a functional organization of the medial temporal lobe memory system: Role of the parahippocampal and medial entorhinal cortical areas. *Hippocampus, 18,* 1314–1324.

Gagliardo, A., Ioale, P., Savini, M., Dell'Omo, G., & Bingman, V. P. (2009). Hippocampal-dependent familiar area map supports corrective re-orientation following navigational error during pigeon homing: A GPS-tracking study. *European Journal of Neuroscience, 29,* 2389–2400.

Gilestro, G. F., Tononi, G., & Cirelli, C. (2009). Widespread changes in synaptic markers as a function of sleep and wakefulness in Drosophila. *Science, 324,* 109–112.

Izumi, Y., Tokuda, K., & Zorumski, C. F. (2008). LTP inhibition by low-level NMDA receptor activation involves calcineurin, nitric oxide and p38 MAP kinase. *Hippocampus, 18,* 258–265.

Izumi, Y., & Zorumski, C. F. (2008). Direct cortical inputs erase LTP at Schaffer collateral synapses. *Journal of Neuroscience, 28,* 9557–9563.

Jones, T. S. G. (1993). Entorhinal-hippocampal connections: A speculative view of their function. *Trends in Neuroscience, 16,* 58–64.

Kempermann, G. (2008). The neurogenic reserve hypothesis: What is adult hippocampal neurogenesis good for? *Trends in Neurosciences, 31,* 163–169.

Klausberger, T., & Somogyi, P. (2008). Neuronal diversity and temporal dynamics: The unity of hippocampal circuit operations. *Science, 321,* 53–57.

Lewis, C. M., Baldassarre, A., Committeri, G., Romani, G. L., & Corbetta, M. (2009). Learning sculpts the spontaneous activity of the resting human brain. *Proceedings of the National Academy of Sciences (USA), 106,* 17558–17563.

Lisman, J. E. (1999). Relating hippocampal circuitry to function: Recall of memory sequences by reciprocal dentate-CA3 interactions. *Neuron, 22,* 233–242.

Lopes Da Silva, F. H., Witter, M. P., Boeijinga, P. H., & Lohman, A. H. M. (1990). Anatomic organization and physiology of the limbic cortex. *Physiology Reviews, 70*, 453–511.

Lubenov, E. V., & Siapas, A. G. (2009). Hippocampal theta oscillations are travelling waves. *Nature, 459*, 534–538.

Malenka, R. C., & Bear, M. F. (2004). LTP and LTD: An embarrassment of riches. *Neuron, 44*, 5–21.

Manns, J. R., Howard, M. W., & Eichenbaum, H. (2007). Gradual changes in hippocampal activity support remembering the order of events. *Neuron, 56*, 530–540.

Martin, S. J., Grimwood, P. D., & Morris, R. G. (2000). Synaptic plasticity and memory: An evaluation of the hypothesis. *Annual Review of Neuroscience, 23*, 649–711.

Molle, M., & Born, J. (2009). Hippocampus whispering in deep sleep to prefrontal cortex–for good memories? *Neuron, 61*, 496–498.

Muzzio, I. A., Kentros, C., & Kandel, E. (2009). What is remembered? Role of attention on the encoding and retrieval of hippocampal representations. *Journal of Physiology (London), 587*, 2837–2854.

Nakashiba, T., Buhl, D. L., McHugh, T. J., & Tonegawa, S. (2009). Hippocampal CA3 output is crucial for ripple-associated reactivation and consolidation of memory. *Neuron, 62*, 781–787.

Nakashiba, T., Young, J. Z., McHugh, T. J., Buhl, D. L., & Tonegawa, L. (2008). Transgenic inhibition of synaptic transmission reveals role of CA3 output in hippocampal learning. *Science, 319*, 1260–1264.

Olney, J. W. (2003). Excitoxicity, apoptosis and neuropsychiatric disorders. *Current Opinion in Pharmacology, 3*, 101–109.

Peyrache, A., Khamassi, M., Benchenane, K., Wiener, S. I., & Battaglia, F. P. (2009). Replay of rule-learning related neural patterns in the prefrontal cortex during sleep. *Nature Neuroscience, 12*, 919–926.

Sacktor, T. C. (2011). How does PKMζ maintain long-term memory? *Nature Reviews Neuroscience, 12*, 9–15.

Sahay, A., & Hen, R. (2007). Adult hippocampal neurogenesis in depression. *Nature Neuroscience, 10*, 1110–1115.

Singer, A. C., & Frank, L. M. (2009). Rewarded outcomes enhance reactivation of experience in the hippocampus. *Neuron, 64*, 910–921.

Somogyi, P., & Klausberger, T. (2005). Defined types of cortical interneuron structure space and spike timing in the hippocampus. *Journal of Physiology (London), 562*, 9–26.

Song, H., Stevens, C. F., & Gage, F. H. (2002). Neural stem cells from adult hippocampus develop essential properties of functional CNS neurons. *Nature Neuroscience, 5*, 438–445.

Tamminga, C. A., Stan, A. D., & Wagner, A. D. (2010). The hippocampal formation in schizophrenia. *American Journal of Psychiatry, 167*, 1178–1193.

Tononi, G., & Cirelli, C. (2006). Sleep function and synaptic homeostasis. *Sleep Medicine Reviews, 10*, 49–62.

Van der Werf, Y. D., Altena, E., Schoonheim, M. M., Sanz-Arigita, E. J., Vis, J. C., De Rijke, W., et al. (2009). Sleep benefits subsequent hippocampal functioning. *Nature Neuroscience, 12*, 122–123.

Van Strien, N. M., Cappaert, N. L. M., & Witter, M. P. (2009). The anatomy of memory: An interactive overview of the parahippocampal-hippocampal network. *Nature Reviews Neuroscience, 10*, 272–282.

Wierzynski, C. M., Lubenov, E. V., Gu, M., & Siapas, A. G. (2009). State-dependent spike-timing relationships between hippocampal and prefrontal circuits during sleep. *Neuron, 61*, 587–596.

Witter, M. P., Wouterlood, F. G., Naber, P. A., & Van Haeften, T. (2000). Anatomical organization of the parahippocampal-hippocampal network. *Annals of the New York Academy of Science, 911*, 1–24.

Zorumski, C. F. (2005). Neurobiology, neurogenesis and the pathology of psychopathology. In C. F. Zorumski & E. H. Rubin (Eds.), *Psychopathology in the genome and neuroscience era* (pp. 175–187). Washington, DC: American Psychiatric Publishing.

7

Network Dysfunction
Stress, Psychiatric Disorders,
and the Hippocampus

As emphasized in Chapter 6, the hippocampus is a node with very high external connectivity and dynamic internal structure. This region is critical for the operations of several intrinsic connectivity networks (ICNs), including the default network and networks involved with explicit memory formation and emotions. The hippocampus is also intimately tied to motivational processing systems in ventral tegmental area (VTA)–nucleus accumbens–prefrontal cortex (PFC) pathways.

In this chapter, we will consider what happens to the hippocampus in psychiatric disorders and how hippocampal changes may affect overall brain function. We will compare evidence from studies of depression to observations in other psychiatric disorders, particularly schizophrenia and stress-related disorders. Many of these studies involve humans, but we also will extrapolate from work using rodent models of psychosocial stress. Because there are no definitive rodent models for human psychiatric illnesses, some of this discussion will be speculative. Nonetheless, many brain regions have similar organization across species, and insights from rodent studies can be instructive when thinking about network dysfunction in humans. We will point out areas where this is already happening.

As a result of the unique structure and function of the hippocampus, as well as the quality and quantity of human and animal data regarding the role of the hippocampus in psychiatric illnesses, we are able to use this structure to demonstrate specific principles regarding network operations and psychiatric disorders, emphasizing how cellular, synaptic, and network changes may conspire to produce psychiatric symptoms and illness. While we are focusing on the hippocampus to make specific points, we emphasize that no psychiatric disorder is mediated strictly by hippocampal dysfunction. In fact, no single brain region is responsible for any psychiatric disorder. These illnesses reflect dysfunction within and across brain networks; therefore, multiple regions and multiple networks are likely involved.

PSYCHIATRIC DISORDERS AND STRUCTURAL CHANGES IN THE HIPPOCAMPUS

In this section, we will briefly review studies examining changes in hippocampal structure in several major psychiatric illnesses, highlighting changes observed in major depression. We are using major depression as an example because many, but not all, studies using structural magnetic resonance imaging (MRI) have reported that one or both hippocampi are smaller in subjects with depression compared to matched controls. Based on meta-analyses, which combine data from numerous studies for the purpose of statistical analysis, it is clear that the available structural imaging studies of depression are heterogeneous with regard to age and gender of subjects, age of onset of depression, course of illness, and response to treatment. This heterogeneity makes interpreting the data more difficult. Despite these limitations, meta-analyses indicate that individuals with major depression exhibit about 8% to 10% reduction in hippocampal size bilaterally. Fewer studies have examined people with bipolar disorder, but the trends are similar. It is not yet clear whether changes in specific hippocampal subregions account for the smaller hippocampal volumes in depressed subjects.

To put the findings in depression in perspective, it is helpful to compare them with observations in other neuropsychiatric disorders. Subjects with Alzheimer's disease exhibit about 24% reduction in hippocampal volume, whereas subjects with the syndrome of mild cognitive impairment exhibit about 12% shrinkage. In schizophrenia, meta-analyses indicate that there is about 5% to 7% reduction in hippocampal volumes, and a recent meta-analysis concluded that there is about a 7% decrease in hippocampal size in subjects with posttraumatic stress disorder. Thus, the degree of hippocampal shrinkage in major depression is much less than Alzheimer's disease but similar to that seen in mild cognitive impairment, posttraumatic stress disorder, and schizophrenia. Several studies suggest that the changes in hippocampal volume observed in depression correlate with problems in explicit memory processing, including difficulties with hippocampus-dependent recollection. This strongly suggests that there are functional correlates to the structural abnormalities. One of the larger of these studies reported data from a cohort of more than 8,000 individuals in a general practice setting and provided support for the idea that depressed subjects have problems with declarative memory. Other recent studies have reported that depressed individuals have impaired spatial navigation that correlates with abnormal hippocampal function.

It is important to know whether the changes in hippocampal volume observed in depressed subjects occur prior to the development of clinical symptoms or during the course of the illness. The timing of hippocampal volume loss with respect to the appearance of clinical symptoms and functional deficits varies across studies. Some studies suggest that defects are present early in the disorder, while others suggest that they arise over the course of illness, particularly when individuals remain ill or untreated for long periods. For example, in the large general practice study mentioned above, defects in declarative memory correlated with the length of time the individuals had been depressed, suggesting that the state of being depressed may have a cumulative adverse effect on memory function. Consistent with this, Yvette Sheline and colleagues found that changes in left hippocampal volume correlated with the duration of depression in women and that depressed women treated with antidepressants had larger hippocampal volumes than depressed women who received less effective or no treatment. This latter observation raises the possibility that treatment with antidepressant medications may have a neuroprotective (or neurorestorative) effect. These results further suggest that progressive changes in memory function and hippocampal atrophy may occur over the course of the illness. Other studies, however, found that hippocampal atrophy was not related to the number of depressive episodes, duration of remissions, or hospitalizations. There may be gender differences in these effects, and some evidence suggests that men, but not women, with first episodes of depression have smaller hippocampal volumes. The duration of those first depressive episodes did not predict hippocampal size. Some data indicate that women with depression and histories of physical and sexual abuse during childhood have smaller hippocampi than depressed women without histories of abuse, suggesting that childhood trauma may be an environmental factor affecting both hippocampal development and risk for depression.

Only a limited number of studies have examined the microscopic anatomy of the hippocampus in subjects with psychiatric disorders, and, like the neuroimaging data described earlier, these studies present conflicting results. Some evidence suggests that there are changes in synapses and dendrites in depressed subjects, while other work suggests a decrease in the number of neurons or astrocytes, a type of glial cell that is important for maintaining synaptic function and brain homeostasis. In a study using postmortem brain tissue from 11 subjects with bipolar disorder, Francine Benes and colleagues found about a 40% decrease in the number of non-pyramidal neurons (GABAergic inhibitory interneurons) in the CA2 region of the hippocampus but no change in the number of pyramidal (excitatory) neurons. Similar trends were observed in area CA3. This group subsequently found changes in synaptic markers in a class of fast-spiking CA2 interneurons that express the calcium binding protein, parvalbumin. As noted in Chapter 6, these interneurons help to regulate the excitability of pyramidal neurons and the generation of brain rhythms that organize the output and connectivity of pyramidal neurons and brain regions. Results from the Benes studies suggest that changes in the internal processing and longer-range connectivity of the hippocampus are likely to occur in persons with bipolar disorder and possibly depression. We will return to this theme later in the chapter. Importantly, structural changes and cell loss are not restricted to the hippocampus in depressed subjects, and decreases in the densities of glia and neurons, including pyramidal neurons, have been reported in the amygdala, subgenual anterior cingulate cortex (ACC), lateral PFC, and orbitofrontal cortex.

CAUSES OF HIPPOCAMPAL CHANGES IN PSYCHIATRIC ILLNESSES

The studies outlined above support the idea that the hippocampus is involved in the pathology of mood, psychotic, and stress-related disorders and that structural changes can be present at illness onset in some individuals, can progress with illness duration in some individuals, and can be associated with stressful life experiences. Thus, it is important to understand how these changes occur and whether they can be reversed or perhaps prevented. At the present time, animal studies provide the bulk of the available data and extrapolation to humans is speculative.

Because depression and psychosocial stress are associated with excessive secretion of glucocorticoid hormones (e.g., cortisol) that render hippocampal neurons vulnerable to toxic insults, there is interest in determining whether stress steroids are causative factors. Data supporting this hypothesis come from studies in rodents. Also, a role for glucocorticoids in hippocampal shrinkage would be consistent with studies that link illness duration and volume loss, an association that has been found in some but not all studies. One substance that could mediate stress-related shrinkage is glutamate, a neurotransmitter and excitotoxin that contributes to neuronal damage in a number of neurodegenerative conditions. Glucocorticoids enhance the toxicity of glutamate in the hippocampus, providing a potential tie between stress and excitotoxicity. The role of glutamate-induced excitotoxicity in depression would be most consistent with microscopic studies showing neuronal loss. Another interesting idea is that volume loss reflects decreases in key growth factors such as brain-derived neurotrophic factor (BDNF) that help to sustain neuronal structure and function. There is increasing evidence for a role of BDNF in mood disorders, both in terms of the pathogenesis of the illness and the effects of treatments. Table 7-1 lists possible causes of structural brain changes in depression. It is important to note that all of these are speculative at present.

There is also interest in determining whether the hippocampal changes associated with psychiatric disorders reflect a problem in brain development. While multiple mechanisms could contribute to developmental injury, the effects of early life stressors (e.g., abuse and neglect) and/or exposure to neurotoxins have received considerable research interest. A developmental insult would be consistent with data showing structural changes and cell loss early in the course of illness, even at the onset of the disorder in some individuals; this would be particularly true for those who develop the illness early in life (childhood and adolescence). In such instances, the developmental brain changes could predispose an individual to illness.

Based on studies in rodents, it appears that the developmental period during which synapses are being formed (called "synaptogenesis") is a time when neurons are highly vulnerable to damage by toxin or drug exposure. This effect has been most clearly demonstrated with agents that depress brain activity such as alcohol, anticonvulsant medications, and general anesthetics, but it also likely extends to environmental toxins such as lead. John Olney and colleagues found that exposure to depressant drugs for several hours during synaptogenesis is sufficient to destroy

Table 7-1 Possible Causes of Structural Brain Changes in Depression

Glucocorticoids (stress hormones)
Decreased brain-derived neurotrophic factor (BDNF)
Glutamate-mediated excitotoxicity
Developmental abnormalities

millions of neurons in widespread areas of the rodent forebrain. The damage is caused by "apoptosis," a process in which neurons (or other cells) destroy themselves by activating intracellular "death programs" within their own biochemical machinery. Apoptosis results in a form of cellular "suicide," and it is a mechanism by which the body rids itself of damaged or unneeded cells. Some cells undergo apoptosis normally during development, and this is a necessary mechanism for shaping and tuning the healthy brain. Depressant drugs (i.e., agents that inhibit neuronal activity) greatly increase this process when administered during synaptogenesis, resulting in massive amounts of cell loss (10-fold or greater) in some brain regions (Fig. 7-1). Interestingly, rodents experiencing this type of drug-induced developmental insult are not grossly impaired, meaning that they mature to adolescence and adulthood with similar growth and sensorimotor function compared to littermate controls. However, these animals exhibit defects in learning and memory, hippocampal synaptic function, and perhaps stress responses as they reach adolescence and adulthood. They are also more tolerant of alcohol than control littermates, showing markedly less behavioral sedation even with very high acute blood levels of alcohol.

As already noted, the period of synaptogenesis is a time when the mammalian forebrain is highly sensitive to damage inflicted by toxin or drug exposure. In humans, synaptogenesis extends from the third trimester of pregnancy through the first few years of postnatal life. While there are reasonable concerns that this type of apoptotic damage could occur following exposure to clinically used drugs such as anesthetics, anticonvulsant medications, or sedatives, prenatal exposure to alcohol likely

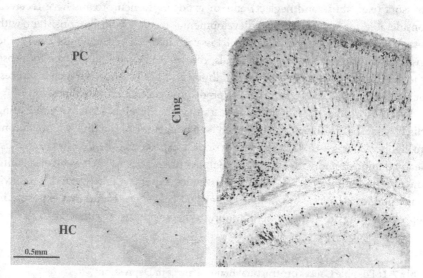

Figure 7-1 Developmental apoptosis. The figure demonstrates the marked increase in cell death (apoptosis) following alcohol exposure during synaptogenesis and highlights changes in parietal cortex (PC), cingulate cortex (Cing), and rostral hippocampus (HC) in 7-day-old mice 8 hours after treatment with either saline (left) or ethanol (right). These brain sections were stained with antibodies to activated caspase-3, a marker of apoptosis. Darkly stained cells are dying. (This photo is courtesy of John Olney, Washington University in St. Louis.)

represents the greatest risk in terms of the general population. Based on studies examining the doses of alcohol required to trigger apoptosis in various species, it appears that pregnant women can likely reach toxic levels by drinking moderate amounts over a several-hour period. Intrauterine ethanol exposure has been associated with fetal alcohol syndrome, one of the most common causes of non-familial mental retardation. In addition to its effects on cognitive function, there is some evidence that individuals with fetal alcohol syndrome are at increased risk of major psychiatric disorders (depression, psychosis, and substance abuse) as they mature to adulthood. Furthermore, development of the highest brain centers in PFC may not be complete until late adolescence or early adulthood, raising the possibility that early drug abuse or drug exposure may have adverse effects on behavior, mood, and high-level cognition via apoptotic mechanisms even when drug exposure begins in adolescence.

THE STRESSED HIPPOCAMPUS: LESSONS FROM ANIMAL MODELS

How changes in hippocampal structure result in the dysfunction leading to depression and other psychiatric disorders is difficult to study. As mentioned earlier, experiments in animals, particularly rodents, can provide important clues as to what might occur in humans. In Chapter 6, we reviewed how the hippocampus normally processes information and highlighted how information flows within the trisynaptic pathway (Fig. 7-2). To study the influence of stress on hippocampal function, Raag Airan, Karl Deisseroth, and colleagues exposed rats to repeated bouts of mild stress. The stressors included things like altering their light/dark cycles, dampening their bedding, or displacing objects in their home cages. Over a period of several weeks, the rats showed physiological signs of stress, including changes in grooming behavior and glucocorticoid secretion. After the stress exposure, the animals were studied in a forced swim test, a test used as a rodent model for detecting "depression-like" behaviors.

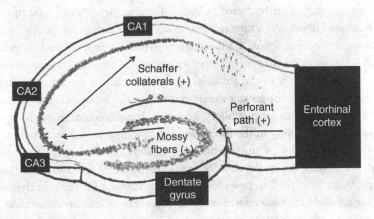

Figure 7-2 Hippocampal slices and the trisynaptic pathway. The diagram depicts information flow from entorhinal cortex to dentate gyrus and the trisynaptic hippocampal pathway.

Rodents that are stressed tend to give up and become immobile in this test sooner than non-stressed animals. Antidepressant medications have long been known to increase swimming times in this model, which has led to the use of the forced swim test as an experimental way to identify potential new antidepressant drugs. In the Deisseroth study, rats exposed to chronic mild stress exhibited greater immobility compared to controls, supporting the idea that they had a "depressed" phenotype.

These findings are consistent with other rat models of chronic stress and depression. What makes the Deisseroth group's studies unique is that these researchers prepared brain slices from the ventral hippocampus of stressed and non-stressed rats and examined hippocampal function using high-speed voltage-sensitive dyes (VSDs) to monitor activity flow within the hippocampus. Hippocampal slices are a type of *in vitro* preparation in which the hippocampus is dissected from a rodent and cut into transverse sections typically 200 to 500 μm thick. These brain sections remain viable for hours and maintain the entire glutamate-using trisynaptic pathway discussed in Chapter 6, including the perforant path inputs to dentate gyrus, the mossy fiber inputs to CA3, and the Schaffer collateral inputs to CA1 (see Fig. 7-2). This preparation has been a standard method for studying hippocampal physiology for more than 30 years. An intriguing feature of the Deisseroth study was the use of VSDs to monitor the flow of electrical activity through the hippocampus. VSDs are fluorescent molecules that interact with cell membranes and emit light in response to voltage changes across the cell membrane. Stimulation of a glutamate pathway causes depolarization (excitation) of the receiving neurons; this depolarization is accompanied by a change in light emission by the VSD that can be detected using specialized microscopes. In effect, VSDs provide a type of functional neuroimaging at the cellular level; as brain regions are excited, they emit a glow that can be quantified and analyzed in term of intensity and degree of spread. While there are experimental limitations in using and interpreting results with VSDs, the method represents a state of the art way to study activity percolation within and between brain regions.

Deisseroth and colleagues found that activity propagation through the hippocampus was substantially altered in stressed rodents when compared to control rats. The altered information flow resulted in an "input–output mismatch" in which there was a decrease in inputs via the dentate gyrus but an increased output from area CA1. Importantly, changes in activity propagation from dentate gyrus to CA1 were a reliable predictor of the animals' performance in the forced swim test: the lower the propagation, the greater the immobility in the behavioral test. Perhaps of even greater importance for psychiatry, both the hippocampal activity changes and the behavioral immobility in the forced swim test were reversed by antidepressant medications but not by an antipsychotic medication. Moreover, the birth of new neurons (neurogenesis) in the dentate gyrus was required for these effects of the antidepressants. This finding provides one line of support for the idea that neurogenesis is involved in some effects of antidepressants, at least in rodents. We will return to this topic later in the chapter. Figure 7-3 presents a schematic diagram of these findings.

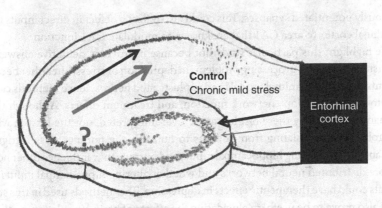

Control
Chronic mild stress

Entorhinal
cortex

?

Figure 7-3 Hippocampal input/output mismatch and chronic mild stress. The diagram depicts changes found by Airan and colleagues when they examined the effects of chronic mild stress on hippocampal function. Behavioral stress resulted in an input/output mismatch in which inflow to the dentate gyrus was diminished while output from area CA1 was enhanced.

What does an input–output mismatch mean for hippocampal information processing? Answers to this question are more speculative, but reasonable hypotheses can be generated based on the known biology of the hippocampus. The diminished inflow suggests that the hippocampus is having problems digesting new data and converting new inputs from cortex into new memories, resulting in a type of learning defect. At the same time, output from the hippocampus back to the cortex via area CA1 is enhanced, suggesting that "old" information already stored in hippocampal circuits is being repeatedly sent to the cortex. This combination suggests that the hippocampus could be having problems correcting errors because updated learning is diminished. This scenario could result in stress-related memories and contextual fear being included repeatedly in messages sent from the hippocampus to the cortex. Although it may be an overly simplistic interpretation, it is also possible that this input–output mismatch is related to the clinical finding that depressed and stressed patients have trouble getting recurrent depressive thoughts out of their heads and have difficulty incorporating new knowledge that might convince them that their reiterative negative thinking is inaccurate or inappropriate. They also have a propensity for incorporating depressive memories into new and ongoing events in their lives.

How the defects in hippocampal input–output arise is unknown. At the level of the dentate, the failure of inputs to propagate could reflect problems with long-term synaptic plasticity, perhaps resulting from defects in mechanisms contributing to long-term potentiation (LTP), stress-induced metaplasticity, or excessive inhibition of dentate granule cells. Stress and glucocorticoid secretion is known to hamper LTP induction and to alter inhibitory tone in some brain regions. Alternatively, the dentate inflow problem could reflect diminished inputs from entorhinal cortex via the perforant path, implying an upstream processing problem. At the other end of the trisynaptic pathway, the sustained output from area CA1 could reflect problems with homeostatic synaptic resetting, including perhaps defects in depotentiation of previously potentiated synapses. This could also reflect a defect in direct inputs from entorhinal cortex to area CA1 that are known to modulate CA1 function.

We highlight this particular study not because it provides definitive answers to understanding neural processing problems in depression or stress, but rather because it points to ways that animal models and sophisticated neuroscience methods can be used to probe behaviors, network function, and treatment effects. Although there are many reasons why these results can be over-interpreted, not the least of which are problems extrapolating from rodents to humans, the findings raise intriguing ideas about how altering hippocampal inputs and outputs may influence other nodes in more distributed neural networks and whether altering hippocampal inputs and outputs could have therapeutic effects in depression. The methods used in this study could also prove to be useful in elucidating the effects of brain stimulation methods, such as electroconvulsive therapy, transcranial magnetic stimulation, and deep brain stimulation. Similarly, these types of studies could also help us understand how learning (psychotherapy) or lifestyle interventions (sleep hygiene and exercise) may have beneficial effects in depression.

As noted in Chapter 6, the hippocampus does not act alone, and it is important to understand how changes in hippocampal function alter information processing in more distributed neural networks. Using mouse models of human illnesses, Joshua Gordon's laboratory has been examining how genetic abnormalities associated with anxiety and psychosis alter synchronization of activity between hippocampus and PFC. Mice with deletion of serotonin 1A receptors show increased stress and anxiety-like behaviors and a marked increase in synchronous activity linking ventral (but not dorsal) hippocampus and medial PFC. In contrast, mice with a chromosomal deletion analogous to the human 22q11.2 deletion that is associated with schizophrenia exhibit impaired working memory (a common cognitive defect in schizophrenia) and diminished synchrony of hippocampal-PFC activity. The importance of these latter studies is that they provide a basis for understanding how cellular and synaptic mechanisms can contribute to inter-regional processing problems and higher-order defects in brain function that accompany psychiatric disorders.

RECENT HUMAN STUDIES IN MOOD AND PSYCHOTIC DISORDERS

As previously noted, changes in hippocampal structure reported in subjects with major depression are associated with problems in memory processing. These findings alone strongly support the idea that depression is much more than emotional dysfunction and that problems with cognition are major contributors to mood disorders. Unfortunately, structural imaging studies tell us nothing about what is happening within the hippocampus of depressed persons or within the networks involved in depression. Advances in imaging the functional connectivity of the human brain at rest and during cognitive tasks offer hope of unraveling some of these issues.

We will start by considering what happens to processing within the default-mode ICN. As we have described previously, the default-mode ICN reflects the coordinated activity of a group of brain regions, including the hippocampus, that shows high activity when the brain is not engaged in doing specific tasks. This high basal activity is believed to involve a focus on intrapersonal information, including mood, autobiographical memories, abstract thoughts, and perhaps future planning. When attention is shifted to a task, activity in the default ICN diminishes as task-oriented ICNs are brought on line. Because patients with a range of psychiatric disorders exhibit preoccupation with their own thoughts and internal worlds, there is considerable interest in determining whether defects in default-mode processing are associated with these illnesses. While data are still preliminary, it appears that depressed individuals have significant problems in default-mode activity. Some evidence indicates that there is enhanced basal connectivity within the network, specifically between the subgenual ACC and certain thalamic nuclei, and that this enhanced connectivity correlates with the duration of the current depressive episode. Depressed individuals also appear to have difficulties shifting out of the default mode when doing specific tasks, particularly when the tasks involve negative emotional content. Yvette Sheline and colleagues found that depressed subjects showed increased activity in the hippocampus, parahippocampus, entorhinal cortex, and amygdala compared to controls when dealing with negative visual stimuli. Other related regions, including medial PFC, superior temporal gyrus, hypothalamus, and periaqueductal gray, also showed significant differences compared to controls. These studies suggest that processing within the default system is abnormal in depression and that depressed individuals may be "stuck" in an internally focused mode of processing.

While it is always a stretch to compare human and animal studies, the overactivity of the default network at baseline and during tasks in depressed individuals is not dissimilar to the findings in the stressed rodents described previously. There, CA1 hippocampal output remained elevated in the face of diminished processing of new information. Given the connectivity of the hippocampus with the cortex and other sites within the default network, this overactive hippocampal output could contribute to excessive activity observed in other regions of the default network, including the subgenual ACC, an area that gets input from the hippocampus.

What causes overactivity within the default network in depression? Why do depressed individuals have difficulty shifting out of the default mode? Answers to these critical questions may go a long way toward unraveling the network defects that underlie depression and perhaps other psychiatric disorders. There are also likely to be multiple paths into and out of these abnormal states, and understanding these paths might help subtype illnesses and define more targeted treatment strategies. In some cases defects may reside in the default ICN itself, while in other cases defects in other ICNs may result in altered default-mode function. Recent studies offer tentative support for both possibilities.

Bradley Peterson, Myrna Weissman, and colleagues studied individuals at varying degrees of risk for major depression based on family histories. High-risk individuals had depression in multiple generations of their families, while low-risk individuals had no family history of depression. Using structural neuroimaging, Peterson and colleagues found that high-risk individuals had thinning of their neocortex across a range of areas, including inferior and medial frontal cortex, somatosensory and motor cortex, dorsal/inferior parietal cortex, inferior occipital and posterior temporal cortex, and precuneus/cingulate cortex. Some of these areas are part of the default ICN and others are not. Importantly, the degree of cortical thinning correlated with measures of the severity of current depressive symptoms as well as problems with cognitive inattention and visual memory for social and emotional stimuli. Furthermore, cortical thickness appeared to mediate the associations among familial risk for depression, cognitive inattention, and clinical symptoms. The authors concluded that familial risk for depression in this carefully selected cohort derives from diminished cortical gray matter in the right (nondominant) hemisphere, which results in problems focusing attention and difficulties with visual memory (a type of memory handled by the right hemisphere). Those individuals who developed clinical depression also had thinning in the left cerebral hemisphere. With respect to the default ICN, an intriguing aspect of this work is that *inattention* was a strong predictor of mood and anxiety symptoms. Recall that focusing attention on a task is associated with exit from default-mode processing. Thus, we speculate that inattention in these subjects resulted in problems shifting out of default-mode processing, perhaps leading to hippocampal and network overactivity. Figure 7-4 presents our interpretation of the results described by Peterson and colleagues.

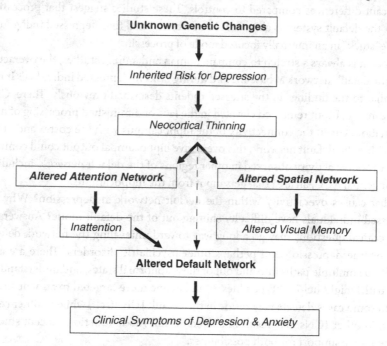

Figure 7-4. Cortical thinning and depression. The diagram provides a schematic depiction of the results reported by Bradley Peterson and colleagues. As-yet-unknown genetic changes in individuals at high familial risk for depression (probably in conjunction with environmental variables) result in thinning of neocortex. These cortical changes result in problems with focusing attention and processing spatial memories. The inattention may result in problems with default network processing and may play a role in clinical symptoms of depression and anxiety.

Another recent study by Christine Esslinger and colleagues used functional neuroimaging to examine how a single nucleotide polymorphism (SNP) in a gene linked to psychosis (psychotic mood disorders and schizophrenia) affects functional brain connectivity. In this study, the gene of interest codes for a protein of unknown function (called a zinc-finger protein) that may help to regulate the expression of other genes. Control subjects without this genetic risk factor showed evidence of strong connectivity between the left and right dorsolateral PFC (dlPFC) (areas involved in working memory) but no connectivity between right dlPFC and left hippocampus. Subjects with one psychosis-linked SNP, who are at moderately increased risk of illness, showed an increase in right dlPFC and left hippocampal connectivity, while those with two risk alleles (at highest risk of illness) showed even greater dlPFC and hippocampal connectivity as well as diminished connectivity between right and left dlPFC. Subjects at highest risk also showed increased connectivity of the amygdala to the hippocampus and to regions of PFC, providing a conduit for emotions to play a greater role in cognitive processing. We believe this study is important for at least two reasons. First, a genetic risk factor for psychiatric disorder was associated with changes in cerebral connectivity involving the hippocampus. Second, the connectivity changes were not specific for a single psychiatric illness; instead, they tracked with risk for psychosis, crossing the clinical boundaries of mood disorders and schizophrenia. This finding adds to a growing literature raising questions about how we categorize current psychiatric phenotypes.

To understand circuitry defects associated with illness at cellular and synaptic levels, it will be important to combine analyses based on functional connectivity with studies examining how information is processed within and across brain regions. This will be difficult to accomplish in humans, given limits of neuroimaging resolution and the inaccessibility of live tissue for physiological, cellular, and molecular studies. An alternative approach used by Francine Benes and colleagues is to study gene expression in postmortem tissue and to draw inferences about how synaptic networks may function. We mentioned previously that the Benes group found that subjects with bipolar disorder have a decreased number of GABAergic interneurons in the CA2 region of the hippocampus. Recently, this group used a highly specialized procedure to isolate specific cells (called laser capture microdissection) in combination with gene-expression profiling to examine the hippocampal trisynaptic pathway of subjects with bipolar disorder and schizophrenia. They analyzed changes in gene expression in major intracellular biochemical cascades, including cascades involved in glucose metabolism, energy production, cell-cycle regulation, synaptic function, and neurogenesis, in specific layers of the hippocampus in different subfields (CA1, CA2, and CA3). In subjects with bipolar disorder, they found diminished expression of a number of important genes in interneurons in the stratum oriens layer of area CA3/2 (the layer where the axons of the pyramidal neurons exit), but they observed enhanced gene expression in this same region of area CA1. Interneurons in the stratum radiatum layer (the layer where inputs from other hippocampal regions synapse) and pyramidal neurons showed more limited changes in gene expression, although metabolic and cell-cycle gene expression was increased in CA1 pyramidal neurons.

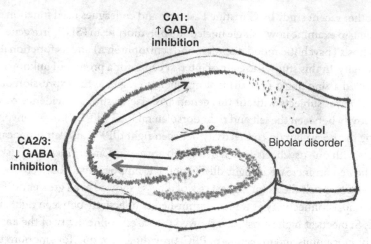

Figure 7-5 Bipolar disorder and hippocampal information flow. The diagram illustrates changes in hippocampal information flow that have been proposed for individuals with bipolar disorder based on changes in gene expression. (This figure is derived from data reported by Francine Benes and colleagues.)

Interestingly, the pattern of gene expression was different in subjects with schizophrenia, with low expression in interneurons in stratum oriens of both CA3/2 and CA1 and limited changes in pyramidal neurons in either region.

From these observations, Benes and colleagues suggested that feed-forward excitation through the hippocampus is attenuated at the level of CA1 as a result of increased activity of the stratum oriens interneurons in subjects with bipolar disorder. In schizophrenia, trisynaptic flow and output may be increased because of underactivity of the CA1 interneurons. Figures 7-5 and 7-6 present schematic

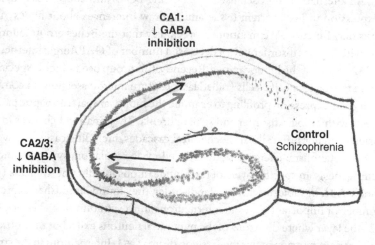

Figure 7-6 Schizophrenia and hippocampal information flow. The diagram illustrates changes in hippocampal information flow that have been proposed for individuals with schizophrenia based on changes in gene expression. (This figure is derived from data reported by Francine Benes and colleagues.)

depictions of these results with possible implications for hippocampal information flow. The strength of this study is its use of sophisticated methods to investigate gene expression and to dissect potential changes in the activity of important synaptic pathways. Unlike the studies conducted by Deisseroth and colleagues in rodents, however, drawing firm conclusions about hippocampal information flow is much less direct and more speculative using this approach. For example, it is unclear whether the increased "activity" of CA1 stratum oriens interneurons in subjects with bipolar disorder results in a decrease in pyramidal neuron firing, or represents an attempt by these interneurons to compensate for pyramidal neuron overactivity (as manifested by the increased expression of metabolic genes in CA1 pyramidal neurons). Nonetheless, this work demonstrates an approach for using cellular and molecular methods to understand network dynamics in humans with psychiatric disorders.

Recent data using high-resolution functional imaging methods indicate that subjects at risk for schizophrenia have abnormally elevated cerebral blood volume in area CA1. These changes correlate with the presence of psychotic symptoms and provide indirect support for the results the Benes group found in schizophrenia. Furthermore, altered blood volume in area CA1 predicted progression from a prodromal (prepsychotic) state to psychosis. Another recent study found that deactivation of the parahippocampal gyrus in subjects with schizophrenia occurred just prior to the onset of auditory hallucinations. These latter findings are consistent with altered inflow of information into the hippocampus and suggest that changes in functional activity within hippocampal circuits may drive problems in distinguishing new and old information, resulting in symptom generation. Carol Tamminga and colleagues have suggested that altered function of the hippocampus in schizophrenia could result in a decrease in pattern separation in the dentate gyrus but an enhancement in pattern completion in area CA3. This would lead to an inappropriate blending of memories and possible recall of incorrect memories and cognitive error generation. Taken together, these studies suggest that changes in hippocampal function occur early in psychosis and are likely drivers of symptom and illness progression.

Interestingly, the hippocampus has strong reciprocal connections with the VTA and influences the release of dopamine. Increased hippocampal output in schizophrenia could contribute to the increased dopaminergic activity thought to be associated with schizophrenia. In turn, dopamine acting on D1-type receptors promotes consolidation of LTP in the hippocampus. Thus, enhanced dopamine release would provide a way for psychotic "memories" to become more persistently entrenched in brain circuits.

The studies outlined here highlight a variety of approaches to investigate how brain systems process information in healthy humans, in humans with psychiatric disorders, and in animal models. Advances in neurosciences, biomedical engineering, and genetics are contributing to increasingly sophisticated studies that are providing information that is applicable to clinical systems neurosciences; these advances have the potential to lead to better understanding of the interrelationships between synaptic biology and functional connectivity. Ultimately, these studies should help to expand our understanding of clinical symptoms and disorders.

CAN DEFECTS IN CONNECTIVITY BE CORRECTED? POTENTIAL THERAPEUTIC TARGETS

Network analysis has the potential to uncover new principles in psychiatric therapeutics. For example, if hippocampal abnormalities are important in cognitive, emotional, and motivational symptoms, then strategies to influence hippocampal function have therapeutic potential. In the rodent stress model, it appears that treatments that enhance hippocampal inflow and/or regulate CA1 output could be beneficial. The ability to achieve this clinically is not as far-fetched as it may seem. Over the past decade, animal studies have repeatedly shown that many treatments for depression enhance the birth or maturation of new neurons in the dentate gyrus. This enhanced neurogenesis is observed with most, if not all, available classes of antidepressant medications, but it is seen much less consistently (or not at all) with antipsychotic or anxiolytic medications. Similarly, brain stimulation methods, including electroconvulsive therapy and vagus nerve stimulation, enhance neurogenesis, although it is not clear whether transcranial magnetic stimulation and deep brain stimulation have this effect. Learning also increases neurogenesis, and since psychotherapy is a form of learning, neurogenesis might contribute to the effects of this form of treatment. Interestingly, certain lifestyle interventions, including voluntary exercise and diet (caloric restriction), that may help depression also increase dentate neurogenesis. Some factors that make depression worse, including stress and abused drugs like ethanol, impair neurogenesis. Stress reduction and avoidance of excess alcohol are beneficial for both depressed patients and neurogenesis.

These observations have led to studies examining whether neurogenesis is critical for the behavioral effects of antidepressants and, if so, how neurogenesis helps to improve symptoms. Rodent studies have provided evidence that dentate neurogenesis is important for some, but not all, of the behavioral changes produced by antidepressant medications. Rene Hen's laboratory used genetic manipulations and irradiation of the hippocampus to show that neurogenesis is required for antidepressant-mediated behavioral changes in two mouse models: novelty suppressed feeding and chronic unpredictable stress. In these studies, irradiation of the hippocampus was used to inhibit the generation of new cells. By itself, irradiation had no effect on behavior or CA1 hippocampal synaptic function, but it prevented changes in behaviors produced by antidepressants. Similar results were obtained by Deisseroth's laboratory using the chronic mild stress model. In these studies, hippocampal irradiation prevented the effects of antidepressant medications both on behavior in the forced swim test and the altered propagation of electrical activity in the hippocampus. The latter finding provides a possible physiological signature for the effects of neurogenesis on this neural system in the chronic stress model. This study also demonstrated that inhibiting neurogenesis in non-stressed rats was neither necessary nor sufficient to produce a "depressed" phenotype. This suggests that defects in neurogenesis *per se* do not produce depression-like behaviors; rather, neurogenesis is a mechanism by which the network can heal itself.

Eric Kandel's laboratory provided an interesting twist on this story using a behavioral intervention. They examined ways to teach rodents "learned safety," allowing them to recognize when they were in an environment where bad things (like shocks) never happen to them. This type of behavioral conditioning has "antidepressant" effects in the forced swim test and in the model of chronic uncontrollable stress. The magnitude of the effects produced by the learned safety behavior rivaled the effects of antidepressant drugs. Inhibiting dentate neurogenesis impaired both the ability of the animals to learn the safety signal and the ability of learned safety to improve behavior in the stress models. This result provides support for the idea that neurogenesis may be involved in both learning and the beneficial aspects of some forms of psychotherapy, or at least behavioral interventions. It is less clear whether other forms of hippocampal-dependent learning (e.g., non-emotion-based spatial learning) helps stressed phenotypes or whether aversive forms of learning (e.g., fear conditioning) hinder neurogenesis and stress reactivity.

WHAT ABOUT OTHER BRAIN REGIONS AND NETWORKS?

Taken together, the studies described above provide support for the hypothesis that at least some effects of antidepressant treatments require the birth and maturation of new neurons in the dentate gyrus. However, depression and other disorders are not simply hippocampal illnesses, and we have already highlighted the involvement of complex but incompletely understood networks in their biology (Chapter 5). We have emphasized the hippocampus in this chapter because much more is known about its biology, and it does play a role in depression and other psychiatric illnesses. We would also emphasize that the involvement of the hippocampus in an illness largely ensures that a disorder will affect cognition, emotion, and motivation, given the role of the hippocampus as a key hub for integrating information across these aspects of the mind. Also, the role of neurogenesis in antidepressant treatment is largely a hippocampal-centric phenomenon, so understanding how neurogenesis affects hippocampal physiology is important.

The hippocampus, however, is not the end of the story. Work in both the Kandel and Hen laboratories emphasize that all effects of antidepressants are not mediated simply by increases in dentate neurogenesis. For example, Kandel and colleagues found changes in gene expression in the amygdala and other brain regions with their learned safety behavioral intervention, and the circuitry of learned safety also involves the dorsal striatum. Thus, there is considerable interest in determining how other brain regions, presumably those that are part of mood-regulating ICNs, are altered in stress and depression. One example is work in Eric Nestler's laboratory examining anxiety and depressive behaviors in a rodent model of social defeat.

These studies found changes in the shell region of the nucleus accumbens that alter neuronal excitability via changes in the function of certain potassium channels; these changes correlate with anxiety-like behaviors exhibited by stressed mice. Beyond these studies, there is a need to understand the connections and dynamics of the depression network that have been highlighted in human imaging studies, particularly the role of key nodes in frontal cortex such as the subgenual ACC. Again, our major point is that depression and other psychiatric disorders are not the products of dysfunction in single brain regions; they are problems of higher-order and interdependent neural circuits. Although complex, the biology of these networks can be solved, and the lessons provided by studies in the hippocampus serve as a model for future work.

Points to Remember

The hippocampus is a critical node in brain function. Considerable evidence indicates changes in hippocampal structure and function across a range of psychiatric disorders. The hippocampus is only one region involved in the biology of psychiatric disorders, however, and it may not be the principal site of dysfunction in any specific psychiatric disorder. Nevertheless, the hippocampus is highly susceptible to the effects of acute and chronic stress, and this may be a common theme across illnesses.

There are no ideal animal models for psychiatric disorders; all have significant limitations. Nonetheless, studies of chronic stress and social defeat in rodents provide methods for untangling some of the neural circuitry and information-processing problems that contribute to behavioral changes associated with human illnesses. Animal models can also provide information about synaptic and molecular mechanisms that can be targeted to treat psychiatric disorders. How those mechanisms influence network function will be critical for understanding their roles in depression and other disorders.

Neurogenesis in the dentate gyrus plays a role in at least some behavioral effects of antidepressant treatments in rodents. Finding ways to harvest the plasticity engendered by neurogenesis is a potential avenue for new and innovative treatments in psychiatry. Importantly, depression (or at least the stress phenotype in rodents) does not result from defective neurogenesis, yet enhanced neurogenesis helps to improve hippocampal network function and behavior. Medications are only one way to influence dentate neurogenesis, and rehabilitative efforts using learning and lifestyle changes can complement or extend the effects of somatic treatments.

Sophisticated research tools are being developed for use in animal models, and some of these may eventually be utilized in humans. These tools are leading to rapid advances in our understanding of how brain regions interact in health and in psychiatric disorders. Understanding neural systems approaches to the brain will be crucial for understanding the development and mechanisms of future therapeutic modalities.

SUGGESTED READINGS

Airan, R. D., Meltzer, L. A., Roy, M., Gong, Y., Chen, H., & Deisseroth, K. (2007). High-speed imaging reveals neurophysiological links to behavior in an animal model of depression. *Science, 317,* 819–823.

LeDoux, J. (2002). *Synaptic self: How our brains become who we are.* New York: Viking Press.

Santarelli, L., Saxe, M., Gross, C., Surget, A., Battaglia, F., Dulawa, S., et al. (2003). Requirement of hippocampal neurogenesis for the behavioral effects of antidepressants. *Science, 301,* 805–809.

Sheline, Y. I., Barch, D. M., Price, J. L., Rundle, M. M., Vaishnavi, S. N., Snyder, A. Z., et al. (2009). The default mode network and self-referential processes in depression. *Proceedings of the National Academy of Sciences (USA), 106,* 1942–1947.

OTHER REFERENCES

Adhikari, A., Topiwala, M. A., & Gordon, J. A. (2010). Synchronized activity between the ventral hippocampus and the medial prefrontal cortex during anxiety. *Neuron, 65,* 257–269.

Becker, S., & Wojtowicz, J. M. (2006). A model of hippocampal neurogenesis in memory and mood disorders. *Trends in Cognitive Sciences, 11,* 70–76.

Benes, F. M. (2007). Searching for unique endophenotypes for schizophrenia and bipolar disorder within neural circuits and their molecular regulatory mechanisms. *Schizophrenia Bulletin, 33,* 932–936.

Benes, F. M., Lim, B., Matzilevich, D., Sugguraju, S., & Walsh, J. P. (2008). Circuitry-based gene expression profiles in GABA cells of the trisynaptic pathway in schizophrenics versus bipolars. *Proceedings of the National Academy of Science (USA), 105,* 20935–20940.

Botteron, K. N., Raichle, M. E., Drevets, W. C., Heath, A. C., & Todd, R. D. (2002). Volumetric reduction in left subgenual prefrontal cortex in early onset depression. *Biological Psychiatry, 51,* 342–344.

Bremner, J. D., Narayan, M., Anderson, E. R., Staib, L. H., Miller, H. I.., & Charney, D. S. (2000). Hippocampal volume reduction in major depression. *American Journal of Psychiatry, 157,* 115–118.

Campbell, S., Marriott, M., Nahmias, C., & MacQueen, G. M. (2004). Lower hippocampal volume in patients suffering from depression: A meta-analysis. *American Journal of Psychiatry, 161,* 598–607.

Cornwell, B. R., Salvadore, G., Colon-Rosario, V., Latov, D. R., Holroyd, T., Carver, F. W., et al. (2010). Abnormal hippocampal functioning and impaired spatial navigation in depressed individuals: Evidence from whole-head magnetoencephalography. *American Journal of Psychiatry, 167,* 836–844.

David, D. J., Samuels, B. A., Rainer, Q., Wang, J.-W., Marsteller, D., Mendez, I., et al. (2009). Neurogenesis-dependent and -independent effects of fluoxetine in an animal model of anxiety/depression. *Neuron, 62,* 479–493.

Diederen, K. M., Neggers, S. F., Daalman, K., Blom, J. D., Goekoop, R., Kahn, R. S., et al. (2010). Deactivation of the parahippocampal gyrus preceding auditory hallucinations in schizophrenia. *American Journal of Psychiatry, 167,* 427–435.

Esslinger, C., Walter, H., Kirsch, P., Erk, S., Schnell, K., Arnold, C., et al. (2009). Neural mechanisms of a genome-wide supported psychosis variant. *Science, 324,* 605.

Famy, C., Streissguth, A. P., & Unis, A. S. (1998). Mental illness in adults with fetal alcohol syndrome or fetal alcohol effects. *American Journal of Psychiatry, 155,* 552–554.

Frodl, T., Meisenzahl, E. M., Zetzsche, T., Born, C., Groll, C., Jager, M., et al. (2002). Hippocampal changes in patients with a first episode of major depression. *American Journal of Psychiatry, 159,* 1112–1118.

Frodl, T. S., Koutsouleris, N., Bottlender, R., Born, C., Jager, M., Scupin, I., et al. (2008). Depression-related variation in brain morphology over 3 years. *Archives of General Psychiatry, 65,* 1156–1165.

Gilbertson, M. W., Shenton, M. E., Ciszewski, A., Kasai, K., Lasko, N. B., Orr, S. P., et al. (2002). Smaller hippocampal volume predicts pathologic vulnerability to psychological trauma. *Nature Neuroscience, 5,* 1242–1247.

Gorwood, P., Corruble, E., Falissard, B., & Goodwin, G. M. (2008). Toxic effects of depression on brain function: Impairment of delayed recall and the cumulative length of depressive disorder in a large sample of depressed outpatients. *American Journal of Psychiatry, 165,* 731–739.

Grimm, S., Boesiger, P., Beck, J., Schuepbach, D., Bermpohl, F., Walter, M., et al. (2009). Altered negative BOLD responses in the default-mode network during emotion processing in depressed subjects. *Neuropsychopharmacology, 34,* 932–943.

Harrison, P. J. (2002). The neuropathology of primary mood disorder. *Brain, 7,* 1428–1449.

Hercher, C., Turecki, G., & Mechawar, N. (2009). Through the looking glass: Examining neuroanatomical evidence for cellular alterations in major depression. *Journal of Psychiatry Research, 43,* 947–961.

Izumi, Y., Kitabayashi, R., Funatsu, M., Izumi, M., Yuede, C., Hartman, R. E., et al. (2005). A single day of ethanol exposure during development has persistent effects on bi-directional plasticity, NMDA receptor function and ethanol sensitivity. *Neuroscience, 136,* 269–279.

Kempermann, G. (2008). The neurogenic reserve hypothesis: What is adult hippocampal neurogenesis good for? *Trends in Neurosciences, 31,* 163–169.

Lisman, J. E., Coyle, J. T., Green, R. W., Javitt, D. C., Benes, F. M., Heckers, S., et al. (2008). Circuit-based framework for understanding neurotransmitter and risk gene interactions in schizophrenia. *Trends in Neuroscience, 31,* 234–242.

Nestler, E. J., Barrot, M., DiLeone, R. J., Eisch, A. J., Gold, S. J., & Monteggia, L. M. (2002). Neurobiology of depression. *Neuron, 34,* 13–25.

Olney, J. W., Young, C., Wozniak, D. F., Jevtovic-Todorovic, V., & Ikonomidou, C. (2004). Do pediatric drugs cause developing neurons to commit suicide? *Trends in Pharmacological Sciences, 25,* 135–139.

Peterson, B. S., Warner, V., Bansal, R., Zhu, H., Hao, X., Liu, J., et al. (2009). Cortical thinning in persons at increased familial risk for major depression. *Proceedings of the National Academy of Science (USA), 106,* 6273–6278.

Pittenger, C., & Duman, R. S. (2008). Stress, depression and neuroplasticity: A convergence of mechanisms. *Neuropsychopharmacology, 33,* 88–109.

Pollak, D. D., Monje, F. J., Zuckerman, L., Denny, C. A., Drew, M. R., & Kandel, E. R. (2008). An animal model of a behavioral intervention for depression. *Neuron, 60,* 149–161.

Raichle, M. E., & Snyder, A. Z. (2007). A default mode of brain function: A brief history of an evolving idea. *Neuroimage, 37,* 1083–1090.

Rogan, M. T., Leon, K. S., Perez, D. L., & Kandel, E. R. (2005). Distinct neural signatures for safety and danger in the amygdala and striatum of the mouse. *Neuron, 46,* 309–320.

Sahay, A., & Hen, R. (2007). Adult hippocampal neurogenesis in depression. *Nature Neuroscience, 10,* 1110–1115.

Sapolsky, R. M. (2000). Glucocorticoids and hippocampal atrophy in neuropsychiatric disorders. *Archives of General Psychiatry, 57,* 925–935.

Schobel, S. A., Lewandowski, N. M., Corcoran, C. M., Moore, H., Brown, T., Malaspina, D., et al. (2009). Differential targeting of the CA1 subfield of the hippocampal formation by schizophrenia and related psychotic disorders. *Archives of General Psychiatry, 66,* 938–946.

Smith, M. E. (2005). Bilateral hippocampal volume reduction in adults with post-traumatic stress disorder: A meta-analysis of structural MRI studies. *Hippocampus, 15,* 798–807.

Sheline, Y., Gado, M. H., & Kraemer, H. C. (2003). Untreated depression and hippocampal volume loss. *American Journal of Psychiatry, 160,* 1516–1518.

Sheline, Y., Sanghavi, M., Mintun, M., & Gado, M. (1999). Depression duration but not age predicts hippocampal volume loss in women with recurrent major depression. *Journal of Neuroscience, 19,* 5034–5043.

Sheline, Y., Wang, P., Gado, M., Csernansky, J., & Vannier, M. (1996). Hippocampal atrophy in recurrent major depression. *Proceedings of the National Academy of Sciences (USA), 93,* 3908–3913.

Shi, F., Liu, B., Zhou, Y., Yu, C., & Jiang, T. (2009). Hippocampal volume and asymmetry in mild cognitive impairment and Alzheimer's disease: Meta-analyses of MRI studies. *Hippocampus, 19,* 1055–1064.

Sigurdsson, T., Stark, K. L., Karayiorgou, M., Gogos, J. A., & Gordon, J. A. (2010). Impaired hippocampal-prefrontal synchrony in a genetic mouse model of schizophrenia. *Nature, 464,* 763–767.

Song, H., Stevens, C. F., & Gage, F. H. (2002). Neural stem cells from adult hippocampus develop essential properties of functional CNS neurons. *Nature Neuroscience, 5,* 438–445.

Tamminga, C. A., Stan, A. D., & Wagner, A. D. (2010). The hippocampal formation in schizophrenia. *American Journal of Psychiatry, 167,* 1178–1193.

Videbech, P., & Ravnkilde, B. (2004). Hippocampal volume loss and depression: A meta-analysis of MRI studies. *American Journal of Psychiatry, 161,* 1957–1966.

Vythilingam, M., Heim, C., Newport, J., Miller, A. H., Anderson, E., Bronen, R., et al. (2002). Childhood trauma associated with smaller hippocampal volume in women with major depression. *American Journal of Psychiatry, 159,* 2072–2080.

Wallace, D. L., Han, M.-H., Graham, D. L., Green, T. A., Vialou, V., Iniguez, S. D., et al. (2009). CREB regulation of nucleus accumbens excitability mediates social isolation–induced behavioral deficits. *Nature Neuroscience, 12,* 200–209.

Warren-Schmidt, J. L., & Duman, R. S. (2006). Hippocampal neurogenesis: Opposing effects of stress and antidepressant treatment. *Hippocampus, 16,* 239–249.

Whitfield-Gabrieli, S., Thermenos, H. W., Milanovic, S., Tsuang, M. T., Faraone, S. V., McCarley, R. W., et al. (2009). Hyperactivity and hyperconnectivity of the default network in schizophrenia and in first-degree relatives of persons with schizophrenia. *Proceedings of the National Academy of Sciences (USA), 106,* 1279–1284.

Wright, I. C., Rabe-Hesketh, S., Woodruff, P. W., David, A. S., Murray, R. M., & Bullmore, E. T. (2000). Meta-analysis of regional brain volumes in schizophrenia. *American Journal of Psychiatry, 157,* 16–25.

Zorumski, C. F. (2005). Neurobiology, neurogenesis and the pathology of psychopathology. In C.F. Zorumski & E. H. Rubin (Eds.), *Psychopathology in the genome and neuroscience era* (pp. 175–187). Washington, DC: American Psychiatric Publishing.

8

Genetics, Epigenetics, and Plasticity

Understanding dysfunction in intrinsic connectivity networks (ICNs) provides a rational basis for relating psychiatric symptoms and disorders to brain physiology. Knowledge at the network level is critical for determining how symptoms and disorders develop and for devising treatments to improve functional outcomes for patients. This is particularly true for treatment efforts aimed at restoring function, which we have termed "rehabilitative" strategies. However, network-level analysis does not address the molecular, cellular, and synaptic mechanisms that lead to dysfunction. That level of understanding will require studies examining synaptic activity and the role of specific molecules in synaptic physiology and pathophysiology. These molecular and synaptic approaches offer the hope of identifying potential targets for drug development and other therapeutic methods such as neurostimulation. Understanding how molecular changes disrupt neural connections and higher-level network organization will provide a deeper understanding of emotional, cognitive, and motivational processing, and ultimately of what goes wrong in psychiatric disorders. In this chapter, we will discuss selected aspects of genetics and molecular neuroscience that are germane to thinking about psychiatric illnesses. Our goal is not to provide a comprehensive review of current knowledge in genetics and epigenetics but rather to provide a framework for thinking about ways molecular and systems neuroscience can work in concert to improve psychiatric diagnosis and treatment.

GENETICS AND PSYCHIATRY

Many if not most human behaviors and psychiatric disorders are heritable, meaning that they run in families and have at least some genetic basis. These behaviors and disorders are complexly inherited, however; they are not the product of single genes but likely involve the contribution of many genes. Gene expression can be altered by life events, which geneticists call the "environment." Estimates of the heritability of psychiatric symptoms and disorders are often based on twin studies, taking advantage of the fact that monozygotic (identical) twins share all of their genes (have identical nuclear DNA) while dizygotic (fraternal) twins share half of their segregating DNA sequence variation (but not necessarily half of their genes). Twins also share some, but not all, environmental experiences. Twin studies are used to assess the amount of variation in expression of a trait or disorder that can be accounted for by genetics and by different categories of environmental factors.

Genetic epidemiologists attempt to separate environmental exposures shared by twins from environmental exposures unique to each twin. The estimation of shared versus unique environment can have considerable variability because of the difficulties involved in measuring critical elements in the environment, including the timing and degree of various exposures. While behavioral traits can vary widely in the degree to which they are determined by genetic versus environmental factors, many traits appear to be about half determined by genetic factors and about half determined by environmental influences. Shared environmental influences often play less of a role than environmental influences uniquely experienced by an individual twin. Put another way, shared family life seems to have less effect on the development of behavioral traits than genes and unique environmental exposures, such as the influence of an individual's own group of friends. Interestingly, peer groups seem to have a stronger influence earlier in life, during childhood and adolescence, and as individuals mature, genetics plays a bigger role in ongoing development. Therefore, not only are genes and environment both important, but the age at which individuals are exposed to various environmental influences can also make a big difference in determining later development.

The number of genes contributing to psychiatric disorders is unknown, but it is possible, perhaps likely, that for some disorders tens, maybe hundreds or more, are involved. In this scenario, each gene contributes relatively little to risk, with less than a few percent of the variance in the expression of a psychiatric illness explained by any of the genes identified to date. Many of the genetic variations associated with psychiatric disorders are single nucleotide polymorphisms (SNPs). SNPs represent places in the human genome where single bases of DNA have been altered ("mutated"). These changes typically have small effects on the function or expression of a gene; most are in non-coding regions of genes, so they don't affect the structure of the encoded protein. SNPs are found throughout the genome. Some SNPs are located in regulatory regions of genes (e.g., promoters) and may influence the degree to which the gene is expressed. Other SNPs occur in regions of a gene that code for proteins and can, in some cases, change the amino acid composition and function of the expressed protein. The great majority of SNPs associated with psychiatric illnesses are found in non-coding regions of genes, and little is known about the way these SNPs actually affect gene expression or cell function. SNPs are by definition relatively common, occurring in at least 1% of the population.

The association of specific SNPs with psychiatric disorders falls under a "common disease–common variant" hypothesis of genetic inheritance, which states that common variations in genes may contribute to the etiology of commonly occurring illnesses. In this case, "common" typically refers to things occurring in about 1% or more of the population. There are rarer, structural changes in genes that also affect gene expression or the function of the resulting protein products. Some of these changes, called "copy number variations" (CNVs), result from microdeletions or microduplications of DNA. An example of a CNV associated with psychiatric illness is the chromosome 22q11.2 microdeletion associated with cognitive impairment and schizophrenia (velo-cardio-facial/DiGeorge syndrome) that we mentioned when discussing mouse model studies in Chapter 7. Although CNVs occur less frequently than SNPs, they can be extremely helpful in identifying proteins and signaling molecules contributing to psychiatric disorders. CNVs are often relatively recent mutations from an evolutionary standpoint, and while any given CNV is rare in an individual, they are fairly common across the entire human population. For example, some estimates suggest that almost all humans have at least one CNV of about 100 kilobases (kb) in their genome and that about 5% to 8% of the population have relatively large CNVs of 500 kb or more. Research exploring how CNVs contribute to common illnesses is in its infancy, but it is possible that major insights into the molecular biology of psychiatric disorders will come from this approach. Importantly, these rarer genetic changes could help to explain why certain severe illnesses such as schizophrenia and autism persist and possibly increase in the population despite the fact that people with these disorders have relatively few offspring. Also, rarer genetic variants may prove to be important in helping to explain how specific protein networks and signaling pathways contribute to pathogenesis. These rarer mutations may also help us to understand why the same mutations can lead to different phenotypes in different individuals and why different genes in the same chemical pathways can lead to similar illness manifestations.

To put SNPs, CNVs, and psychiatric genetics into perspective, it is important to have some idea about what is being learned from studies of the human genome. It is estimated that the human genome contains about 3.3 billion base pairs. To many of us, one of the surprises from the human genome project was how few genes humans actually have. It had been thought that humans would have about 100,000 genes (a gene being a region of the genome that codes for a protein). As the human genome project progressed, it became clear that humans have only about 25,000 genes; this is not as many as some plants, and not many more than certain flies or worms. This number, however, is deceptively low because it doesn't reflect complexities that can be achieved by alternative splicing (a way that parts of genes can be cut and pasted together) and a host of other mechanisms, including segmental duplications and mutations. All humans have highly similar genomes, with only about 0.1% differences accounting for human genetic diversity. This is a small percentage, but within a genome of more than 3 billion base pairs, it results in about 3 million differences in nucleotides among humans. Chimpanzees, our closest animal relatives, differ from humans by about 2% of their genome. Fewer than 200 genes are thought to be uniquely human, and despite their potential importance, we understand little about their function.

The distribution of SNPs throughout the human genome, coupled with major advances in gene sequencing technology, now allows the entire genome of an individual to be scanned and genetic associations determined. These genome-wide association studies (GWAS) have become the norm for studying common human illnesses, and they are helping to identify some common loci involved in psychiatric disorders. Importantly, genetic loci do not necessarily identify specific genes, since most of the human genome does not code for genes (less than 5% is thought to code for proteins). Nonetheless, these loci may be important via their effects on gene expression. When studying the role of common genetic variants, very large samples (e.g., 5,000 to more than 30,000 cases and controls) can be required to provide sufficient statistical power to detect meaningful associations. This requirement for large sample sizes reflects the wide distribution of genetic variants in the population and the fact that in common illnesses, each individual genetic locus contributes very little to overall risk. With advances in technology and diminishing costs, we are now entering an era in which GWAS is being replaced by individual whole-genome sequencing. How this will influence psychiatric genetics remains to be seen, but the paucity of major findings from GWAS has been sobering, if not humbling.

What are we learning about the genetics of psychiatric disorders? First, it is clear that psychiatric disorders are complexly inherited. Thus, having certain genes increases the likelihood of developing specific disorders, and the more associated genes an individual inherits, the higher the liability. However, the risk is never 100%. For example, schizophrenia occurs in about 1% of the population and is thus a common disorder. Having a parent or a sibling with schizophrenia increases a person's risk to about 15%. Having two parents with schizophrenia increases the risk to about 50%. Similarly, having a dizygotic (fraternal) twin with schizophrenia confers a risk of about 15%, while having a monozygotic (identical) twin increases the risk to about 50%. Thus, genetics plays a significant role in the illness, but it cannot account for all of the risk. Using different statistics, less than 10% of the relatives of a person with schizophrenia also have the disorder, and about two-thirds of people with schizophrenia do not have any relative with the disorder. Second, it is at present not clear whether current psychiatric diagnoses are the appropriate phenotypes to study genetically. An increasing number of studies are showing that psychotic disorders such as schizophrenia and bipolar disorder, which were once thought to be distinct diagnostic entities, share genetic risk. This observation has prompted a search for "endophenotypes," underlying traits that are more quantitative (i.e., more measurable and normally distributed in the population) and more closely aligned with genetics and neurobiology. These endophenotypes include traits that run in unaffected family members and might include patterns of neural activity observed in functional imaging or electroencephalographic studies, or even manifestations of illness that transcend diagnostic categories (e.g., patterns of cognitive defects, such as defects in working memory or attention). The endophenotypic approach might be an area that would benefit from a better understanding of ICNs, although it is still unclear whether better understanding of disease-modified ICNs will generate meaningful endophenotypes. Third, psychiatric genetics has been plagued by difficulty in replicating findings from one study to the next. This has been a problem in the field for decades and remains a serious concern. A recent example has been the failure of large-scale meta-analyses to uphold the much-touted finding that certain forms of the serotonin transporter gene are associated with major depression in the context of life stressors. This problem with replication reflects an issue we have already mentioned in relation to GWAS approaches: the need for very large sample sizes, including replication samples, in order to overcome limits in statistical power and phenotypic uncertainty. Recent studies have also highlighted the importance of considering genetic sensitivity to the environment in understanding psychiatric disorders.

Why has it been so difficult to uncover genes responsible for psychiatric disorders, and, when candidate genes have been identified, why have the findings not held up to replication? Kathleen Merikangas, Neil Risch, and colleagues have described several factors that contribute to these issues. The first involves the phenotype problem already discussed and the heterogeneity and poor overall validity of many current diagnostic categories. Because the biological mechanisms underlying any psychiatric disorder have not been clearly identified, psychiatric disorders are validated using clinical criteria initially proposed by Eli Robins and Samuel Guze about 40 years ago. These criteria include clear clinical descriptions, delimitation from other disorders, a characteristic natural history (does the illness follow a chronic or episodic course?), and family history (does the same illness tend to run in the same families?); underlying pathophysiological mechanisms based on laboratory studies (biomarkers) are the elusive "gold standard" for establishing validity.

Other contributors to poor reliability of genetic studies include the variable penetrance (variable expression) of some genes. A further complication is the way environmental variables interact with genes to alter gene expression. We will deal with this in greater detail later when we discuss epigenetic factors. Genetic heterogeneity and genetic pleiotropy, the ability of one gene to have several phenotypic expressions, add to the problem. The importance of genetic pleiotropy in psychiatric genetics has been highlighted graphically in a recent study examining the role of microdeletions (CNVs) on chromosome 15 in determining risk for generalized epilepsy. The same microdeletions associated with epilepsy not only predict risk for seizures but are also associated, in the same families, with multiple psychiatric phenotypes, including schizophrenia, autism, mental retardation, and even panic disorder. This type of phenotypic heterogeneity has important implications for psychiatric genetics and greatly confounds analyses of current diagnostic categories. Importantly, these studies demonstrate that pleiotropy is not just the bane of psychiatry and certainly crosses into common neurological disorders. This has led some to wonder whether efforts to identify important genetic pathways in common illnesses would be better served by examining genetic findings in the context of symptom groups and endophenotypes rather than or in addition to current diagnostic categories.

Despite major problems, progress is being made, and genetic approaches offer one of the best hopes for identifying cellular mechanisms and meaningful targets for therapeutic drug development. For example, recent studies of schizophrenia used combined samples from multiple large studies to increase analytic power, resulting in GWAS data on 8,000 affected individuals and 19,000 controls. Results from this analysis revealed the importance of a major histocompatibility locus on chromosome 6, suggesting the possibility that infections or immune reactions contribute to illness risk. This finding is consistent with two other large studies showing a role for the same major histocompatibility locus. Interestingly, these findings provide some support for older studies suggesting a role for perinatal infections or immune responses in the pathogenesis of schizophrenia. One recent study used a polygenic (multi-gene) analytic approach taking into account shared risk with bipolar disorder.

This study found that common genetic variants involving thousands of small effect alleles may account for up to one-third of the variance in schizophrenia. Finally, there is evidence for the possible involvement of rarer structural variants (CNVs) that affect key neural signaling pathways and that implicate a role for neural development in the pathogenesis of psychotic illnesses. These observations tie genetic findings to specific biochemical pathways involved in neuronal signaling and provide support for earlier work identifying a role for genes regulating the function of the glutamate neurotransmitter system in schizophrenia. Candidate genes include neuregulin-1, a protein involved in synaptic organization; G72, a protein that helps to regulate co-factors that activate the NMDA class of glutamate receptors; and calcineurin, a protein phosphatase that plays an important role in certain forms of glutamate-mediated synaptic plasticity. Other genes linked to psychotic illnesses, such as DISC-1 (disrupted in schizophrenia gene) and neurogranin, also appear to affect synaptic function and neurodevelopment. At the present time, over 40 genes have been linked to schizophrenia and all are of small effect size.

It is important to put the difficulties encountered in psychiatric genetics in the context of other common illnesses. For example, much progress has been made in studying molecular and network mechanisms contributing to Alzheimer's disease. Several major genes with clear involvement in the disorder have been identified, including mutations in genes for β-amyloid, presenilin-1, and presenilin-2. Mutations in these three genes, however, account for only a small percentage of Alzheimer's disease cases, and they are most germane to rarer, early age of onset, highly familial forms of the disorder. A specific allele of the apolipoprotein E (ApoE) gene located on chromosome 19 is a risk factor for late-onset Alzheimer's disease, but even here the percentage of cases explained is relatively small. Beyond this, progress in identifying important genes associated with sporadic late-onset forms of Alzheimer's disease, the most common forms of the disorder, has been slow . . . much like the progress in psychiatry.

EPIGENETICS, THE ENVIRONMENT, AND PSYCHIATRY

Although clinical genetics usually focuses on the contribution of specific genes to risk for illness, it is important to keep in mind that the roles of genes are not to generate illnesses. Rather, they are tools that underlie an organism's plasticity, resilience, and adaptability. Genes have allowed humans to survive and thrive in their environments, and the environment plays a big role in determining which genes are expressed and where they are expressed in the brain and body. Thus, gene–environment interactions are important in illnesses. Indeed, gene–environment interactions are critical for most aspects of life in complex organisms.

Genes and the environment interact in multiple ways. This provides a great deal of flexibility for navigating the protracted period of human development and also contributes to our ability to learn and remember. One of the major ways gene–environment interactions are expressed appears to involve epigenetic processes. Epigenetic changes are lasting and sometimes heritable changes in gene expression that occur without changes in DNA sequence. Hence, epigenetic changes are *not* mutations in the classic sense. These changes typically involve the structure of chromatin, a chemical complex consisting of tightly packaged DNA and histone proteins. Histones are basic (charged) proteins that interact with DNA and help to compress the huge molecules of DNA so that they can be stored in the nucleus of every cell of the body (all 3.3 billion base pairs). The primary unit of chromatin is the nucleosome, a complex of 147 base pairs of DNA wrapped around a core histone complex of eight protein subunits. Importantly, when DNA is packed in a tight ("closed") configuration, gene expression is inactive. When the complex undergoes certain chemical modifications, it opens up structurally, allowing gene expression to proceed. These chemical modifications include a variety of chemical "tags" usually placed on either the DNA or the histones; these tags target particular sections of DNA for reading. Tags can include acetyl groups, methyl groups, ubiquitin, and phosphate groups, among others. In the case of histone changes, these modifications are referred to as "chromatin remodeling." Epigenetic changes occur *after* the histone (or DNA) is synthesized and are thus called "posttranslational" modifications.

A major goal of current genetic research is to identify epigenetic modifications in the human genome and to determine how these modifications affect gene expression. This research has resulted in the sequencing of what is being termed the human "epigenome." To put the importance of epigenomic research in perspective, it is instructive to consider what happens in monozygotic twins who share all of their nuclear DNA. Some evidence indicates that about one-third of monozygotic twins differ significantly in their patterns of DNA methylation and histone acetylation. These differences are greater with aging and in twins who have lived in different environments. Thus, monozygotic twins can be markedly different when epigenetic modifications are taken into account. While multiple processes likely contribute to these differences, it is important to note that epigenetic changes, like DNA, are subject to mutation over time, and simple random chemical instability can result in significant differences in the epigenome of even monozygotic twins. Table 8-1 presents an overview of how genetic and epigenetic changes are thought to contribute to psychiatric disorders.

Table 8-1 Genetics, Epigenetics, and Common Illnesses

Genetics → mutations → phenotypic inheritance
SNPs (common illness, common variants)
- Multiple genes, each with small effect

CNVs (rarer structural variants)
- Fewer variants with larger effects on function

Epigenetics → environmental modifications of gene expression → phenotypic variability
Posttranslational modification of histones and DNA (e.g., acetylation, methylation, phosphorylation)

Based on findings in animal models, histone acetylation is increasingly recognized as a possible mechanism for controlling gene expression in neuropsychiatric disorders. During acetylation, an acetyl group from acetyl-coenzyme A (acetyl-CoA) is transferred to the amino (N) terminus of a histone protein, neutralizing its charge. This transfer is accomplished by enzymes called histone acetyltransferases (HATs) and usually results in increased gene expression. Acetylation is a dynamic process, and other enzymes, called histone deacetylases (HDACs), remove acetyl groups from histones. Deacetylation is typically associated with diminished gene expression. These actions create a type of yin and yang system for regulating chromatin structure and gene expression. At least 12 different HDACs have been identified; they fall into two major families and three classes of enzymes. Importantly, HDACs are targets for certain drugs that might have psychotropic actions based on their ability to reverse the effects of behavioral stress in rodents. We will discuss some of these studies later. There is also evidence suggesting that epigenetic mechanisms may contribute to several human neurocognitive disorders. Rubenstein-Taybi syndrome, a rare disorder associated with characteristic physical and behavioral traits, is associated with increased histone acetylation resulting from changes in the function of cyclic AMP response element binding (CREB) protein (CBP). CBP has HAT activity and is regulated via the adenylate cyclase-CREB messenger system. Rett syndrome, a complex disorder that includes mental retardation and autistic features, is associated with diminished histone acetylation. This syndrome involves mutations in the MECP2 gene whose product binds to CpG ("cytosine-phosphate-guanine") islands in DNA and recruits HDACs to that genetic locale. CpG islands are major regulators of gene expression via chemical modifications. Fragile X syndrome is another developmental syndrome involving cognitive impairment. It is associated with increased DNA methylation and histone acetylation. There is also some evidence that adult-onset disorders such as Alzheimer's disease and schizophrenia involve epigenetic changes. In studies to date, changes associated with schizophrenia have included increased DNA methylation in the vicinity of the gene that codes for "reelin," an extracellular matrix protein involved in synapse formation and development. Also, valproate, an anticonvulsant mood stabilizer, is an inhibitor of class I and II (group 1) HDACs, although it is uncertain whether this activity contributes to its antiepileptic and mood-stabilizing properties. Class III HDACs are referred to as sirtuins (named after the yeast protein SIR2 [silent information regulator-2]). The sirtuins are unique in that they require nicotinamide adenine dinucleotide (NAD^+) as a co-substrate and are activated by resveratrol, a polyphenol in red wine that has been touted as a potential anti-aging and anti-neurodegenerative treatment. The sirtuins are also thought to be important mediators of the ability of caloric restriction (diet) to extend life expectancy in a variety of species, perhaps via effects on the expression of genes involved in energy metabolism.

Many environmental factors, including diet, exercise, oxidative stress, and aging, among many others, can cause effects via epigenetic mechanisms. Epigenetic mechanisms are also involved in learning and synaptic plasticity. For example, David Sweatt and colleagues showed that a particular histone in the CA1 region of the hippocampus is acetylated during contextual fear conditioning in rodents. Interestingly, the changes in histone acetylation associated with contextual fear conditioning are blocked by another behavioral paradigm that results in latent inhibition of fear. This suggests that different behavioral experiences can have positive and negative effects on histone acetylation and that context is important in determining the chemical events. Furthermore, in the CA1 region of hippocampal slices, Sweatt's group found that class I and II HDAC inhibitors enhance long-term potentiation (LTP), providing a potential synaptic correlate for the effects on contextual fear conditioning. The effects of HDAC inhibition on LTP required gene transcription, providing a tie between histone acetylation, synaptic plasticity, and gene expression. In the model proposed to underlie these effects, the HAT, CBP, is thought to play a key role.

Other studies have linked behavioral stress to epigenetic changes, and these observations have potential relevance for understanding the biology of psychiatric disorders. For example, in a model of chronic social defeat, a possible animal model for stress and depression, Eric Nestler's group showed that rodents exhibit persistent decreases in the expression of specific transcripts of the gene for brain derived neurotrophic factor (BDNF) in the hippocampus. BDNF is an important growth factor that regulates synaptic development and synaptic plasticity. Changes in the expression of BDNF transcripts involved increased histone methylation. Interestingly, both the changes in gene expression and the behavioral effects of social defeat stress were reversed by imipramine, an antidepressant; imipramine treatment also resulted in increased acetylation at specific promoter regions of the BDNF gene and depressed the activity of HDAC5, providing a potential mechanism for the enhanced acetylation. This study raises the possibility that agents that alter histone methylation and acetylation might have antidepressant actions, and more recent studies by Nestler's group found that specific HDAC inhibitors have antidepressant effects in rodent models. Interestingly, effects on HDAC function may vary from region to region in the brain. For example, the Nestler group found that chronic social defeat diminished HDAC5 function in the nucleus accumbens; this was associated with enhanced behavioral responses to stressors. Similar changes were observed with chronic cocaine exposure, suggesting that changes in chromatin structure could contribute to the lasting nature of a variety of psychiatric problems, including addictive disorders. These studies also suggest mechanisms by which the operations of key ICNs can be altered by environmental conditions and stressors, and propose a way by which addictive drugs can result in long-term mood changes (see Chapter 2). Sorting out how similar behavioral stress leads to different epigenetic effects and potentially to different psychiatric conditions is an area of active research interest.

The process of neurodevelopment also involves epigenetic changes, and this may hold major significance for psychiatry, given data suggesting that early abuse and neglect predispose individuals to a host of psychiatric disorders later in life. Michael Meaney and colleagues found that the type of nurturing that rat pups receive from their mothers has long-term effects on stress responses; these effects are mediated by epigenetic changes. Not only do these effects last into adulthood, but they also appear to alter behavioral responses to stress even in second- and third-generation rodents, suggesting cross-generational transmission. Pups who received more nurturing from their mothers (meaning lots of licking, grooming, and arched back nursing) have lower stress responses in adulthood, and their offspring have lower stress responses than animals that received less nurturing. When pups from highly nurturing mothers were fostered by low-nurturing mothers, this difference was reversed. Pups reared by highly nurturing mothers showed altered DNA methylation and altered histone acetylation in regulatory regions of the glucocorticoid receptor gene in the hippocampus. These changes were associated with differences in both the behavioral stress responses and the hypothalamic-pituitary-adrenal (HPA) axis hormonal responses to stress. Interestingly, the enhanced stress responses in rodents exposed to low nurturing were reversed by HDAC inhibitors. These findings have important implications not only because early development may play a role in determining risk for psychiatric disorders but also because longstanding changes in behavior and gene expression are potentially reversible via manipulation of epigenetic changes.

A recent study provided tentative support for the idea that these findings in rats pertain to humans. This postmortem study found that suicide victims with histories of childhood abuse had epigenetic changes when compared to suicide victims without childhood abuse or to control subjects. The changes included increased methylation in a neuron-specific hippocampal promoter for glucocorticoid receptors. Taken together, these studies have implications for understanding the impact of parent–child, particularly mother–child, interactions during postnatal development. Women with young children are at increased risk for depression, and there is evidence that children of depressed mothers are at increased risk for psychiatric problems early in life. Some of the risk in the children likely reflects genetic risks for psychiatric disorders (i.e., having a depressed mother), but environmental difficulties encountered by depressed parents in caring for their children may also contribute. Importantly, these risks may be diminished by effective treatment of the mother's depression and by targeting high-risk adolescent offspring with cognitive behavioral interventions.

STRESS, ALLOSTASIS, AND PSYCHIATRY

The epigenetic changes associated with social defeat and early life rearing raise important questions about the mechanisms underlying the role of stress in psychiatric disorders. On one hand, the idea that stress is involved in psychiatric illnesses is a truism: certain disorders are diagnosed on the basis of adverse life events (e.g., posttraumatic stress disorder, acute stress disorder, and adjustment disorders). Nonetheless, the statement that stress "causes" psychiatric disorders is complex and fraught with misunderstanding. One of the major problems encountered when considering a causative role for stress is defining the term. In general, "stress" refers to a fairly vague group of behavioral and physiological responses to life circumstances. As discussed by Jeansok Kim and David Diamond, stress is defined not by parameters in the environment, but rather by the way an organism perceives and responds to the environment. Also, while the brain is the primary organ mediating behavioral stress responses, there are numerous bodily and neurochemical changes that occur

Table 8-2 Stress and Mind

Arousal (motivational component)
Brain stem, midbrain, hypothalamus
Aversion (emotional component)
Extended amygdala
Uncontrollability (cognitive component)
Prefrontal cortex

with stress. These responses, however, are not unique to psychosocial stress. For example, glucocorticoid hormones (cortisol) are elevated in stressful conditions, and this is one of the markers used to identify a "stress" response. These hormones, however, are also increased by exercise, eating, and sex, among other behaviors, and are thus more likely to be part of general adaptation systems than markers of adverse life events.

Kim and Diamond emphasize that stress has three major components. First, a stressful event evokes *arousal*—an enhanced level of alertness in response to a perception. This process likely involves several neurotransmitter systems, including catecholamines (norepinephrine, dopamine, and epinephrine), serotonin, endogenous opiates (enkephalins), and glucocorticoids, among others. Again, arousal is not unique to stress; it is more of a general alerting system than a specific stress response. Secondly, stress is perceived as *aversive*, something to be avoided. In this regard, stress responses overlap with the negative primary emotions of fear, sadness, and anger. Finally, stress also involves an estimation of how *controllable* a situation is. Stress is perceived as being difficult or impossible to manage. Thus, stress, like other psychiatric phenomena, has components affecting all aspects of the mind: motivation (arousal), emotion (aversiveness), and cognition (perceived control) (Table 8-2).

The involvement of all three aspects of the mind suggests that the state of an individual's brain networks when experiencing "stress" has a lot to do with how a person responds to a given situation. For example, as with other emotions, the capacity to withstand stress benefits greatly from top-down control over autonomic and neuroendocrine functions. This highlights a major problem in defining stress as a "cause" of any psychiatric disorder: having a preexisting psychiatric illness is stressful by itself and leaves individuals more vulnerable to ongoing and future stressors. This has been substantiated by Carol North and colleagues in their studies of the psychiatric outcomes of individuals exposed to major disasters, such as the terrorist attacks in Oklahoma City and New York. The individuals at greatest risk for psychiatric problems following these attacks had more psychiatric problems antedating the traumatic events. Also, in studies of major disasters, psychiatric problems typically arise early following the traumatic event, with almost all occurring within the first month. Delayed stress disorders, in which symptoms first appear 6 months or longer after an isolated event, were not observed, largely dispelling a popular myth that a stressful experience can leave a person vulnerable for long periods of time and have repercussions at any time in the future. More persistent and repeated traumatic exposures, such as those experienced by rescue workers following the September 11 attack, may have mental health consequences that develop later in some individuals, perhaps reflecting dose–effect and time–effect relationships—but again, preexisting psychiatric problems, including mood, personality, and substance-abuse problems, contribute significantly. It is also important to note that some research indicates that having a psychiatric disorder increases the probability that individuals will experience adverse events in the future. For example, the presence of a substance-abuse disorder or a psychotic disorder increases risk for accidents and violence. In the case of psychosis, affected individuals are more likely to be the victims of violence than the perpetrators.

This discussion is not meant to indicate that major traumas and chronic stressors do not take a significant toll on the body and brain. Rather, stress is a complex and multifaceted phenomenon, and there are longitudinal aspects to stress vulnerability. Bruce McEwen has discussed this cogently in the context of what he refers to as "allostasis." Broadly defined, allostasis refers to the body's ability to adjust its set points in order to maintain the balance (homeostasis) of fundamental physiological systems like temperature, oxygenation, electrolytes, and acid–base regulation. Allostasis is a broad form of physiological coping that allows the body to adjust appropriately to demands, including the generation of memories for events, altered immune function, changes in energy stores, and maintenance of efficient cardiovascular function. Regular exercise can be used as an example to explain the relationship between stress and allostasis. Acutely, exercise stresses the body, involving changes in heart rate, respiration, temperature, and glucocorticoid release, as well as placing demands on muscles and joints. These changes are not necessarily good in the short run, and injuries and heart attacks can occur during exercise. Over time, however, regular exercise has substantial health benefits affecting many bodily systems, including the brain. This situation is not unique to exercise. In fact, life without any stressors is probably not healthy; repeated exposures to milder and more controllable stress lead to a state of resilience (sometimes called "hormesis") in which the body and brain are able to respond more appropriately and effectively to major stressors because of the benefits accrued from handling repeated minor challenges.

The body does pay a price for frequent exposures to stress, particularly those exposures that are perceived as involuntary and uncontrollable. McEwen refers to this as "allostatic load," a term that emphasizes the wear and tear that results from being forced to adapt repeatedly to aversive physical and/or psychosocial situations. At some point, an organism reaches "allostatic overload," when brain and body systems begin to break down and show signs of illness in response to stress. Signs of allostatic overload include impaired memory, excessive anxiety and low mood, altered immune function (including chronic inflammation and arthritis), obesity, muscle wasting, and atherosclerotic changes. The cumulative nature of allostatic overload underscores the potential importance of uncontrollable stressors early in development. For example, there is evidence that children reared under unfavorable

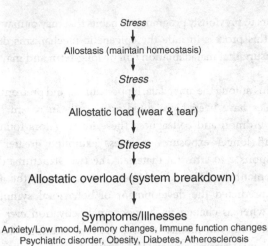

Stress
↓
Allostasis (maintain homeostasis)
↓
Stress
↓
Allostatic load (wear & tear)
↓
Stress
↓
Allostatic overload (system breakdown)
↓
Symptoms/Illnesses
Anxiety/Low mood, Memory changes, Immune function changes
Psychiatric disorder, Obesity, Diabetes, Atherosclerosis

Figure 8-1 Stress and allostasis. The diagram depicts the relationships between stress, allostatic load, and the development of psychiatric symptoms and illnesses. (Adapted from the work of Bruce McEwen.)

socioeconomic conditions are at increased risk of several chronic diseases as they age. Recent studies suggest that individuals raised in such environments develop altered glucocorticoid and pro-inflammatory signaling responses that persist throughout life and may predispose the individuals to chronic medical and psychiatric illnesses via allostatic mechanisms. Similarly, a recent study found significant epigenetic changes (diminished methylation) in genes regulating immune function in individuals with posttraumatic stress disorder. These epigenetic changes appeared to affect susceptibility to infections with cytomegalovirus. Figure 8-1 presents an overview of allostatic changes that can lead to illness.

How do brain mechanisms contribute to allostasis? It is believed that repeated psychosocial stressors can lead to allostatic overload in the amygdala and its targets, resulting in emotional hyperreactivity. This results in dysfunction of the HPA stress system and symptoms of illness. Some of the neurochemical changes associated with this allostatic sequence, including changes in monoamine transmitters and glucocorticoids, can lead to cellular damage and atrophy of neuronal dendrites along with other physical and functional changes in the brain. The hippocampus is particularly affected and exhibits smaller size, dendritic changes, diminished synaptic plasticity, and decreased neurogenesis in the dentate gyrus. In Chapter 7, we discussed changes in hippocampal function following chronic mild stress in rodents. These various hippocampal changes may partially result from the abnormal amygdala activity together with the effects of stress-related neuromodulators and stress-related release of the transmitter glutamate. Similar changes in structure and function are thought to occur in the fronto-striatal circuits required for behavioral flexibility. In animal models of chronic stress, rodents become more habit-driven and stereotyped in their behaviors, even when such behaviors are maladaptive. In effect, the sequence leading from stress to allostatic overload can be viewed as a defective form of learning/plasticity: the brain learns inappropriate responses to the load and defers to previously programmed habits that may or may not be adaptive. Key changes in this process include the epigenetic mechanisms discussed earlier; these changes ensure that maladaptation will be long-term and may even be passed on to offspring.

The interactions among the amygdala, hippocampus, and prefrontal cortex (PFC) in stress responses have been highlighted graphically in recent human imaging studies by Roee Admon and colleagues. These investigators found that military recruits who had longer exposures to stress exhibited greater amygdala and hippocampal responses to stressful material. The two structures differed in their temporal involvement, however. The degree of reactivity in the amygdala *before* stress exposure predicted the development of behavioral symptoms following stressful events, whereas changes in hippocampal activation *over time* correlated with increases in symptom intensity. Also, the hippocampus showed enhanced functional connectivity to ventromedial PFC (vmPFC) as a result of stress, a change that was also predicted by the degree of amygdala reactivity prior to stress. Interestingly, greater functional connectivity of hippocampus to vmPFC after stress predicted having fewer stress-related symptoms, possibly reflecting greater cognitive control and extinction of fear-based learning. This study highlights the key roles of the amygdala as an early and automatic processor of stress responses and the hippocampus as a modulator of stress responses and symptoms over time. The involvement of the hippocampus also likely contributes to the engagement of expanding neurocircuitry in stress behaviors, a theme that seems to recur in multiple psychiatric disorders.

MOLECULES, NETWORKS, AND TREATMENTS

The biochemical mechanisms underlying the genetic, epigenetic, and allostatic effects discussed in this chapter are complex, and describing these mechanisms as well as specific related findings identified in psychiatric disorders is beyond the scope of this text. Instead, we will highlight the importance of these mechanisms and the ways they interface with, and likely influence, the function of brain networks that underlie psychiatric disorders. Results from genetic and epigenetic studies offer the hope of identifying new and more specifically targeted pharmacological treatments for neuropsychiatric disorders. For example, it is reasonable to expect that agents targeting the complex network of molecules involved in synaptic function could be useful for treating certain disorders, particularly if the drugs could be directed to specific brain regions and networks involved in illness. Such targeting might be accomplished via regional specificity in gene expression or nanotechnology strategies. Recent studies using focused ultrasound and magnetic targeting of chemotherapeutic nanoparticles in combination with magnetic resonance monitoring in rats with brain tumors provide an early proof-of-concept for this approach. Similarly, studies of HDAC inhibitors in animal stress models suggest that epigenetic changes can be manipulated and might be targets for drug development, provided that particular brain regions of interest could be effectively targeted.

As a caveat, it is at present unclear how effective highly specific treatments will be for many common neuropsychiatric disorders. For example, Brian Roth and colleagues have considered whether the goal in developing new antidepressant treatments should be the creation of "magic bullets" that are highly specific or "magic shotguns" that target many systems. They suggest the latter might be the more appropriate conceptual strategy. Treatment of partial complex epilepsy serves as a useful example. Here, drugs targeting numerous mechanisms underlying neuronal excitability are available to treat the disorder. For example, there are anticonvulsants that specifically enhance GABAergic inhibition (barbiturates and benzodiazepines), inhibit sodium channels (phenytoin, lamotrigine), and inhibit certain glutamate-activated channels (felbamate). The sodium channel inhibitors also preferentially diminish release of glutamate, providing another way to decrease excitability. All of these drugs are effective at doing what they were designed to do, but they are not that effective as monotherapies for partial complex seizures. The most effective treatment strategies combine several drugs with different mechanisms, although outcomes are still less than optimal. In fact, outcomes are so poor with polypharmacotherapy that neurosurgical ablation of seizure foci has become the norm for treating the large population of refractory patients with partial complex seizures.

The situation is somewhat similar with psychiatric disorders, where current treatments are not effective for a substantial minority of individuals. Also, most available psychiatric drugs target the same or overlapping transmitter systems, restricting treatment options. Having a broader array of targets based on results from genetic and epigenetic studies could be a major advance, even though individual treatments might not be adequate as monotherapies. This could create a type of "rational polypharmacy" for treating refractory psychiatric disorders while minimizing the side effects and complications that can accompany some current "irrational" polypharmacy approaches (e.g., combining drugs of the same class or drugs with very similar mechanisms of action). Ultimately, however, it will be important to understand how therapeutic approaches affect the function of ICNs. In terms of rational combinations of therapeutic approaches, the judicious use of well-selected pharmacological or neurostimulation methods together with psychotherapeutic and rehabilitative strategies might be the most appropriate strategy.

The potential for developing new therapeutic avenues to treat psychiatric disorders based on genetic and epigenetic approaches may not be as far-fetched as it sounds. Earlier, we described the potential role of epigenetic changes in several human neurocognitive developmental disorders. The genes involved in many of these disorders are becoming much better characterized, leading to the generation of transgenic animal models that are being used to study the influence of genetic defects and epigenetic changes on synaptic and network function. For example, mental retardation syndromes associated with Down syndrome and Rett syndrome result from different genetic mechanisms. Yet in animal models of both of these disorders, some evidence suggests an imbalance in the ratio of GABAergic inhibition to glutamatergic excitation. In the Down syndrome model, diminishing excessive inhibition with drugs that inhibit GABA-A receptors can prevent and even reverse learning problems and synaptic plasticity defects. Similarly, in a fragile X animal model, there is excessive activation of a specific type of metabotropic glutamate receptor that participates in hippocampal synaptic plasticity. Treatment of these mice with an inhibitor of the overactive glutamate receptor (called "mGluR5") reverses changes in plasticity and learning defects. This finding is already leading to clinical trials in humans with this disorder. In tuberous sclerosis, changes in a protein kinase regulating mitochondrial and synaptic function called "mammalian target of rapamycin" (mTOR) contribute to seizures and cognitive impairment. In an animal model of the disorder, rapamycin, an inhibitor of mTOR, improves the defects. The point of this discussion is that these mental retardation syndromes, once thought to be hopeless from a therapeutic standpoint, are now becoming targets for innovative and previously unanticipated treatments. How these treatments continue to evolve and how they interface with cognitive rehabilitative efforts could be highly instructive for psychiatry. In this light, studies in a number of animal models of neurodevelopmental and neurodegenerative disorders have shown benefits from environmental enrichment (i.e., more complex and challenging, but non-stressful, living and learning circumstances), even in aged animals.

Studies of allostasis also highlight potential approaches for treating psychiatric disorders and emphasize the role of psychotherapy (constructive learning) and lifestyle variables in the therapeutic and rehabilitative process. Perhaps even more importantly, these studies point to ways that certain psychiatric disorders may be prevented. Studies involving the offspring of depressed mothers might be the most vivid example of this. Research is increasingly drawing attention to the role of neurodevelopment in the genesis of mood, anxiety, substance-abuse, and psychotic disorders, including very early identification of children at high risk and with symptoms of disorder. Exposure to childhood abuse and neglect increases risk for a variety of illnesses, including heart disease, certain cancers, respiratory disorders, obesity, and multiple psychiatric disorders. Importantly, it appears that the risks associated with childhood stress are not specific for any single disorder, but rather increase risk for many common disorders. While the etiology of these disorders is complex and includes genetic loading, an abusive environment is a significant contributor. Thus, opportunities for prevention exist via environmental enrichment strategies, including efforts directed at improving parent–child interactions. In addition, healthier lifestyles along with protection from abuse can help to diminish allostatic load via improved diet, weight management, stress reduction, relaxation techniques, exercise, and opportunities for constructive learning.

Interestingly, many of the strategies outlined increase neurogenesis in the dentate gyrus and presumably enhance hippocampal synaptic function and plasticity. The value of positive interpersonal interactions and social support in human life also makes it important to find ways to improve social networks as a way to diminish allostatic load. A person's ability to control his or her own life circumstances is an important concept in this regard. Studies in rodents suggest that "voluntary" exercise and "forced" exercise (treadmill running) may have different effects on behavior and brain function. Lifestyle strategies in humans should be tailored to the abilities of individual patients, an approach that lies at the heart of all effective rehabilitative and psychotherapeutic strategies. The earlier these strategies are implemented the better; intervention early in development, before health problems become manifest, is ideal. However, even when started in adulthood or later in life, lifestyle and enrichment interventions can be useful, highlighting the ongoing plasticity of the brain.

Points to Remember

Genetic and epigenetic mechanisms provide a basis for developing new molecular targets for altering network function in the brain and treating psychiatric disorders.

From a genetic perspective, psychiatric disorders are complex, reflecting the involvement of multiple genes and the effects of environmental variables on gene expression. Because each individual gene contributes only a small amount to the overall risk of developing a psychiatric disorder, environmental influences often are the most important (and potentially controllable) factors in determining whether illness will develop.

The identification of rare genetic variants (e.g., duplications and deletions) associated with psychiatric syndromes has the potential to clarify the genetics of these disorders and to point to molecular networks that can be targeted for therapeutic purposes.

Epigenetic studies provide a way for understanding how environmental exposures translate into symptoms and disorders. Epigenetic changes interface with allostatic mechanisms and contribute, at least in part, to the effects of the stressful aspects of the environment on humans. To say that stress causes psychiatric disorders is overly simplistic and at times naïve, given the complex interplay among genetic, epigenetic, and allostatic loads.

SUGGESTED READINGS

Arnsten, A. F. T. (2009). Stress signaling pathways that impair prefrontal cortex structure and function. *Nature Reviews Neuroscience, 10*, 410–422.

Kim, J. J., & Diamond, D. M. (2002). The stressed hippocampus, synaptic plasticity and lost memories. *Nature Reviews Neuroscience, 3*, 453–462.

Levenson, J. M., & Sweatt, J. D. (2005). Epigenetic mechanisms in memory formation. *Nature Reviews Neuroscience, 6*, 108–118.

McEwen, B. S. (2007). Physiology and neurobiology of stress and adaptation: central role of the brain. *Physiological Reviews, 87*, 873–904.

Meaney, M. J., & Szyf, M. (2005). Maternal care as a model for experience-dependent chromatin plasticity? *Trends in Neurosciences, 28*, 456–463.

Petronis, A. (2010). Epigenetics as a unifying principle in the aetiology of complex traits and diseases. *Nature, 465*, 721–727.

Tsankova, N., Renthal, W., Kumar, A., & Nestler, E. J. (2007). Epigenetic regulation in psychiatric disorders. *Nature Reviews Neuroscience, 8*, 355–367.

OTHER REFERENCES

Admon, R., Lubin, G., Stern, O., Rosenberg, K., Sela, L., Ben-Ami, H., et al. (2009). Human vulnerability to stress depends on amygdala's predisposition and hippocampal plasticity. *Proceedings of the National Academy of Science (USA), 106,* 14120–14125.

Alarcon, J. M., Malleret, G., Touzani, K., Vronskaya, S., Ishii, S., Kandel, E. R., et al. (2004). Chromatin acetylation, memory and LTP are impaired in CBP +/− mice: A model for the cognitive deficit in Rubinstein-Taybi syndrome and its amelioration. *Neuron, 42,* 947–959.

Attia, J., Ioannidis, J. P. A., Thakkinstian, A., McEvoy, M., Scott, R. J., Minelli, C., et al. (2009). How to use an article about genetic association. A. Background concepts. *Journal of the American Medical Association, 301,* 74–81.

Bayes, A., van de Lagemaat, L., Collins, M. O., Croning, M. D. R., Whittle, I. R., Choudhary, J. S., et al. (2011). Characterization of the proteome, diseases and evolution of the human postsynaptic density. *Nature Neuroscience, 14,* 19–21.

Borelli, E., Nestler, E. J., Allis, C. D., & Sassone-Corsi, P. (2008). Decoding the epigenetic language of neuronal plasticity. *Neuron, 60,* 961–974.

Caspi, A., Hariri, A. R., Holmes, A., Uher, R., & Moffitt, T. E. (2010). Genetic sensitivity to the environment: The case of the serotonin transporter gene and its implications for studying complex diseases and traits. *American Journal of Psychiatry, 167,* 509–527.

Caspi, A., & Moffitt, T. E. (2006). Gene–environment interactions in psychiatry: Joining forces with neuroscience. *Nature Reviews Neuroscience, 7,* 583–590.

Covington, H. E., Maze, I., LaPlant, Q. C., Vialou, V. F., Ohnishi, Y. N., Berton, O., et al. (2009). Antidepressant actions of histone deacetylase inhibitors. *Journal of Neuroscience, 16,* 11451–11460.

Dias-Ferreira, E., Sousa, J. C., Melo, I., Morgado, P., Mesquita, A. R., Cerqueira, J. J., et al. (2009). Chronic stress causes frontostriatal reorganization and affects decision making. *Science, 325,* 621–625.

Ehninger, D., Li, W., Fox, K., Stryker, M. P., & Silva, A. J. (2008). Reversing neurodevelopmental disorders in adults. *Neuron, 60,* 950–960.

Evans, G. W., & Schamberg, M. A. (2009). Childhood poverty, chronic stress and adult working memory. *Proceedings of the National Academy of Science (USA), 106,* 6545–6549.

Feder, A., Nestler, E. J., & Charney, D. S. (2009). Psychobiology and molecular genetics of resilience. *Nature Reviews Neuroscience, 10,* 446–457.

Fraga, M. F., Ballestar, E., Paz, M. F., Ropero, S., Setien, F. Ballestar, M. L., et al. (2005). Epigenetic differences arise during the lifetime of monozygotic twins. *Proceedings of the National Academy of Sciences (USA), 102,* 10604–10609.

Hackman, D. A., Farah, M. J., & Meaney, M. J. (2010). Socioeconomic status and the brain: Mechanistic insights from human and animal research. *Nature Reviews Neuroscience, 11,* 651–659.

Hardy, J., & Singleton, A. (2009). Genomewide association studies and human disease. *New England Journal of Medicine, 360,* 1759–1768.

Henckens, M. J. A. G., Hermans, E. J., Pu, Z., Joels, M., & Fernandez, G. (2009). Stressed memories: How acute stress affects memory formation in humans. *Journal of Neuroscience, 29,* 10111–10119.

Insel, T. R. (2010). Rethinking schizophrenia. *Nature, 468,* 187–193.

International Schizophrenia Consortium. (2009). Common polygenic variation contributes to risk of schizophrenia and bipolar disorder. *Nature, 460,* 748–752.

Karayiorgou, M., Simon, T. J., & Gogos, J. A. (2010). 22q11.2 microdeletions: Linking DNA structural variation to brain dysfunction and schizophrenia. *Nature Reviews Neuroscience, 11,* 402–416.

Kendler, K. S. (2005). Psychiatric genetics: A methodologic critique. *American Journal of Psychiatry, 162,* 3–11.

Korzus, E., Rosenfeld, M. G., & Mayford, M. (2004). CBP histone acetyltransferase activity is a critical component of memory consolidation. *Neuron, 42,* 961–972.

Levenson, J. M., O'Riordan, K. J., Brown, K. D., Trinh, M. A., Molfese, D. L., & Sweatt, J. D. (2004). Regulation of histone acetylation during memory formation in the hippocampus. *Journal of Biological Chemistry, 279,* 40545–40559.

Liston, C., McEwen, B. S., & Casey, B. J. (2009). Psychosocial stress reversibly disrupts prefrontal processing and attentional control. *Proceedings of the National Academy of Sciences (USA), 106,* 912–917.

Liu, H.-L., Hua, M.-Y., Yang, H.-W., Huang, C.-Y., Chu, P.-C., Wu, J.-S., et al. (2010). Magnetic resonance monitoring of focused ultrasound/magnetic nanoparticle targeting delivery of therapeutic agents to the brain. *Proceedings of the National Academy of Sciences (USA), 107,* 15205–15210.

Luby, J. L. (2009). Early childhood depression. *American Journal of Psychiatry, 166,* 974–979.

Lupien, S. J., McEwen, B. S., Gunnar, M. R., & Heim, C. (2009). Effects of stress throughout the lifespan on the brain, behavior and cognition. *Nature Reviews Neuroscience, 10,* 434–445.

Manolio, T. A., Collins, F. S., Goldstein, D. B., Hindorff, L. A., Hunter, D. J., McCarthy, M. I., et al. (2009). Finding the missing heritability of complex diseases. *Nature, 461,* 747–753.

Mattson, M. P. (2008). Hormesis and disease resistance: Activation of cellular stress response pathways. *Human and Experimental Toxicology, 27,* 155–162.

McClellan, J., & King, M-C. (2010). Genetic heterogeneity in human diseases. *Cell, 141,* 210–217.

McGowan, P. O., Sasaki, A., D'Alessio, A. C., Dymov, S., Labonte, B., Szyf, M., et al. (2009). Epigenetic regulation of the glucocorticoid receptor in human brain associates with childhood abuse. *Nature Neuroscience, 12,* 342–348.

Miller, G. E., Chen, E., Fok, A. K., Walker, H., Lim, A., Nicholls, E. F., et al. (2009). Low early-life social class leaves a biological residue manifested by decreased glucocorticoid and increased proinflammatory signaling. *Proceedings of the National Academy of Sciences (USA), 106,* 14716–14721.

Merikangas, K. R., & Risch, N. (2003). Will the genomics revolution revolutionize psychiatry? *American Journal of Psychiatry, 160,* 625–635.

Nemeroff, C. B. (2004). Neurobiological consequences of childhood trauma. *Journal of Clinical Psychiatry, 65*(Suppl. 1), 18–28.

North, C. S., Nixon, S. J., Shariat, S., Mallonee, S., McMillen, J. C., Spitznagel, E. L., et al. (1999). Psychiatric disorders among survivors of the Oklahoma City bombing. *Journal of the American Medical Association, 282,* 755–762.

Paus, T., Keshavan, M., & Giedd, J. N. (2008). Why do many psychiatric disorders emerge during adolescence? *Nature Reviews Neuroscience, 9,* 947–957.

Ramocki, M. B., & Zoghbi, H. Y. (2008). Failure of neuronal homeostasis results in common neuropsychiatric phenotypes. *Nature, 455,* 912–918.

Renthal, W., Maze, I., Krishnan, V., Covington, H. E., III, Xiao, G., Kumar, A., et al. (2007). Histone deacetylase 5 epigenetically controls behavioral adaptations to chronic emotional stress. *Neuron, 56,* 517–529.

Robins, E., & Guze, S. B. (1970). Establishment of diagnostic validity in psychiatric illness: Its application to schizophrenia. *American Journal of Psychiatry, 126,* 983–987.

Roozendaal, B., McEwen, B. S., & Chattarji, S. (2009). Stress, memory and the amygdala. *Nature Reviews Neuroscience, 10,* 423–433.

Roth, B. L., Sheffler, D. J., & Kroeze, W. K. (2004). Magic shotguns versus magic bullets: Selectively non-selective drugs for mood disorders and schizophrenia. *Nature Reviews Drugs Discovery, 3,* 353–359.

Schwabe, L., & Wolf, O. T. (2009). Stress prompts habit behavior in humans. *Journal of Neuroscience, 29,* 7191–7198.

Shi, J., Levinson, D. F., Duan, J., Sanders, A. R., Zheng, Y., Pe'er, I., et al. (2009). Common variants on chromosome 6p22.1 are associated with schizophrenia. *Nature, 460,* 753–757.

Shin, L. M., & Liberzon, I. (2010). The neurocircuitry of fear, stress and anxiety disorders. *Neuropsychopharmacology Reviews, 35,* 169–191.

Stefansson, H., Ophoff, R. A., Steinberg, S., Andreassen, O. A., Cichon, S., Rujescu, D., et al. (2009). Common variants conferring risk of schizophrenia. *Nature, 460,* 744–747.

Tsankova, N. M., Berton, O., Renthal, W., Kumar, A., Neve, R. L., & Nestler, E. J. (2006). Sustained hippocampal chromatin regulation in a mouse model of depression and antidepressant action. *Nature Neuroscience, 9,* 519–525.

Uddin, M., Aiello, A. E., Wildman, D. E., Koenen, K. C., Pawelec, G., de los Santos, R., et al. (2010). Epigenetic and immune function profiles associated with posttraumatic stress disorder. *Proceedings of the National Academy of Sciences (USA), 107,* 9470–9475.

Van Praag, H. (2009). Exercise and the brain: Something to chew on. *Trends in Neuroscience, 32,* 283–290.

Walsh, T., McClellan, J. M., McCarthy, S. E., Addington, A. M., Pierce, S. B., Cooper, G. M., et al. (2008). Rare structural variants disrupt multiple genes in neurodevelopmental pathways in schizophrenia. *Science, 320,* 539–543.

Wang, H.-X., Karp, A., Herlitz, A., Crowe, M., Kareholt, I., Winblad, B., et al. (2009). Personality and lifestyle in relation to dementia incidence. *Neurology, 72,* 253–259.

Weaver, I. C., Cervoni, N., Champagne, F. A., D'Alessio, A. C., Sharma, S., Seckl, J. R., et al. (2004). Epigenetic programming by maternal behavior. *Nature Neuroscience, 7,* 847–854.

Weissman, M. M., & Olfson, M. (2009). Translating intergenerational research on depression into clinical practice. *Journal of the American Medical Association, 302,* 2695–2696.

9

Conceptualizing Causes
of Psychiatric Disorders

Determining the "cause" of an illness is complicated. Cause can be considered from multiple perspectives, including the roles of genes, environment, and brain mechanisms. Even when the cause of an illness is determined at a genetic or biochemical level, the pathway leading from cause to symptoms might not be understood. For instance, a particular genetic defect might be discovered to cause a specific disorder; however, understanding how the genetic defect leads to specific symptoms may remain a mystery until research elucidates the biological impact of the genetic defect and the specific effect that defect has on the brain. Huntington's disease is a good example. A specific mutation in the gene for the huntingtin protein has been associated with the illness for about 20 years. Nevertheless, scientists are still unraveling what this protein does and how mutations result in the clinical phenotype.

Determining cause may be a correlative exercise. For example, if a patient develops recurrent bouts of hypothyroidism and experiences slowed thinking and depression with each bout, then it is likely that a diminished level of thyroid hormone is "causing" the depression. This idea is further supported if treatment with thyroid hormone results in remission of depressive symptoms. However, this does not tell us how low thyroid function produces depression. Similarly, if a person has a stroke involving Broca's area in the brain and develops an expressive aphasia, we know that the stroke "caused" the aphasia, but we don't know exactly how damage to this brain region causes this type of aphasia and its attendant symptoms. The hope is that better understanding of the brain's intrinsic connectivity networks (ICNs) will help to clarify these issues and allow researchers to better define clinically relevant pathophysiologies of brain disorders.

Some psychiatric disorders are said to be "due to medical illnesses." DSM-IV has specific codes for such illnesses (e.g., depression due to hypothyroidism). For these disorders, the precipitating cause is thought to be known. The reason why the precipitating cause leads to the specific behaviors is usually not clear; however, if the primary medical condition is effectively treated, then the psychiatric symptoms may improve, although this is not always the case. Many medical disorders can influence the brain either directly or indirectly and can lead to behavioral changes.

The causes of primary psychiatric disorders are difficult to elucidate largely because there are often no clear, well-understood structural, biochemical, or synaptic abnormalities. Rather, psychiatric disorders most likely reflect changes in brain networks and connectivity, with or without changes in specific cell types in specific brain regions. In contrast, many neurological illnesses, like strokes or brain tumors, have clear-cut structural abnormalities that are observable with routine brain imaging studies. In other cases, specific changes in cellular chemistry or neuronal excitability are observed. For instance, lysosomal storage diseases involve the accumulation of abnormal lipids in the brain and other tissues; these lipids have been identified and the primary causes for many of these disorders have been established. Similarly, many muscle disorders can be characterized on the basis of microscopic changes found in muscle biopsies. Several rare types of seizure disorders run in families, and genetic studies have identified the role of certain "channelopathies" as underlying causative mechanisms. Channelopathies typically result from mutations in specific ionic channels that alter neuronal excitability and lead to various forms of seizures. Even in neurological disorders, however, there is often a significant gap in understanding how specific biochemical or molecular defects result in particular symptoms in a given disorder or patient. For example, knowing that there is a defect in a sodium or calcium channel in a type of epilepsy does not necessarily translate into understanding how the molecular and biophysical defect results in the network dysfunction underlying generalized seizures or other clinical manifestations. In some cases, the known physiological changes are even counterintuitive. For example, the change in ion channel function sometimes suggests the opposite effect on neuronal excitability when taken at face value. Thus, we would emphasize that both neurology and psychiatry will benefit from further understanding of the operations of brain systems in conjunction with associated molecular, cellular, and synaptic mechanisms. To date, primary psychiatric illnesses have no clearly identified structural pathology, laboratory correlates, or molecular mechanisms. Without such findings, it is difficult to develop rational descriptions of illness pathophysiology. It seems increasingly clear, however, that the clinical phenotype of primary psychiatric disorders reflects complex dysfunctions of neural circuits, which can be best conceptualized as defects in inter- and intra-network function.

As discussed previously in this book, the human mind can be described in terms of the integration of cognitive, emotional, and motivational functions. To accomplish these functions, a finite number of ICNs have evolved. Each ICN has its own internal computational capability and functionally unites a number of brain regions in order to serve specific forms of information processing, integration, and interpretation. As noted earlier, some brain regions serve as highly connected nodes within and across processing networks. This means that they may participate in several ICNs, depending on how they are functionally wired. It is likely that these highly connected nodes integrate information across many inputs. In addition, some of these nodes may have specialized internal wiring that allows them to perform specific types of computational processing. The beautiful and unique circuitry of the hippocampus is an example of such an important nodal structure (as discussed in Chapter 6). Examining causes of primary psychiatric disorders in terms of malfunctioning ICNs is, in our opinion, a critical approach for understanding the causes and functional defects in many of these disorders.

Table 9-1 Types of Abnormalities

Developmental abnormalities
Connectivity abnormalities—later in life
Substance-induced abnormalities
Abnormalities from traumatic brain injury
Abnormalities due to defects in brain metabolism
Age-related abnormalities

In this chapter, we will focus on the "causes" of primary psychiatric disorders and not address the causes of those psychiatric symptoms "due to medical illnesses." We will explore six categories of abnormalities that we hope provide a framework to organize thinking and future research to determine "cause": developmental abnormalities, abnormalities of ICN connectivity that develop later in life, abnormalities resulting from exogenous or endogenous substances, abnormalities resulting from brain damage, abnormalities resulting from problems in brain energy use, and abnormalities due to aging (Table 9-1). These are not the only possible categories of "cause," but they reflect kinds of brain changes that can help us think about the ways "lesions" (chemical, structural, or functional) can result in clinical problems.

DEVELOPMENTAL ABNORMALITIES

Most common medical disorders involve genetic predispositions that are unmasked by environmental challenges. For example, most cancers are associated with some form of genetic predisposition, but it is the combination of genetic predisposition plus environmental exposure (e.g., cigarette smoking, asbestos) that ultimately results in illness. What do we mean by "genetic predisposition?" Humans have about 25,000 genes that code for proteins—the major building blocks of our organs, including our brains. Each gene may have subtle differences in chemical sequence from person to person. These differences are called mutations when relatively large sections of a gene are affected and single nucleotide polymorphisms (SNPs) when only isolated base pairs are affected. These variations may have no effect on function or may lead to differences, both subtle and large, in how genes are expressed and how cells develop, grow, live, interact, and die. Since most genes have only subtle variations in their makeup, most individuals are dealt a hand of "normal" genes that vary just a bit from their neighbors. Combinations of particular genes may have additive influences on various cell functions, however. If a person happens to have certain variations in a group of genes that regulate the development of several functionally related proteins, then it is possible that this person may have a different vulnerability to disturbances involving the function of those proteins. Genetic vulnerability or genetic resilience may be a matter of random sorting of individual genes that have subtle differences in different individuals. Also, over generations, some genes (or gene regions) tend to cluster together and are inherited together, making the assortment of these genes less random in some segments of the population. This is called "linkage disequilibrium" in genetic terms. This is one reason why some families and groups of people have higher risks of certain illnesses.

While genetic inheritance is complex, understanding environmental contributors to illness may be even more daunting, particularly when considering the interaction of environmental risks with genetic risks. What do we mean by "environmental challenges"? Humans are exposed to a broad array of environments. Historically in the field of psychiatry, psychological stressors have been highlighted for study (Chapter 8); however, many forms of environmental variations are potential modifiers of our development and behavior, some being more "stressful" than others. For example, significant variations in nutrition may influence development. The degree of social interaction and the amount and quality of play during childhood may be very important for social development. The amount of exercise a person gets throughout life can be a major environmental consideration. The amount of time spent watching TV, working or playing on computers, talking on cell phones, and using other modern devices may have a substantial impact on current and future behaviors. Various environmental circumstances are likely to influence individuals differently depending on their genetic makeup. How people adapt to their individual environments is likely related to aspects of their temperament and character, and thus to their core personality.

As we have already mentioned, people differ substantially in both genetic makeup and environmental exposure. How does this relate to developmental abnormalities? What does it mean when we say that schizophrenia may be a developmental disorder with genetic and environmental contributions? Certain illnesses likely result from a combination of genetic effects and environmental perturbations that occur during brain development. This is certainly true for disorders that declare themselves during early childhood, such as attention-deficit/hyperactivity disorder and some autistic disorders. It is also likely to be true for disorders that don't become clinically apparent until adolescence. Schizophrenia is an example of a disorder that typically becomes symptomatic during teenage years or early adulthood. Many if not all persons with this illness have abnormalities that were programmed during fetal or early childhood development. Structural and functional brain changes have been found in persons with this illness, including changes that antedate the onset of psychosis. These structural changes include decreased volume in specific regions of the cerebral cortex and hippocampus as well as increased volume of the ventricular system of the brain, sometimes present at the onset of clinical symptoms; changes in neuropsychological function are also observed early in the illness course. In addition to changes in gross brain structure, microscopic changes suggesting abnormalities in the number and connectivity of cells in certain brain regions have been discovered. Since these changes are not accompanied by gliosis, a reactive overgrowth of glia typically observed following brain injury, it is likely that the abnormalities occurred during early development and are not the result of ongoing neuronal destruction.

The brain continues to grow and to form different patterns of connections as individuals mature to adolescence and adulthood. In particular, some of the ICNs that are found in children change as the children become adolescents and young adults. This biologically programmed but environmentally influenced progression into adolescence may explain why clinical symptoms of illnesses like schizophrenia don't become fully evident until adolescence or early adulthood. Something that goes wrong during early development may not show up until abnormal programs are played out during the changes in brain connectivity that occur as a child's brain becomes a teenager's brain. This may lead to abnormalities that interfere with the efficient functioning of one or more ICNs. Such developmental abnormalities may involve specific nodal structures, such as regions in the prefrontal cortex, parietal cortex, or hippocampus. When a nodal structure doesn't develop or function properly, abnormal processing in multiple brain systems and dysfunction across all aspects of mind may occur. The importance of this concept is highlighted by recent advances in network science demonstrating that failure of a key node within one network can result in cascading failures across *interdependent* networks. Such effects, particularly when they occur during neurodevelopment, also may interfere with the correct wiring between brain regions, leading to functional disconnections among regions. ICNs with abnormal wiring may not be able to process information in the manner necessary for normal cognitive, emotional, or motivational function. It is also important to emphasize that defects in functional connectivity among brain networks do not necessarily imply structural changes within these networks, as highlighted by functional connectivity between contralateral regions of visual cortex or amygdala that lack direct anatomical projections.

Although we have not yet discovered the specific abnormalities that result in illnesses like schizophrenia or autism, it is important to understand the concepts underlying how genes can interact with environment to produce altered brain development. Thomas Insel, Director of the National Institute of Mental Health, has emphasized the importance of understanding the developmental progression of certain mental disorders as individuals proceed from early developmental insults through a sometimes latent period in childhood that precedes the onset of clinical symptoms. By the time clinical symptoms are manifest in illnesses such as schizophrenia, the brain has already undergone substantial changes. The more researchers are able to elucidate specific defects and clarify the consequences of those defects, the more likely we will be able to develop specific treatments. Some of these treatments may directly target a group of genetic defects that influence particular developmental pathways (for example, targeting defects in neurotransmitter release in illnesses such as schizophrenia). In the immediate future, however, it is more likely that treatments will be rehabilitative in nature, focusing on the earliest brain systems that are functioning abnormally. Young brains are highly plastic, and this offers significant opportunity for intervention. If we know that certain regions of the brain haven't developed correctly, then behavioral, pharmaceutical, social, exercise-oriented, or task-oriented interventions can be developed. Far from being nonspecific, these types of early interventions may be the most effective strategies for diminishing or even preventing the adverse consequences of illnesses. It is already known that intervening early in young children with autism may allow for substantial developmental gains. This probably results from helping the brain develop "work-arounds" for existing deficits.

A recent study examining early intervention in 81 subjects at ultra-high risk for schizophrenia provides an early proof-of-concept for this approach. In this study, high-risk subjects were treated with long-chain omega-3 polyunsaturated fatty acids (PUFAs) for 12 weeks and followed for an additional 40 weeks. Over this time, about 28% of placebo-treated controls progressed to psychosis, compared to about 5% in the PUFA-treated group. How these effects are achieved at a neurosystems level is unknown, but it is unlikely that the treatment simply corrected a "PUFA deficiency." Also, while it is still too early to know whether these preliminary findings sustain and generalize, this is an exciting direction for research. As humans age, their brains become more difficult, but not impossible, to influence. Nevertheless, we are learning that there may be ways to help older brains regain some flexibility or plasticity. For example, there is evidence that even in older rodents (and humans), environmental enrichment, loosely defined as living in a more stimulating non-stressful situation with more things to do, can help to restore cognitive function and learning. Some evidence suggests that computer-based neurocognitive training over a 2-year period can help preserve gray-matter volumes in hippocampus, parahippocampal gyrus, and fusiform gyrus in subjects with early schizophrenia. Pharmacological strategies that enhance synaptic plasticity may help humans learn new strategies to deal with specific anxieties, so beneficial effects of these approaches may not be restricted to any one illness or set of illnesses.

ABNORMALITIES OF ICN CONNECTIVITY THAT DEVELOP LATER IN LIFE

When we described dementia of the Alzheimer's type (DAT) and behavioral variant frontotemporal dementia (bvFTD) in Chapter 2, we indicated that the clinical phenotypes of these two disorders may involve an initial breakdown of specific ICNs: the default ICN in the case of DAT and the emotional-salience ICN in the case of bvFTD. Phenotypes of many and perhaps most psychiatric illnesses are likely related to dysfunction in specific ICNs or to defects in brain regions that serve as major hubs and influence the function of several ICNs. If this is true, then specific psychiatric illnesses may become clinically apparent when an ICN or highly connected node becomes disrupted. Support for this idea comes from recent studies examining the functional connectivity of brain networks in individuals who are clinically normal despite exhibiting fibrillar amyloid burden in their brains based on positron emission tomographic (PET) imaging of Pittsburgh Compound B, an *in vivo* marker for brain amyloid deposition. These individuals have significant changes in connectivity in the default network, including early changes involving the hippocampus. Importantly, while connectivity changes in these individuals have already begun, they have not progressed to the point of producing significant cognitive impairment. Thus, these individuals have preclinical neural circuitry abnormalities that place them at high risk for developing clinical Alzheimer's disease. Going forward, it will be important to know whether these individuals develop DAT and which brain changes accompany the progression from amyloid deposition to symptomatic dysfunction. In this way, it may be possible to link specific changes in ICN function to illness manifestations.

It is logical that the vulnerability to disruption of an individual ICN may reflect the functional integrity of that ICN. ICNs are composed of various brain regions that function together in order to perform specific information-processing tasks. The interconnectedness of various ICNs and the robustness of those connections may vary among individuals. In some people, the structures involved in a particular ICN may be strongly bound together; in other individuals, these connections may be less stable. The degree of stability is likely influenced by genetics and brain development, which varies in every individual, as well as by ongoing synaptic plasticity resulting from life experiences. Over the course of development, it appears that functional brain connectivity shifts from a more local processing mode to a more distributed organization in which distant brain sites are incorporated into computational processing. In other words, earlier in life connectivity is driven by anatomical proximity among regions, while in adulthood connectivity reflects functional relationships. Importantly, however, brains of both children and adults maintain small-world properties and, despite differences in connectivity, process information efficiently but in different ways. It is at present unclear why brain networks undergo this developmental change, but understanding how this occurs could help to explain ICN vulnerabilities and how development affects illness expression.

During the developmental transition, less stable ICNs are likely to be more susceptible to interference from environmental insults, and factors that affect the establishment of longer-range connectivity can greatly affect functional organization. Using a medical analogy, some persons with diabetes can easily tolerate high blood sugar without mental consequences such as depressive, anxiety, or cognitive symptoms. Other persons are more susceptible to depression or memory problems during periods of poor glucose control. Perhaps the ICNs regulating mood and cognition are more easily disrupted by variations in insulin and blood sugar in these individuals. Similarly, the dopamine system may be intimately involved in one or more ICNs. Differences in this system may explain why some individuals are much more prone than others to develop an "addiction" to gambling and why some individuals are more likely than others to develop serious emotional turmoil when a friendship goes awry.

How various ICNs connect with each other and use energy to maintain their processing may also be a critical consideration. For example, we previously noted that the default ICN is a major consumer of brain energy; its high activity and energy demand also appear to be mechanisms that contribute to its susceptibility to attack in Alzheimer's disease. Recent studies indicate that the default system may be distinguished primarily by its high rate of aerobic glycolysis rather than by its overall energy use. Aerobic glycolysis involves glucose use beyond that needed for oxidative phosphorylation and has been referred to as the "Warburg effect" when seen in cancer cells. This form of glycolysis is less efficient but faster from an energy production standpoint, and it may be critical for maintaining high excitatory synaptic drive and plasticity. Understanding the mechanisms underlying the differences in susceptibility to various environmental exposures of different individual ICNs, including how insults affect energy use, could allow us to develop therapies that may make susceptible ICNs more resilient to various insults. Interestingly, effective psychotherapies might accomplish just this; they may provide tools by which ICNs can either strengthen themselves or develop "work-arounds" that allow other ICNs to compensate for the ill effects of more susceptible brain systems.

While we have drawn a distinction between disorders resulting from *developmental abnormalities* and disorders resulting from *abnormalities of ICN connectivity that develop later in life*, we acknowledge that this distinction is highly arbitrary. The protracted nature of human brain development almost ensures the likelihood of a continuum. Recall, for example, that full maturation of the prefrontal cortex does not occur until early adulthood. The degree to which an ICN becomes a resilient, functional system is strongly influenced by developmental events. ICNs might vary in "strength" from person to person. "Strong" ICNs have affiliated structural nodes that are resilient to insults encountered during life and are wired together in a manner that leads to efficient synchronous activity. Some people may have weaker (more susceptible) ICNs because certain environmental exposures during development, some of which may have been subtle, interfered with the development of the nodes and the connections between key nodes. We emphasize abnormalities in ICN connectivity as a cause for psychiatric illness because brain networks mimic the structure and connectivity of small-world networks (Chapter 3) and are critically dependent on the function of major highly connected hubs. This protects overall brain function against failure from random insults, but it leaves systems vulnerable if highly connected nodes are disrupted or dysfunctional.

As a clinical example, we would cite the case of fetal alcohol exposure. In Chapter 7, we noted that exposure to moderate doses of alcohol during the equivalent of the last trimester of pregnancy in humans can lead to marked increases in programmed (apoptotic) cell death of neurons throughout the forebrain of rodents and non-human primates (see Fig. 7-1). Importantly, a dramatic increase in neuronal apoptosis occurs with exposure to levels of ethanol similar to those achieved during a single episode of binge drinking in humans. Although cell death is a normal part of development and helps to shape the connections within and among brain regions, drugs such as alcohol substantially increase the degree of and alter the timing of cell death, which can result in fetal alcohol syndrome, one of the most common causes of cognitive impairment in children. Some data suggest that significant exposure to alcohol *in utero* may also increase the risk for mood and psychotic illnesses later in life. It may be more appropriate to suggest that there is a continuum of toxic effects resulting from fetal alcohol exposure. It is possible that the increased cell death caused by gestational exposure to alcohol leads to ICNs with weaker connections, making these ICNs more susceptible to breakdown or environmental influences later in life. Based on the findings with fetal alcohol exposure, we also wonder, more speculatively, about the effects of adolescent alcohol and drug use on the maturation of neocortex and executive function. There is evidence from animal studies that adolescent alcohol exposure is associated with poor decision-making and risk-taking behavior in adulthood, even in animals that had no further exposure to ethanol after adolescence. These findings strengthen the argument that causes of illness related to ICN connectivity may be part of a continuum with developmental causes of psychopathology.

ABNORMALITIES RESULTING FROM EXOGENOUS OR ENDOGENOUS SUBSTANCES

While we would argue that psychiatric disorders are not the result of "chemical imbalances," it is clear that accumulation of certain external and internal chemicals can disrupt the smooth functioning of ICNs. We have mentioned the ravages that can accompany fetal alcohol exposure, but what about exposure to exogenous substances later in life? Similarly, the accumulation of certain endogenous substances can also disrupt ICN function.

Exogenous Substances

Again we emphasize substance-abuse disorders because they represent clear examples of external substances that disrupt neural systems and specific ICNs. As described in earlier chapters, addicting drugs can reset the brain's reward system and lead to long-lasting altered function across multiple brain systems. Persistent use of these drugs is associated with restructuring the connections between various brain regions, likely as a result of synaptic plasticity. These structural and functional changes create a situation where the brain's reward system doesn't function correctly unless the drug is present, and this leads to drug-seeking behavior. Instead of the usual state of homeostasis, a state of allostasis develops. As described in Chapter 8, an allostatic state reflects the effects of repeated wear and tear on a system, in this case resulting from chronic drug use. The result of allostatic load is somewhat akin to a person needing to run fast on a treadmill in order to stay in the same place. Over time, the system can't keep up and malfunctions. This malfunctioning initially involves neurons within a specific region (ventral tegmental area–nucleus accumbens) and its connections. As substance abuse progresses, emotional and cognitive circuits are engaged, resulting in an expanding sphere of clinical symptoms that ultimately involve all aspects of the mind (Chapter 5). We believe this progression from dysfunction in a single ICN to broader dysfunction of neural networks is a recurrent theme in psychiatric disorders.

While drugs of abuse are highly instructive, there are numerous other exogenous substances to which humans are exposed that also result in brain dysfunction. These include heavy metals (e.g., lead, mercury), other environmental toxins (pesticides, solvents), and infectious agents (viruses, bacteria, fungi), among many others. Many therapeutic drugs also have adverse effects on brain function and produce side effects that alter cognition and mood. Examples include drugs affecting the function of multiple neurotransmitters, particularly anti-muscarinic agents (scopolamine and others), NMDA receptor antagonists (ketamine and nitrous oxide), and GABA-enhancing drugs (barbiturates, anesthetics, and benzodiazepines). The various exogenous agents can have a host of effects on brain function, but how they actually produce mental dysfunction is not well understood in many (if not most) cases. The ability of many drugs and exogenous agents to induce delirium (a state of acute confusion) is a reminder of how delicate the homeostatic balance between normal and dysfunctional can be, particularly in the elderly or individuals with preexisting brain lesions.

In considering how exogenous agents produce complex mental changes, an instructive example involves the effects of NMDA receptor antagonists such as ketamine and phencyclidine (PCP). The biophysical mechanisms underlying the actions of these drugs are fairly well understood and involve blockade of NMDA ion channels. This means that although they allow glutamate to bind to the NMDA receptor, their presence prevents ions from flowing through the channel. Because NMDA receptors are involved in the synaptic plasticity underlying learning and memory, PCP and related drugs have adverse effects on cognition, producing a form of amnesia in which it is difficult to learn new information while under the influence of the drug. This is beneficial in anesthesia, where recollection of events occurring during surgery is unwanted, but leads to complex behavioral problems when the drugs are abused. Perhaps more surprising is the fact that these drugs can induce an acute psychotic state that is similar to primary psychotic disorders like schizophrenia. Based on work by John Olney and colleagues, it appears that the psychotomimetic effects of these drugs may involve disinhibition in a complex circuit that includes posterior cingulate and retrosplenial cortex, anterior thalamus, basal forebrain cholinergic neurons, brain-stem adrenergic and serotonergic neurons, and perhaps hippocampus and other limbic regions. While the acute effects of PCP result from the blockade of NMDA ion channels, the more complex psychotic state appears to involve increased release of excitatory transmitters as a result of decreased interneuron-mediated GABAergic inhibition. Perhaps related to their psychotomimetic effects, PCP-like drugs also induce pathological changes in cingulate cortex pyramidal neurons involving formation of intracellular vacuoles in endoplasmic reticula and mitochondria. The psychotomimetic effects are consistent with the idea that hypofunction of NMDA receptors contributes to psychosis and indicate that even agents with well-understood cellular mechanisms of action can produce complex cellular and neurocircuitry changes that underlie changes in mental function. Studies of PCP-induced intracellular vacuoles have also led to treatment strategies that prevent these effects and perhaps prevent psychotic symptoms. These strategies include dampening network disinhibition with anti-muscarinic or GABA-enhancing agents, or modulating monoaminergic tone. Interestingly and perhaps paradoxically, ketamine (and other NMDA receptor antagonists) also appear to have acute antidepressant effects, raising questions about relationships among mood states and psychosis.

Endogenous Substances

Some illnesses result from abnormal accumulation of internally generated substances. For example, in Chapter 2 we described the effects of the abnormal accumulation of beta-amyloid. Beta-amyloid is a substance that is normally synthesized and removed from our central nervous system. When too much amyloid is produced or too little existing amyloid is cleared, the elevated levels can lead to synaptic dysfunction, neuronal damage, and disconnectivity. This damage leads to gradual and progressive functional impairments that are recognized phenotypically as DAT. In DAT, accumulation of an abnormal amount of a normal substance gums up the works of a key ICN: the default system. It is likely that the default system interacts with many other ICNs. Thus, it is no surprise that a primary interruption in a major system results in the development of an illness with diverse mental symptoms.

Prion-related disorders such as Creutzfeld-Jacob dementia (CJD) and "mad cow disease" are examples of other illnesses that involve abnormal accumulation of a brain substance. Prions are proteins that are normal constituents of certain brain cells. Occasionally, the prion polypeptide folds into an abnormal shape, and when it does so, it can induce other prion proteins to misfold. These misfolded proteins form a template that encourages the accumulation of abnormally folded prion sheets. The sheets of abnormal prion proteins disrupt cellular function and result in neuronal loss. This sequence of events can begin in several ways. Sometimes the initial event is a spontaneous misfolding of a normal, endogenous, prion protein. Rarely, an abnormally folded prion protein enters the body from exogenous sources—for instance, by infecting an open cut with the bodily fluids of a person with a prion disorder or by ingesting contaminated tissue, as seen in the syndromes of kuru and mad cow disease. Very rarely, a genetic mutation leads to prion proteins with a propensity to misfold.

Prion proteins can misfold in different ways that have different impacts on brain function. Most commonly, the misfolding results in a clinical picture of rapidly progressive dementia such as CJD. However, a small number of people who ingest meat from contaminated cows develop mad cow disease. The abnormally folded cow prions act as templates for human prion proteins and promote the formation of abnormal prion sheets. The shape of this template differs from that of the misfolded proteins that accumulate in CJD, and the mad cow prions appear to influence different brain systems than CJD. Mad cow disease typically occurs in younger persons and presents clinically with a psychiatric syndrome that involves mood and psychotic symptoms along with cognitive changes. CJD tends to occur in people in their 50s and is usually a rapidly progressive dementia, leading to death over months to a few years. The fact that mad cow disease has a very specific clinical phenotype suggests that a particular ICN is vulnerable to the toxicity from prions that are misshaped in a particular manner. Why does the misfolding of prion protein by a cow template result in mad cow disease, while a differently shaped misfolding of the same type of protein causes CJD? Further research should help to elucidate the ICNs that each of these prion diseases influences and help us better understand why different

ICNs are susceptible to different shapes of the misfolded proteins. As we better understand the genetics and molecular mechanisms of these disorders and the selective vulnerabilities of various ICNs, more specific treatments for these fatal diseases should become feasible.

We highlight prion disorders because they are clear examples in which abnormal endogenous or exogenous substances result in altered protein folding that leads to cellular dysfunction and neuronal loss. The notion that certain disorders involve abnormally folded proteins is a recurrent theme in the biology of neurodegenerative illnesses and is an area of active investigation. Although some of these disorders initially present with psychiatric symptoms, they progress to involve substantial neurodegeneration involving widespread areas of the brain.

Other neuropsychiatric illnesses attack mitochondria, resulting in disruption of cellular energy production and the generation of endogenous reactive oxygen species (ROS). Examples of ROS include superoxide and peroxy radicals. These chemicals are highly interactive with other cellular chemicals because of their free radical properties. ROS disrupt a variety of cellular functions, including energy metabolism, and often result in neurodegeneration. Mitochondrial dysfunction contributes to aging and a variety of brain illnesses.

ABNORMALITIES RESULTING FROM TRAUMATIC BRAIN INJURY

Traumatic brain injuries are associated with a variety of neurological and psychiatric symptoms. The particular brain regions directly and indirectly influenced by the trauma determine the nature of the symptoms. For instance, blunt trauma on one side of the head can lead to direct injury on the traumatized side and indirect injury on the other side of the brain (called "coup" and "contrecoup" injury, respectively). In addition to the regions directly involved in the injury, disruptions can occur in brain systems and ICNs connected to the directly damaged regions. Traumatic brain damage can lead to multiple functional abnormalities, including paralysis, seizures, mood changes, and psychotic symptoms. Recent data indicate that more than 50% of individuals who experience traumatic brain injury meet criteria for major depression over the ensuing 6 months, and this is associated with a high degree of comorbid anxiety.

Bilateral damage to the hippocampus or areas near the hippocampus can result in an amnesic syndrome in which new declarative memories can no longer be formed. A person with such damage lives continuously in the present moment and has an inability to learn new information. He or she cannot process and remember new life experiences, including people and places encountered subsequent to the injury. Memories generated months and years prior to the accident are generally recalled well. Interestingly, and consistent with the fact that the hippocampus is not involved in all types of memory formation, individuals with this amnesic syndrome can form implicit memories, including procedural and emotional memories. Nonetheless, they remain extremely handicapped in their daily lives. Unfortunately, little can be done to treat the learning deficit specifically, particularly if there is bilateral structural damage to the hippocampus. Loss of a major hub like the hippocampus has catastrophic consequences for overall brain function.

As we learn more about the overall functioning of the brain, we will gain a better understanding of the varied symptoms and syndromes that can result from traumatic brain injuries. One important area for consideration involves the mechanism(s) by which the effects of direct trauma lead to the longer-term sequelae of head injuries. In other words, even in circumstances where the initial injury appears to be relatively mild, there can be longer-term effects on mental function that reflect changes in the function and connectivity of ICNs. The development of psychiatric symptoms along with persistent and sometimes subtle cognitive impairment can result in protracted periods of recovery and disability following traumatic brain injury, even when gross neurological manifestations may have improved substantially. Thus, rehabilitative efforts are often needed well beyond the initial injury to help reestablish cognition and other mental functions.

ABNORMALITIES RESULTING FROM DEFECTS IN BRAIN METABOLISM

The brain continuously requires glucose and oxygen. Despite its relatively small size, the brain uses about 20% of cardiac output and bodily energy supplies to maintain efficient function. Although certain neurological illnesses result from malfunctioning mitochondria, the primary energy-generating powerhouses of cells, we will concentrate on the much more common reason for energy interference encountered in clinical psychiatry: vascular disease. With respect to psychiatric illnesses, vascular disease can be organized into two major categories: acute vascular insults (strokes) and more chronic vascular conditions, including "silent" infarcts and syndromes resulting from the narrowing of small vessels.

Acute stroke has similarities to traumatic brain injury. A stroke directly injures the brain regions dependent on the supply of nutrients and oxygen it interrupts, and it also can indirectly influence brain systems that are dependent on input from these directly damaged regions. Thus, psychiatric symptoms can include a full spectrum of acute cognitive, emotional, and motivational changes. Psychotic symptoms may develop depending on the location of the stroke, particularly when attentional networks in the nondominant hemisphere are involved or connections between cognitive processing regions in prefrontal cortex and subcortical emotional processing systems are disrupted. Strokes can also result in longer-term mental dysfunction, including post-stroke depression. Certain post-stroke depressions represent interesting and instructive examples of the ways damage to a specific ICN can result in disrupted function in other ICNs. For example, strokes involving the anterior left (dominant) hemisphere appear to have an increased probability of producing depression. In these cases, the insult is often restricted to prefrontal cortex and its underlying white matter. Thus, ICNs required for higher-order cognition (e.g., language function and perhaps working memory) are affected. Yet, defects in these regions can result in mood symptoms that presumably reflect aberrant activity in emotional ICNs. In some cases, the direct damage may not extend to the emotional ICNs, but their function is altered by loss of key input from the damaged areas and perhaps by defects in the ability to control emotions via top-down processing. In addition, the right (nondominant) hemisphere, lacking input from the left hemisphere, becomes a dominant processing vehicle, and its "detail-oriented" mode of function contributes to symptoms. The point here is that although emotional ICNs may not be directly injured by these strokes, the loss of input and control from the damaged regions has adverse consequences on mood. It is important to emphasize that the altered mood state in post-stroke depression is often not simply a "reaction to illness"; it is the result of complex dysfunction and disconnection among key CNS processing networks. This is not to say that adjustment disorders and other types of mood problems do not occur following a stroke, but rather to highlight how symptom generation can result from altered brain function. Such considerations are critical in planning treatment and rehabilitative strategies.

More chronic vascular compromises may also occur, especially in the aging brain; these are just beginning to be understood. It is clear from brain autopsies that a large percentage of people have "silent" mini-strokes during life. Although these are frequently referred to as "silent," it is likely that certain "silent" strokes are speaking volumes via changes in personality, mood, or other behaviors. For example, neuroimaging studies have found small white-matter hyperintensities in the basal ganglia and other structures of individuals with depressive syndromes in later life. These hyperintensities typically do not result in focal neurological findings (such as weakness or speech problems), but they may predispose individuals to depression and perhaps delirium. As with traumatic brain injury, vascular insults may lead to dysregulation in the supply of nutrients or oxygen to various brain regions. Although safety mechanisms are built into the CNS to allow the brain to tolerate variations in blood flow and oxygen, chronic deficits may have subtle consequences that affect the efficient functioning of ICNs. This may be particularly true for regions or pathways located in highly susceptible regions of the brain where blood flow can be most easily compromised; these regions are called "watershed" areas in the distal vascular fields of specific arteries. Although chronic vascular defects in these regions may not result in gross neurological deficits, they may cause subtle changes in regional function and connectivity that contribute to defects in mental activity.

ABNORMALITIES DUE TO AGING

There are many health issues related to aging. The subspecialties of geriatric medicine and geriatric psychiatry developed because of a perceived need for physicians with specialized expertise in the biological, psychological, and social consequences of aging. Aging can lead to an increased incidence of certain behavioral disorders as a result of factors already discussed. As we live longer, we are more susceptible to disorders that disrupt brain energy such as strokes and diabetes. Similarly, the longer we live, the greater the likelihood of being involved in accidents that result in brain trauma. Psychosocial and environmental challenges that can test the resiliency of our ICNs also increase with aging.

Age-related changes take place in our brains normally. A certain degree of cell loss and atrophy occurs. Changes in neurotransmitter systems develop. Independent of the development of DAT, the microtubule-associated protein *tau* starts to accumulate in brain regions in and around the hippocampus as people enter their 50s. While some areas of the brain continue to develop new cells and new connections well into old age, brain plasticity is unlikely to be as vigorous as in younger years. Certain abilities, such as reading comprehension, are stable well into old age. Other abilities, such as multitasking, become harder. The connectivity of some ICNs probably changes with aging, but this has not been studied in great detail to date. There is also evidence that the strategies used to solve complex tasks change with aging, with older persons tending to be more reactive in their cognitive-control approach and younger persons using more proactive strategies. This likely reflects developmental and age-related changes in brain connectivity.

Interestingly, many aspects of mental health do not deteriorate with age. Life satisfaction can be maintained, and older age is associated with the cognitive equivalent of "wisdom." George Vaillant has referred to this acquisition of wisdom as becoming a "keeper of the meaning," an individual who has developed life schemas and cognitive strategies to see the "big picture" and the context of life events instead of getting lost in details or novelty. Major depressive disorders are not more common in the physically healthy elderly. It is true that there are likely to be subtle changes involving cognition, emotion, and motivation; however, if no major brain illness exists, these age-related changes need not interfere with the ability to enjoy advancing age. Key aspects of successful aging include remaining physically fit, socially involved, and cognitively intact. Recent studies highlight the interdependence of mind and body fitness and emphasize the importance of both physical (cardiovascular condition and muscle strength) and motor (balance and agility) fitness in healthy aging. Both physical and motor fitness contribute to greater executive-control function and more efficient metabolic operation of brain systems. Frontotemporal processing is enhanced in the physically fit, while parietal visuospatial processing is enhanced in those with higher motor fitness.

Two of the most serious concerns with aging are the increased susceptibility to dementias and deliria. Changes in brain structure and brain plasticity probably occur with aging, and these changes make our brains more vulnerable to the cumulative effects of other processes that impair cognition. Older adults become more susceptible to confusion with milder perturbations of brain systems. For example, they are more likely to develop confusion following general anesthesia. About 30% to 50% of individuals in their 80s exhibit accumulation of beta-amyloid in their brains. This increased level of beta-amyloid gradually disrupts brain function and likely drives the marked rise in the incidence and prevalence of DAT in the very old. Why some people develop DAT in their 60s and others in their 90s isn't fully known. Certainly, increases in accumulation of beta-amyloid appear to be age-related. In addition, other changes may be occurring in the aging brain. Vascular changes may cause the brain to be more susceptible to the influence of accumulating beta-amyloid. The strength of connections between ICNs may change with aging. Certain cell types may be more susceptible to chemical or nutritional changes that occur with aging. The age of onset of symptoms associated with DAT may be dependent on an individual's unique balance of genetic makeup, life-long environmental exposures, and age-related structural and chemical changes. The instructive point is that the specific nature of the molecular pathology may not fully correlate with the age of onset or the specific clinical presentation of DAT in an individual. How pathology and brain compensatory mechanisms interact to produce clinical phenotypes is also uncertain, but it will be important to understand this relationship in order to devise strategies to diminish or prevent cognitive deterioration.

It is important to understand what happens to brain ICNs as we get older so we can develop strategies to minimize the consequences of cognitive illnesses with aging. If we can understand how amyloid accumulation is toxic to the brain, we may be able to better protect against DAT. Psychotic symptoms become common as DAT progresses, occurring in about 50% of persons with moderate dementia. Why does this occur, and can we do anything about it? This is an important question because psychotic symptoms have much to do with whether a person is able to live with family or requires nursing home placement. We also have little understanding of what makes the brain increasingly susceptible to delirium as we age.

Points to Remember

We know little about the causes of any primary psychiatric disorder.

Primary psychiatric disorders likely involve disruption of brain ICNs. Which ICNs are affected in various illnesses may reflect the inherent vulnerability of brain systems in specific individuals (genetics) and the intersection of this vulnerability with life events (environment).

ICN dysfunction can occur throughout the life cycle and can be driven by a variety of internal and external causes.

Direct and indirect disruptions of ICNs are frequent consequences of brain trauma and vascular events.

Considering causes of psychiatric disorders in terms of disruptions of brain systems can facilitate research and creative thinking about diagnosis and therapeutic strategies.

SUGGESTED READINGS

Aguzzi, A., & Calella, A. M. (2009). Prions: Protein aggregation and infectious diseases. *Physiological Reviews, 89,* 1105–1152.

Caviston, J. P., & Holzbaur, E. L. F. (2009). Huntingtin as an essential integrator of intracellular vesicular trafficking. *Trends in Cell Biology, 19,* 147–155.

Fair, D. A., Cohen, A. L., Power, J. D., Dosenbach, N. U. F., Church, J. A., Miezen, F. M., et al. (2009). Functional brain networks develop from a "local to distributed" organization. *PLoS Computational Biology, 5,* 1–14.

Guskiewicz, K. M., Marshall, S. W., Bailes, J., McCrea, M., Cantu, R. C., Randolph, C., et al. (2005). Association between recurrent concussion and late-life cognitive impairment in retired professional football players. *Neurosurgery, 57,* 719–726.

McEwen, B. S. (2007). Physiology and neurobiology of stress and adaptation: Central role of the brain. *Physiological Reviews, 87,* 873–904.

Seeley, W. W., Crawford, R. K., Zhou, J., Miller, B. L., & Greicius, M. D. (2009). Neurodegenerative diseases target large-scale human brain networks. *Neuron, 62,* 42–52.

Soong, B.-W., & Paulson, H. L. (2007). Spinocerebellar ataxias: An update. *Current Opinion in Neurology, 20,* 438–446.

Sperling, R. A., LaViolette, P. S., O'Keefe, K., O'Brien, J., Rentz, D. M., Pihlajamaki, M., et al. (2009). Amyloid deposition is associated with impaired default network function in older persons without dementia. *Neuron, 63,* 178–188.

Tau, G. Z., & Peterson, B. S. (2010). Normal development of brain circuits. *Neuropsychopharmacology Reviews, 35,* 147–168.

Teper, E., & O'Brien, J. T. (2008). Vascular factors and depression. *International Journal of Geriatric Psychiatry, 23,* 993–1000.

OTHER REFERENCES

Aguzzi, A., Baumann, F., & Bremer, J. (2008). The prion's elusive reason for being. *Annual Review of Neuroscience, 31,* 439–477.

American Psychiatric Association. (1994). *Diagnostic and statistical manual of mental disorders* (4th ed.). Washington, DC: American Psychiatric Association

Amminger, G. P., Schafer, M. R., Papageorgiou, K., Klier, C. M., Cotton, S. M., Harrigan, S. M., et al. (2010). Long-chain omega-3 fatty acids for indicated prevention of psychotic disorders: A randomized, placebo-controlled trial. *Archives of General Psychiatry, 67,* 146–154.

Benes, F. M. (2007). Searching for unique endophenotypes for schizophrenia and bipolar disorder within neural circuits and their molecular regulatory mechanisms. *Schizophrenia Bulletin, 33,* 932–936.

Biswal, B. B., Mennes, M., Zuo, X.-N., Gohel, S., Kelly, C., Smith, S. M., et al. (2010). Toward discovery science of human brain function. *Proceedings of the National Academy of Sciences (USA), 107,* 4734–4739.

Bombardier, C. H., Fann, J. R., Temkin, N. R., Esselman, P. C., Barber, J., & Dikmen, S. S. (2010). Rates of major depressive disorder and clinical outcomes following traumatic brain injury. *Journal of the American Medical Association, 303,* 1938–1945.

Braver, T. S., Paxton, J. L., Locke, H. S., & Barch, D. M. (2009). Flexible neural mechanisms of cognitive control within human prefrontal cortex. *Proceedings of the National Academy of Sciences (USA), 106,* 7351–7356.

Buldyrev, S. V., Parshani, R., Paul, G., Stanley, H. E., & Havlin, S. (2010). Catastrophic cascade of failures in interdependent networks. *Nature, 464,* 1025–1028.

Cannon, S. C. (2006). Pathomechanisms in channelopathies of skeletal muscle and brain. *Annual Review of Neuroscience, 29,* 387–415.

Caspi, A., & Moffitt, T. E. (2006). Gene–environment interactions in psychiatry: Joining forces with neuroscience. *Nature Reviews Neuroscience, 7,* 583–590.

Corlett, P. R., Honey, G. D., Krystal, J. H., & Fletcher, P. C. (2011). Glutamatergic model psychoses: Prediction error, learning and inference. *Neuropsychopharmacology Reviews, 36,* 316–338.

DiMauro, S., & Schon, E. A. (2008). Mitochondrial disorders in the nervous system. *Annual Review of Neuroscience, 31,* 91–123.

Eack, S. M., Hogarty, G. E., Cho, R. Y., Prasad, K. M. R., Greenwald, D. P., Hogarty, S. S., et al. (2010). Neuroprotective effects of cognitive enhancement therapy against gray matter loss in early schizophrenia. *Archives of General Psychiatry, 67,* 674–682.

Fair, D. A., Cohen, A. L., Dosenbach, N. U. F., Church, J. A., Miezin, F. M., Barch, D. M., et al. (2008). The maturing architecture of the brain's default network. *Proceedings of the National Academy of Sciences (USA), 105,* 4028–4032.

Fair, D. A., Cohen, A. L., Dosenbach, N. U. F., Church, J. A., Miezin, F. M., Schlaggar, B. L., et al. (2009). Functional brain networks develop from a local to distributed organization. *PLoS Computational Biology, 5,* e1000381.

Farber, N. B., Creeley, C. E., & Olney, J. W. (2010). Alcohol-induced neuroapoptosis in the fetal macaque brain. *Neurobiology of Disease, 40,* 200–206.

Hedden, T., Van Dijk, K. R. A., Becker, J. A., Mehta, A., Sperling, R. A., Johnson, K.A., et al. (2009). Disruption of functional connectivity in clinically normal older adults harboring amyloid burden. *Journal of Neuroscience, 29,* 12686–12694.

Herrmann, L. L., Le Masurier, M., & Ebmeier, K. P. (2008). White matter hyperintensities in late life depression: A systematic review. *Journal of Neurology, Neurosurgery and Psychiatry, 79,* 619–624.

Insel, T. R. (2010). Rethinking schizophrenia. *Nature, 468,* 187–193.

Johnson, D. K., Storandt, M., Morris, J. C., & Galvin, J. E. (2009). Longitudinal study of the transition from healthy aging to Alzheimer disease. *Archives of Neurology, 66,* 1254–1259.

Koob, G. F., & Volkow, N. D. (2010). Neurocircuitry of addiction. *Neuropsychopharmacology Reviews, 35,* 217–238.

LeDoux, J. (2002). *Synaptic self: How our brains become who we are.* New York: Viking Press.

Manolio, T. A., Collins, F. S., Cox, N. J., Goldstein, D. B., Hindorff, L. A., Hunter, D. J., et al. (2009). Finding the missing heritability of complex diseases. *Nature, 461,* 747–753.

Meyer-Lindenberg, A. (2010). From maps to mechanisms through neuroimaging of schizophrenia. *Nature, 468,* 194–202.

Milgram, N. W., Siwak-Tapp, C. T., Araujo, J., & Head, E. (2006). Neuroprotective effects of cognitive enrichment. *Ageing Research Reviews, 5,* 354–369.

Nasrallah, N. A., Yang, T. W. H., & Bernstein, I. L. (2009). Long-term risk preference and suboptimal decision making following adolescent alcohol use. *Proceedings of the National Academy of Sciences (USA), 106,* 17600–17604.

Olney, J. W., Labruyere, J., Wang, G., Wozniak, D. F., Price, M. T., & Sesma, M. A. (1991). NMDA antagonist neurotoxicity: Mechanisms and prevention. *Science, 254,* 1515–1518.

Olney, J. W., Young, C., Wozniak, D. F., Jevtovic-Todorovic, V., & Ikonomidou, C. (2004). Do pediatric drugs cause developing neurons to commit suicide? *Trends in Pharmacological Sciences, 25,* 135–139.

Ongur, D., Drevets, W. C., & Price, J. L. (1998). Glial reduction in the subgenual prefrontal cortex in mood disorders. *Proceedings of the National Academy of Sciences (USA), 27,* 13290–13295.

Price, J. L., McKeel, D. W., Jr., Buckles, V. D., Roe, C. M., Xiong, C., Grundman, M., et al. (2009). Neuropathology of nondemented aging: Presumptive evidence for preclinical Alzheimer disease. *Neurobiology of Aging, 30,* 1026–1036.

Querfurth, H. W., & LaFerla, F. M. (2010). Alzheimer's disease. *New England Journal of Medicine, 362,* 329–344.

Raichle, M. E. (2009). A paradigm shift in functional brain imaging. *Journal of Neuroscience, 29,* 12729–12734.

Ridley, M. (2003). *Nature via nurture: Genes, experience, and what makes us human.* New York: HarperCollins Publishers.

Robinson, R. G. (1998). *The clinical neuropsychiatry of stroke.* New York: Cambridge University Press.

Sheline, Y. I., Raichle, M. E., Snyder, A. Z., Morris, J. C., Head, D., Wang, S., et al. (2010). Amyloid plaques disrupt resting state default mode network connectivity in cognitively normal elderly. *Biological Psychiatry, 67,* 584–587.

Silver, J. M., McAllister, T. W., & Arciniegas, D. B. (2009). Depression and cognitive complaints following mild traumatic brain injury. *American Journal of Psychiatry, 166,* 653–661.

Vaillant, G. E., DiRago, A. C., & Mukamal, K. (2006). Natural history of male psychological health, XV: Retirement satisfaction. *American Journal of Psychiatry, 163,* 682–688.

Vaishnavi, S. N., Vlassenko, A. G., Rundle, M. M., Snyder, A. Z., Mintun, M. A., & Raichle, M. E. (2010). Regional aerobic glycolysis in the human brain. *Proceedings of the National Academy of Sciences (USA), 107,* 17757–17762.

Van Os, J., Kenis, G., & Rutten, B. P. F. (2010). The environment and schizophrenia. *Nature, 468,* 203–212.

Voelcker-Rehage, C., Godde, B., & Staudinger, U. M. (2009). Physical and motor fitness are both related to cognition in old age. *European Journal of Neuroscience, 31,* 167–176.

Zhang, D., & Raichle, M. E. (2010). Disease and the brain's dark energy. *Nature Reviews Neurology, 6,* 15–28.

10

Neurotransmitters and Receptors

If systems neuroscience provides a useful basis for understanding psychiatric disorders, why should psychiatrists be concerned about neurotransmitters, receptors, and molecular and cellular neuroscience? We believe that these areas are important for understanding fundamental mechanisms underlying various treatments and possibly for describing the defects that cause psychiatric illnesses. They also form the basis for future and novel developments in psychopharmacology and interventional psychiatry. There is a tendency, however, to use cellular and molecular mechanisms to provide oversimplified explanations of how treatments work. For instance, stating that depression is a "chemical imbalance" and that medication corrects this imbalance is a simplistic metaphor that tells us nothing about how brain function is altered. Similarly, when a research paper demonstrates that a certain disorder is associated with an increased density of a certain type of receptor, this finding may add only a small piece to the "mechanism of illness" puzzle, and it should be put into an appropriate context. A cellular or molecular finding may be the brain's reaction to treatment, a response to a yet-to-be discovered primary defect underlying the illness, or an epiphenomenon resulting from the consequences of the illness. We emphasize that these concerns also pertain to the various neuroimaging findings described throughout this book. Whether any given finding or set of findings is causative, correlative, or restorative can be difficult to discern. Given the complex genetics of psychiatric disorders and the complexities of neural systems involved in generating mind and mental disorders, it would be extraordinary if any single cellular, molecular, or imaging finding represented the primary defect of a major illness. In fact, we would argue that the complex results emerging from psychiatric genetics are telling us that psychiatric disorders are not "molecular" illnesses, but rather problems of neural circuits with multiple paths leading into and out of dysfunction. Thus, we think it is important to be cautious about enthusiastic statements that molecular findings, including genetic findings, explain the illness. This is true not only of human studies but also of studies in which various genes are knocked out of or into mice. In the latter studies, there is a tendency to manipulate a gene's expression, describe a behavioral phenotype, and simplistically extrapolate the phenotype to a complex human disorder. This can make for great press, but most often it will have little impact on clinical thinking or practice.

We suggest that it is important for psychiatrists to understand the concepts and language of neurotransmitters, receptors, and synapses in order to appreciate how these various signaling devices determine the functioning of brain systems involved in illnesses and help us understand how treatments work. A comprehensive understanding of these aspects of neuroscience is impractical and, we believe, unnecessary for clinicians. A conceptual understanding, however, is both feasible and useful. In this chapter, we will first review some basic principles of neurotransmitters and receptors, expanding upon themes introduced in earlier chapters. We will then illustrate the usefulness of understanding these principles by examining the mechanisms underlying a clinically relevant pharmacologic question: why do traditional antidepressants take weeks to work, whereas benzodiazepine anxiolytics work in minutes?

NEUROTRANSMITTERS AND RECEPTORS

There are hundreds of neurochemicals that potentially can act as neurotransmitters or neuromodulators and an even greater number of receptors that respond to these neurochemicals. Evolution can be extremely messy, and if subtle differences in transmitters and receptors provide an advantage in performing a function that is favorable for survival, then that transmitter or receptor is likely to survive and thrive. Learning the exact metabolic pathways of all of the transmitters and receptors would be difficult if not impossible. More importantly, it is not necessary for thinking about clinical illnesses. In this section, we outline some basic principles that we believe are useful for understanding how neurotransmission works.

The Brain Uses a Variety of Neurotransmitters

Many substances with varied chemical structures can serve as neurotransmitters. Biogenic amines such as dopamine, serotonin, and norepinephrine are structurally different from amino acid neurotransmitters such as glutamate and glycine. Amino acids can be slightly modified to form other transmitters such as gamma-aminobutyric acid (GABA). Chains of amino acids (called peptides) can also act as neurotransmitters, and a large number of these are synthesized and stored in the brain. Lipid-soluble substances, such as the endogenous cannabinoids, anandamide and 2-arachidonoyl-glycerol (2AG), can form within cell membranes and can also serve as neurotransmitters. These substances are sometimes generated in postsynaptic cells and diffuse back to specific cannabinoid receptors located on presynaptic membranes, moving in the reverse direction from "typical" neurotransmitters. There, these endocannabinoids influence presynaptic function, including the release of other neurotransmitters like glutamate or GABA. Although we don't usually think of gasses as neurotransmitters, several small-molecular-weight gasses such as nitric oxide (NO) and carbon monoxide (CO) are generated in the brain and can act as neuromodulators, sometimes in a "retrograde" fashion like the endocannabinoids.

Neurotransmitters, hormones, and growth factors differ largely with respect to the distance that they travel from their site of origin to their site of influence. Hormones and growth factors can work in ways that are analogous to neurotransmitters. Some hormones act on receptors on the cell surface, while others cross the

TYPE OF TRANSMISSION (diffuse ⟶ local)
hormonal ⟶ paracrine ⟶ volume transmission ⟶ synapse

TRANSMITTERS (slow ⟶ fast)

neuropeptides	biogenic amines	glutamate, GABA
biogenic amines	neuropeptides	acetylcholine
	purines	serotonin
	glutamate, GABA	
	acetylcholine	
	endocannabinoids	

RECEPTORS (metabotropic ⟶ ion channels)

| high affinity GPCRs | high affinity GPCRs | ionotropic receptors |
| nuclear receptors | | |

Figure 10-1 The transmitter continuum. The diagram depicts a continuum of neurotransmitter effects ranging from diffuse to local and slow to fast, and highlights the types of receptors that are thought to underlie these effects. Abbreviation: GPCRs (G-protein coupled receptors). (This figure is courtesy of Steve Mennerick, Washington University in St. Louis.)

cell membrane and combine with receptors inside the cell to form complexes that enter the cell nucleus and influence gene expression. Various growth factors, including brain derived neurotrophic factor (BDNF), nerve growth factor (NGF), and others, also function in a manner similar to neurotransmitters in that they interact with specific receptors and have a broad array of cellular effects, including effects on gene expression. Figure 10-1 presents an overview of the types of transmitters used in the brain.

Over time, diverse chemical mechanisms have evolved that allow brain cells to communicate and influence each other. The complexities of these systems are such that it would be very difficult to understand the overall function of the brain by examining each individual system. By analogy, we suggest that while it may be useful to study each type of tree and plant in a forest, such an approach is unlikely to describe the overall function of a forest. Similarly, while it is important to understand the existence and general purpose of specific transmitter systems, such understanding is of limited utility in describing the overall picture of how the brain generates the mind and behavior. On the other hand, neurotransmitters and neuronal excitability are the currencies that drive function within and between neural systems. Thus, interventions that influence various transmitter systems can strongly influence neural systems and, therefore, thinking and behavior. Some drugs influence neural systems in beneficial ways, while others have negative effects. For example, antidepressant medications can lead to positive changes and result in a depressed person feeling better, while opiates can not only relieve acute pain but also take over the central reward systems and lead to addictive behaviors. A corollary to this point is that every pharmacological agent ingested by humans has both positive and negative effects; decisions in clinical therapeutics are largely based on an analysis of the risk/benefit ratio.

Although there are many varieties of neurotransmitters and hormones, some seem to have broad influence on a large number of cells, whereas others influence a small number of cells in a very direct and powerful manner. In Chapter 3, we briefly discussed different types of transmitters as belonging to the broad categories of "slow" and "fast" transmitters, and we examined how these transmitters generate their effects. Several transmitters that play a major role in psychiatry, including dopamine, norepinephrine, and serotonin, can be released by neurons in a diffuse manner. One neuron may have thousands of synaptic boutons (terminals), and when that neuron fires an action potential, many packets of neurotransmitter are simultaneously (or nearly simultaneously) released in a broadly distributed manner across regions of the brain to influence many cells. This "slow" type of neurotransmitter functions more like a neuromodulator in that it sets the "gain" of a large number of cells and, in so doing, it changes how easily these cells fire action potentials in response to other transmitters. In this way, the transmitters can influence a variety of cells that may be involved in one or more brain systems. These slower neurotransmitters typically work via chemical second-messenger systems to exert their effects on neuronal excitability. Examples of second messengers include cyclic AMP, cyclic GMP, inositol phosphates, and arachidonic acid, among many others.

Other transmitters have direct and powerful effects on a relatively small number of cells. For instance, one cell may strongly influence 5 to 10 other cells (divergence; see Chapter 6), and each of these "receiving" cells may receive input from another 3 to 5 cells (convergence; see Chapter 6). These direct and powerful cell-to-cell effects are likely involved in fast information transfer and processing. Transmitters like glutamate and GABA act in this manner via the opening of specific ion channels that are part of their receptors. The "slow" transmitters, such as the monoamines, can modulate large regions of neurons by influencing how neurons respond to the more targeted and faster-acting transmitters. They accomplish this by altering the release of the fast transmitters or by changing the electrical and chemical properties of the pre- and postsynaptic neurons, making these neurons more or less responsive to the fast transmitter.

Transmitters Use a Variety of Receptors

Chemical transmitters are the principal source of intercellular information transfer. Transmitters and transmitter-like substances usually influence cells by stimulating specific receptors expressed on cell membranes. Certain hormones (e.g., cortisol, estrogen, and progesterone) are exceptions to this rule. These steroids are lipid-soluble and readily cross cell membranes and bind to intracellular receptors in the cell's cytoplasm. These intracellular steroid–receptor complexes then move to the cell nucleus and alter gene expression. Some steroid hormones can also bind cell membrane receptors for other neurotransmitters and influence how those receptors work. An example is the progesterone derivative, allopregnanolone. This endogenous steroid, called a "neurosteroid" because it can be synthesized in the brain, is a potent and highly effective enhancer of GABA-A receptors and causes GABA to be much more effective at inhibiting neurons. At higher concentrations, allopregnanolone can actually open GABA-A chloride channels in the absence of GABA.

Furthermore, there is evidence that allopregnanolone can be synthesized in excitatory neurons, providing an autocrine (self-acting) way in which a neuron can regulate its own excitability. This is just one demonstration of how complex the topic of neurotransmitters, neuromodulators, and receptors can become.

There are several types of receptors for neurotransmitters and neuromodulators found in cell membranes. Each receptor usually recognizes a specific neurotransmitter; for instance, there are serotonin-specific receptors and glutamate-specific receptors. For each neurotransmitter, there may be several types of receptors that recognize that transmitter. Sometimes, these receptors are given number or letter names such as the 5HT1 (5-hydroxytryptamine [serotonin] type 1), 5HT2, 5HT3 ... receptors, the GABA-A and GABA-B receptors, and the α- and β-adrenergic receptors, or a combination of numbers and letters, such as 5HT1A receptors. Sometimes, receptors are given names based on exogenous chemicals that have been found to bind specifically to the receptor. For instance, there are AMPA, NMDA, and kainate receptors for glutamate, and nicotinic and muscarinic receptors for acetylcholine.

As described in Chapter 3, receptors can be broadly categorized as ionotropic receptors or metabotropic receptors. In general, an ionotropic receptor (also called a "ligand gated ion channel") consists of four or five protein subunits that each traverse the cell membrane three or four times. When stimulated by its neurotransmitter, the portion of the receptor within the cell membrane forms an open pore that spans the entire width of the lipid bilayer membrane. The open channel allows specific ions such as calcium, sodium, potassium, or chloride to flow through the channel. Whether an ion flows into or out of the cell is determined by two factors, a chemical gradient across the membrane (determined by the concentration of the ion on either side of the membrane) and an electrical gradient (the membrane potential [driving force] across the cell membrane). The flow of ions through these channels changes the electrical gradient across the membrane, resulting in either hyperpolarization (the transmembrane voltage becomes more negative) or depolarization (the transmembrane voltage becomes more positive). Most ion channels are permeable to only one or a few ions and show selectivity for either positively charged cations (sodium, potassium, or calcium) or negatively charged anions (chloride). When stimulated, these receptors open quickly, and the consequences of the ionic flow are almost immediate. The cell either depolarizes (is excited) or hyperpolarizes (is inhibited). In addition, the changes in ionic concentration inside the cell may initiate other cellular events. For example, see Chapter 6 regarding the NMDA receptor, calcium, and long-term potentiation (LTP). There are two very important principles to remember regarding ionotropic receptors: the electrical consequences are rapid, and both the immediate and delayed effects are triggered by changes in ion flow across the cell membrane.

Metabotropic receptors also are triggered by the direct binding of a neurotransmitter to a receptor. Metabotropic receptors generally consist of one protein that weaves back and forth through the cell membrane seven times before poking one end (called the carboxy or C-terminus) into the cytoplasm of the cell. In some cases, a functioning metabotropic receptor involves interactions of two of these proteins (a dimer).

When the neurotransmitter binds to the receptor, the receptor changes shape and this triggers sequences of chemical events, referred to as second-messenger cascades, inside the cell. These chemical events can eventually lead to changes in the activity or number of ion channels and membrane receptors, including ionotropic receptors. They also can activate intracellular chemicals that enter the nucleus and influence the production of other cellular chemicals, including new membrane receptors or chemical signals that lead to growth of the neuron itself. More dendrites may form or more synaptic connections may be triggered. Although the initial binding of a neurotransmitter to the receptor on the membrane may be rapid, the various chemical events triggered by stimulation of a metabotropic receptor usually take more time to unfold than the events following stimulation of an ionotropic receptor. In general, metabotropic receptors are coupled to their intracellular messenger systems via GTP-binding proteins (called G-proteins) that are the key initial mediators of intracellular events. Thus, metabotropic receptors are sometimes referred to as "G-protein coupled receptors" (GPCRs). Because activation of a single GPCR can result in the activation of multiple G-proteins and the triggering of a large cascade of cellular events, these receptors are viewed as chemical "amplifiers" through which signals initiated by neurotransmitter binding result in profound and sometimes prolonged changes in the receiving cell, including changes in electrical excitability.

There are other varieties of receptors in addition to these two classes of receptors. For example, the TRK receptors ("tyrosine receptor kinases") bind specific growth factors, such as NGF and BDNF. An activated TRK receptor phosphorylates intracellular proteins at tyrosine residues, resulting in a cascade of changes in the cell that ultimately affect gene expression. As noted previously, some membrane and intracellular receptors bind to hormones. This vast array of transmitters and receptors provides tools that allow neurons to interact with other cells in a variety of ways. As discussed in Chapter 6, learning, memory, and thinking all derive from the ability of neurons to interact with each other and modify their structural and functional connections.

NEUROTRANSMITTERS AND SYNAPSES: COMPLEX SIGNALING DEVICES

Neurotransmitter–receptor systems are actually much more complex than we have indicated in these simple descriptions. Many receptors, including ionotropic receptors, are only one component of intracellular signaling networks that include many other proteins. For example, ionotropic NMDA receptors are likely part of a network involving perhaps 100 or more proteins that are linked either directly or indirectly to the receptor itself. Some of these other proteins use the calcium signals triggered by NMDA receptors to activate chemical reactions, including protein kinases, protein phosphatases, and others. These chemical reactions in turn influence other cellular proteins to drive intracellular changes that result in LTP, long-term depression (LTD), and metaplasticity. In Chapter 3, we described how small-world and scale-free networks in the brain are likely to operate as part of intrinsic connectivity networks (ICNs). An interesting feature of receptor-linked protein networks as well as other intracellular protein networks (e.g., networks governing metabolism and gene expression) is that they also appear to have a scale-free organization, with a few highly connected molecules serving as critical nodes that facilitate the activity of the entire protein network. Also, some molecules within the network, either by their own movement within the cell or by their activation of other proteins, provide longer-range connections within the cell and transmit signals back to the nucleus or to other organelles, giving these protein networks small-world characteristics as well.

Receptors for neurotransmitters are typically found at synapses, the points of close contact between neurons where most intercellular communication occurs. Here, electrical activity (an action potential) in a sending neuron (the presynaptic cell) invades its own nerve terminals (called synaptic boutons) and triggers the calcium-dependent release of neurotransmitter from synaptic vesicles. The nature of the molecular machinery governing release of neurotransmitters from synaptic vesicles is being worked out in exquisite detail and is described by what is referred to as the "SNARE" hypothesis (named after "soluble NSF attachment protein receptors"). In this scheme, specific proteins regulate the uptake and storage of transmitter in vesicles (vesicular transporters), the calcium-dependent docking of vesicles at the cell membrane of the presynaptic terminal, the formation of pores through which the transmitter is actually released into the synaptic cleft (the small space that separates presynaptic and postsynaptic cells), and the recycling of synaptic vesicles for subsequent rounds of neurotransmission. Key molecules in the release of transmitters include v-(vesicle)-SNARES such as VAMP (vesicle-associated membrane protein, also known as synaptobrevin) and the synaptotagmins, and t-(target)-SNARES at cell membranes, including syntaxin and SNAP-25. Other molecules (e.g., Munc proteins) appear to facilitate interactions between vesicles and plasma membranes. Some evidence indicates that the synaptotagmins serve as calcium sensors that link calcium influx into presynaptic terminals to transmitter release. The actual fusion pore through which transmitter is released appears to be formed by a combination of vesicle (perhaps synaptophysin) and plasma membrane proteins.

Once released, the transmitter diffuses across the synaptic cleft to act on specific receptors in the postsynaptic receiving neuron. Transmitter receptors are expressed in both the postsynaptic neuron and the presynaptic neuron. They are also found in regions outside of the synapse (called extrasynaptic receptors) and can be present on non-neuronal cells (glia or blood vessels, for example). All of these receptors have a major impact on how neurotransmitters operate and how the brain functions. Other important synaptic molecules, including extracellular matrix proteins, such as the neurexins, and neuroligans, help hook synapses together physically. In some cases, these molecules involve direct protein–protein interactions between the presynaptic and postsynaptic neurons.

The actions of neurotransmitters are terminated by several processes. These include simple diffusion away from the site of action following unbinding from their receptor. Most transmitters are then taken up into nerve terminals or glia by the actions of specific cell membrane transporters that use ionic gradients to drive movement of the transmitter molecule into the cell. Some transmitters are degraded by specific enzymes; for example, acetylcholine is degraded by acetylcholinesterase.

Some of the genetic findings in neuropsychiatric disorders involve these signaling molecules. A recent study of the human postsynaptic density indicated the presence of over 1,400 proteins at these sites of synaptic contact; over 130 of these already have a link to neurological or psychiatric disorders. The point of this discussion is that the molecular machinery governing presynaptic and postsynaptic function is extremely intricate, and the various proteins involved are subject to genetic mutations that can have profound effects on synaptic function. It is beyond the scope of this text to discuss this cellular machinery in great detail. Based on the simple account we have given, it should be clear that synaptic transmission is likely to involve hundreds of proteins or more. Understanding the detailed role of each of these proteins is complicated and of interest primarily to synaptic neurobiologists. Nevertheless, many of the genes now being linked to psychiatric disorders involve this complex cellular machinery regulating synaptic transmission and synaptic plasticity. Given the complexity, it is extremely difficult for clinicians to keep up to date with the latest findings. Instead, we suggest that clinicians focus on understanding how brain synapses and ICNs work at a more global level and how the treatments they use in everyday practice are likely to alter synaptic function and excitability. It is at this level that we believe the most relevant clinical understanding of drug mechanisms, genetics, and other therapeutic interventions will occur.

TRANSMITTERS, SYNAPSES, AND BRAIN RHYTHMS

To do its job in producing the mind, the brain makes use of electrical, synaptic, and intercellular signals to coordinate activity within local areas and across distributed neural networks. The mechanisms underlying the "mind" are unlikely to reside in the properties of single neurons or single brain regions but rather reflect properties emerging from intraregional and interregional computations. As noted earlier, this is a daunting task, and one way the brain accomplishes this is through rhythmic oscillations in neural activity. Brain activity is known to fluctuate over a range of about 0.01 to 500 Hz (cycles per second). Clinicians are familiar with many of these, including delta (1 to 3 Hz), theta (4 to 7 Hz), alpha (8 to 13 Hz), beta (14 to 30 Hz), and gamma (more than 30 Hz) rhythms. Additionally, very-low-frequency oscillations in resting state BOLD fMRI signals (less than 0.1 Hz) seem to underlie the workings of ICNs. These various rhythms are important because they provide substrates for energy-efficient temporal coordination within and among brain regions, reflecting the interplay of intrinsic cellular properties and circuit properties. As discussed by Pascal Fries, gamma-band synchronization, a rhythm that is disrupted in schizophrenia, seems to play a fundamental role in cross-regional communications within neocortex. This rhythm is thought to provide a means by which the many convergent inputs to a neuron (Chapter 6) can be segmented functionally and selected for use, allowing neurons to overcome the confusion that can arise from having a lot of impinging inputs. An example is the observation that fast gamma oscillations in the CA1 hippocampal region preferentially synchronize with fast gamma inputs coming directly from entorhinal cortex, while slow gamma oscillations in CA1 synchronize with slow gamma oscillations flowing from area CA3 in the trisynaptic pathway. This helps to determine the inputs to which a CA1 neuron pays attention. Rhythms of various frequencies also interact with and modulate each other. An example is the ability of theta rhythms in the hippocampus to influence the effects of gamma-frequency inputs. Here the timing of a gamma input relative to the theta cycle can determine the type of synaptic plasticity that results. Input at the peak of a theta cycle strengthens synaptic connections via LTP, while input at the trough of a cycle results in synaptic weakening via LTD.

Importantly, in a brain with many different neuronal types and transmitters, excitatory (glutamate-using) pyramidal neurons are the principal drivers of local activity. However, it is the interplay of these excitatory neurons with GABAergic interneurons that sculpts output into specific frequencies. Although interneurons are fewer in number than excitatory neurons (only about 10% to 20% of all cortical neurons are interneurons), there is a large diversity among interneurons that provides an amazing degree of flexibility in regulating regional activity. For example, in the CA1 region alone, at least 21 different types of interneurons help to orchestrate the activity of a pyramidal neuron. All of these neurons are also influenced by a diverse array of slow neurotransmitters using mechanisms described above. The yin and yang among transmitter systems and intrinsic neuronal properties ultimately result in network oscillations that foster feed-forward coincidence detection and input gain modulation. In mental terms, coordinated humming across brain regions appears to provide a neural substrate for binding information together in states of alertness, perception, attention, memory, motivation, and mood.

WHY ANTIDEPRESSANTS TAKE TIME TO WORK WHILE BENZODIAZEPINE ANXIOLYTICS ACT QUICKLY

The previous discussion provides an introduction to the world of neurotransmitters. This information is important because many treatments used in psychiatry, including all psychotherapeutic medications, involve manipulation of chemical transmitter or signaling systems. Thus, understanding how these drugs work clinically requires some understanding of how neurons and synapses operate. It is important to emphasize, however, that the phenotypic expressions of psychiatric disorders reflect problems of neural networks. Simplified explanations about how psychotropic drugs work on specific synapses and cells are useful, but they are not mechanistic explanations about the factors underlying aberrant thinking, mood, and motivation.

Clinically, it is well known that antidepressants often take several weeks to work. When a person with major depression is feeling down, he or she cannot just pop an antidepressant and start to feel better within a few minutes, hours, or even days. In contrast, if a person becomes very anxious when traveling by airplane, he or she can take a benzodiazepine-type anxiolytic such as diazepam (Valium) or lorazepam (Ativan) and become much calmer within half an hour. Why is there such a difference in the time it takes these two kinds of drugs to work? Although we don't know the answer for certain, information about transmitters, receptors, and signal transduction can help us better understand the differences between these two categories of medication.

Depression is defined by consistent and persistent changes in mood, thinking, and behavior that typically last for weeks, months, and sometimes years. When a person develops major depressive disorder, brain systems that control attention, reward mechanisms, cognition, and emotion malfunction (Chapter 5), leading to a diverse group of symptoms. Although antidepressants aren't miracle drugs, they can gradually alleviate most if not all symptoms over a period of several weeks to several months. The robustness of the benefit can be augmented with various types of informal and formal psychotherapies as well as lifestyle interventions such as exercise, sleep hygiene, and perhaps diet. What do antidepressants do and why do they take so long to work? For illustrative purposes, we will examine selective serotonin reuptake inhibitors (SSRIs) as one category of antidepressants. Many of the other categories of antidepressants have similar effects.

As noted, one major way that the brain resets itself once a transmitter is released is by removing the transmitter from the synaptic cleft and recycling it for future use. At synapses that use serotonin as their transmitter, a serotonin transporter serves this function and transports released serotonin back into the presynaptic cell. A "transporter" is a membrane protein that uses ions and ionic gradients to drive the uptake of the transmitter; this clean-up function provided by transporters is part of the tightly regulated life cycle of serotonin. SSRI medications block the reuptake of serotonin by the serotonin transporter. In a test tube, this inhibition of reuptake occurs rapidly, as soon as the SSRI binds to the transporter. Therefore, soon after a person takes the medication, more of the serotonin released from the presynaptic terminal by an action potential remains floating in the extracellular synaptic region as a result of the blockade of reuptake. The increased amount of serotonin leads to increased stimulation of the various serotonin receptors (maybe up to 20 different types by present count). The enhanced stimulation of serotonin receptors leads to postsynaptic, intracellular, chemical events that include increased formation of second-messenger molecules within the receiving cell. All of these events occur rapidly. Importantly, however, these second-messenger chemicals then lead to changes of various other intracellular chemicals that influence the genetic apparatus of the neuron to produce diverse effects. Other intracellular modulators, including growth factors, may be produced. The production of growth factors eventually leads to structural changes in the cell, including an increase in cell size and changes in the number of synaptic connections and receptors expressed on the cell surface. These structural changes take time and eventually translate into functional modifications of cellular connections.

Although speculative, it is possible that these cellular changes help to correct specific functional deficits in brain systems that may be perturbed by the underlying cause of the depression. Alternatively, these changes may simply compensate for the defects in cellular/synaptic function. In other words, the drug-induced changes may have nothing to do with the underlying defect that causes depression but rather help to reset cells and ICNs to function more effectively. Support for this latter explanation comes from the finding that SSRIs (and almost all other antidepressant medications and electroconvulsive therapy) increase the generation of new neurons in the dentate gyrus of the hippocampus. Present data suggest that a defect in neurogenesis is probably not the cause of depression, yet the birth and development of new dentate neurons help to correct defects within the hippocampal network and, in turn, within distributed neural circuits (Chapter 6). Importantly, it takes time for structural changes to occur and for new, functionally helpful cellular connections to be established. The effectiveness of antidepressant medications suggests that depression may involve problems with communication between cells in certain brain systems that may be partially remedied by the enhanced growth potential that antidepressants facilitate. The structural modifications that are necessary to mend the abnormal circuitry causing illness take time to correct.

The effects described for SSRIs are not restricted to this class of drugs and likely reflect the actions of most chemical antidepressants as well as other drugs used to treat psychiatric disorders (e.g., antipsychotic medications and mood stabilizers). The brain regions, transmitter systems, specific synapses, and chemical cascades involved differ among drug types, but the principles underlying acute drug effects leading to long-lived changes in neuronal structure and function are shared across drug classes. Furthermore, the same types of long-lived changes are also likely to occur with many classes of abused drugs. Addictive drugs tend to attack the brain's reward and motivation systems, and the longer-lived drug effects associated with their chronic use and abuse are among the reasons that substance-abuse syndromes are so difficult to treat clinically and so prone to relapse.

What about the person who experiences rapid relief of airplane-associated anxiety following ingestion of a benzodiazepine? In this case, the symptoms are acute and are brought on by exposure to a situation that the person finds anxiety-provoking. The anxiety is likely caused by situation-induced stimulation of fear/anxiety circuitry mediated in part by the extended amygdala and modified by activity of other brain regions such as the locus coeruleus (LC) and by the release of the neurotransmitter norepinephrine from the terminals of LC neurons distributed widely throughout the brain. Certain types of GABA receptors (called GABA-A receptors) inhibit the LC and the amygdala and help to keep neurons in these regions in check. As we have noted, GABA-A receptors are ionotropic receptors that respond to the neurotransmitter GABA by opening a channel to the flow of chloride ions. Influx of these negatively charged anions hyperpolarizes the cell, effectively inhibiting the neuron and making it harder for it to fire action potentials (and thus to release its neurotransmitter onto other neurons). Benzodiazepines enhance the activity of GABA-A receptors. When a benzodiazepine enters the brain, it rapidly binds to a portion of the GABA-A receptor complex known as the benzodiazepine binding site (sometimes called the benzodiazepine "receptor" just to make matters more confusing). Once bound, the benzodiazepine rapidly augments the GABA-A receptor's response to GABA; that is, when GABA binds its receptor at a time when the benzodiazepine is also bound to the GABA receptor complex, more chloride is able to enter the cell in response to GABA. This enhanced chloride influx rapidly results in more powerful inhibitory effects on the neuron receiving the GABA signal from the interneurons that release GABA.

Importantly, the effects of benzodiazepines require only that the benzodiazepine bind the GABA-A receptor and that GABA activates its ion channel. Once both GABA and a benzodiazepine are bound, the GABA-A receptor chloride channels open more effectively, hyperpolarizing the neuron; no second messenger, growth factor, or gene expression is needed. Such effects immediately influence the brain regions that are involved in anxiety, including the LC and the amygdala. The anxiety-provoking situation activates the amygdala, an area involved in activating other brain regions that lead to the subjective feeling and the physical manifestations of nervousness (increased heart rate and respiration, and sweating). The benzodiazepine quiets these effects by dampening the activity and output of amygdala neurons. Since the symptoms result from acute activation of this system and benzodiazepines produce immediate changes in GABA channels, the clinical effects of a benzodiazepine are rapid; there is no need for structural changes. Thus, a benzodiazepine can be a "prn" (taken as needed) type of medication, whereas an antidepressant requires continuous and prolonged use in order to be effective.

As we have seen, both SSRIs and benzodiazepines have clear acute effects on neurons and synapses. In the case of the benzodiazepines, the acute actions are all that is needed to provide symptomatic relief: the chloride channels work more effectively as soon as a benzodiazepine is present. In the case of the SSRIs, the acute effects are only the beginning and are not enough to produce significant clinical benefits. Why this is the case is not entirely clear, but the difference between drugs affecting the serotonin and GABA systems highlighted here may have a lot to do with how these transmitter systems influence brain systems. GABA acting at GABA-A receptors is a classic fast neurotransmitter, and serotonin is typically a diffusely acting, slower neuromodulator. All drugs, however, can have long-term effects, including changes in receptor numbers and neuronal structure. Thus, when benzodiazepines are used for longer periods of time to treat chronic anxiety symptoms or insomnia, they also produce compensatory cellular changes that lead to tolerance, dependence, and withdrawal symptoms when suddenly discontinued. This is the reason that the dose of benzodiazepines should be gradually tapered before being discontinued after chronic use. The gradual decrease in dose allows the brain and body to reset more gradually to the absence of the drug. Again, this effect is not unique to benzodiazepines, and gradually tapering the dose of all psychotropic medications used for longer-term treatment is generally recommended when it comes time to discontinue the medication.

In summary, transmitters and receptors are the tools brain cells use to communicate. Such cell-to-cell communications can influence the connectivity between components of neural systems. Changes in the connectivity of neural systems can be important in reversing clinical symptoms of illnesses, but such changes can take time to develop, which contributes to the time lag associated with the effectiveness of certain medications like antidepressants.

Points to Remember

Neurotransmitters vary greatly in chemical structure, ranging from small (low-molecular-weight) molecules to larger (higher-molecular-weight) peptides.

Some neurons release slow-acting neurotransmitters to wide areas of the brain. These slow-acting transmitters help to organize activity within and across regions of the brain and influence the responsiveness of cells to other, more locally acting fast transmitters. In effect, the broadly released neurotransmitters "set the gain" of cells and modulate the way the receiving cells respond to other transmitters.

Some neurotransmitters act more locally and rapidly and convey very specific information to a smaller number of cells.

Two broad classes of neurotransmitter receptors are ionotropic receptors and metabotropic receptors. These two groups have different chemical structures and, in general, work at different speeds.

Psychiatric medications influence neurotransmitters and receptors. Some medications lead to slow, long-term changes in structure and function; other medications acutely influence a particular function for a brief period of time.

SUGGESTED READINGS

Fries, P. (2009). Neuronal gamma-band synchronization as a fundamental process in cortical computations. *Annual Review of Neuroscience, 32,* 209–224.

McClung, C. A., & Nestler, E. J. (2008). Neuroplasticity mediated by altered gene expression. *Neuropsychopharmacology Reviews, 33,* 3–17.

Pittenger, C., & Duman, R. S. (2008). Stress, depression and neuroplasticity: A convergence of mechanisms. *Neuropsychopharmacology Reviews, 33,* 88–109.

Zorumski, C. F., Isenberg, K. E., & Mennerick, S. (2009). Cellular and synaptic electrophysiology. In B. J. Sadock, V. A. Sadock, & P. Ruiz (Eds.), *Kaplan and Sadock's comprehensive textbook of psychiatry* (9th ed., pp. 129–147). Baltimore, MD: Lippincott Williams and Wilkins.

OTHER REFERENCES

Airan, R. D., Meltzer, L. A., Roy, M., Gong, Y., Chen, H., & Deisseroth, K. (2007). High-speed imaging reveals neurophysiological links to behavior in an animal model of depression. *Science, 317,* 819–823.

Bayes, A., & Grant, S. G. N. (2009). Neuroproteomics: Understanding the molecular organization and complexity of the brain. *Nature Reviews Neuroscience, 10,* 635–646.

Bayes, A., van de Lagemaat, L. N., Collins, M. O., Croning, M. D. R., Whittle, I. R., Choudhary, J. S., et al. (2011). Characterization of the proteome, diseases and evolution of the human postsynaptic density. *Nature Neuroscience, 14,* 19–21.

Buzsaki, G., & Draguhn, A. (2004). Neuronal oscillations in cortical networks. *Science, 304,* 1926–1929.

Colgin, L. L., Denninger, T., Fyhn, M., Hafting, T., Bonnevie, T., Jensen, O., et al. (2009). Frequency of gamma oscillations routes flow of information in the hippocampus. *Nature, 462,* 353–357.

Di Marzo, V. (2011). Endocannabinoid signaling in the brain: Biosynthetic mechanisms in the limelight. *Nature Neuroscience, 14,* 9–15.

Grant, S. G. N., & O'Dell, T. J. (2001). Multiprotein complex signaling and the plasticity problem. *Current Opinion in Neurobiology, 11,* 363–368.

Klausberger, T., & Somogyi, P (2008). Neuronal diversity and temporal dynamics: The unity of hippocampal circuit operations. *Science, 321,* 53–57.

Krishnan, V., & Nestler, E. J. (2008). The molecular neurobiology of depression. *Nature, 455,* 894–902.

Madden, D. R. (2002). The structure and function of glutamate receptor ion channels. *Nature Reviews Neuroscience, 3,* 91–101.

McKernan, R. M., Rosahl, T. W., Reynolds, D. S., Sur, C., Wafford, K. A., Atack, J. R., et al. (2000). Sedative but not anxiolytic properties of benzodiazepines are mediated by the $GABA_A$ receptor α1 subunit. *Nature Neuroscience, 3,* 587–592.

Moore, C. I., Carlen, M., Knoblich, L., & Cardin, J. A. (2010). Neocortical interneurons: From diversity, strength. *Cell, 142,* 184–188.

Nemeroff, C. B. (2003). The role of GABA in the pathophysiology and treatment of anxiety disorders. *Psychopharmacology Bulletin, 37,* 133–146.

Nourry, C., Grant, S. G., & Borg, J. P. (2003). PDZ domain proteins: Plug and play. *Science STKE, 179,* RE7.

Ravasz, E., Somera, A. L., Mongru, D. A., Oltvai, Z. N., & Barabasi, A.-L. (2002). Hierarchical organization of modularity in metabolic networks. *Science, 297,* 1551–1555.

Sahay, A., & Hen, R. (2007). Adult hippocampal neurogenesis in depression. *Nature Neuroscience, 10,* 1110–1115.

Sudhof, T. C. (2004). The synaptic vesicle cycle. *Annual Review of Neuroscience, 27,* 509–547.

11

Methods of Determining Diagnosis and Cause

Diagnosis is critical for all fields of medicine, including psychiatry. A valid diagnosis is the best predictor of both the future course of illness and response to various treatments. Thus, one of the primary goals of psychiatric evaluation is to determine the most appropriate diagnosis. A related goal is the determination of the specific biological cause of the diagnosis in an individual patient, to the extent that this is possible given the current state of knowledge. Armed with an accurate diagnosis and specific cause, the clinician can design a treatment regimen that best meets the needs of the patient. We believe that the clinical picture, the phenotypic manifestation of an illness, will be best understood by determining which brain systems are malfunctioning and how they are malfunctioning. This knowledge will be driven by clarifying the anatomy and function of the brain's intrinsic connectivity networks (ICNs) in conjunction with understanding the cellular, synaptic, and molecular mechanisms that result in network dysfunction. As research advances in describing the specific brain mechanisms that result in dysfunction, more specific treatments will be developed. Approaches to determining diagnoses and causes are likely to evolve rapidly as the neurosciences progress. In this chapter, we will focus on methods used to make and validate psychiatric diagnoses. First, we will review current methods, and then we will speculate about approaches that might be used in the future. Once again we will use Alzheimer's disease and frontotemporal dementias as examples of illnesses that provide glimpses into the future for understanding traditional psychiatric symptoms and disorders.

CURRENT METHODS OF DIAGNOSIS

By far the most important tool for establishing a psychiatric diagnosis is the clinical interview and examination of the patient. The clinical interview uses highly complex and sophisticated technology: the skills, intelligence, and experience housed in the brains of well-trained psychiatrists. In our earlier book *Demystifying Psychiatry*, we described typical psychiatric evaluations in some detail. The psychiatrist frequently interviews both the patient and a collateral source familiar with the patient's history and behavior. Collateral information from family or caregivers, as well as from previous psychiatrists and therapists, is of fundamental importance in ensuring that the clinical history is reliable and valid. In these interviews, the clinician asks a variety of questions designed to elicit symptoms and determine the significance of these symptoms with regard to severity, impact on the person's life, and temporal course.

Ultimately, the clinician must judge whether or not the symptoms meet diagnostic criteria summarized in DSM-IV. A mistake often made by inexperienced psychiatrists is to take normal variants of behavior and try to pigeonhole them into clinically relevant categories. A clinically relevant symptom is one that is outside the realm of normal and has significant dysfunction or disability associated with it. As an example, consider sadness immediately following the death of a loved one. This response is almost universal among humans and by itself is not indicative of psychiatric illness. However, a disabling sadness that persists for months or longer following the death of a loved one, particularly when associated with other depressive symptoms, including weight loss, sleep disturbance, and suicidal ideas, strongly suggests a major depression. Some symptoms almost always indicate disorder. For example, intrusive psychotic symptoms associated with dysfunction and disabilities are always outside the realm of normality.

In addition to gathering an in-depth history from the patient and ancillary sources, the clinician conducts a careful examination of the patient. As described in Chapter 1, the psychiatric examination emphasizes evaluation of the patient's appearance, behavior, speech and language, flow of thought, thought content, mood and affect, insight and judgment, and cognitive domains such as attention, memory, orientation, general knowledge, and abstract reasoning. When there is consistency between the information gathered from the history and the signs demonstrated by the patient, a diagnosis can be made based on specific criteria.

DSM-IV is the current standard for making psychiatric diagnoses. The diagnostic criteria in DSM-IV were derived from clinical research and expert clinical opinion. For the most part, the current criteria are based on studies demonstrating that certain symptoms seem to occur together over extended periods of time and have characteristic patterns of fluctuation or consistency. Once psychiatric disorders were defined in this way using specific criteria, epidemiologic studies could be designed to determine the incidence and prevalence of the disorders in the population. It is important to emphasize that the use of diagnostic criteria for categorizing psychiatric disorders was a major advance in the field and the criteria are currently being refined based on advancing research. The criteria in DSM-IV are highly reliable, meaning that for most disorders there is excellent agreement among psychiatrists about the presence or absence of a disorder in individual patients. Establishing the validity of these diagnostic categories has been much more problematic, however. Validity, in this case, refers to the ability of a diagnosis to predict the underlying pathological mechanisms leading to illness. As we have noted throughout this book, pathological validity has not been established for any primary psychiatric disorder and, at present, there are no meaningful biomarkers for any of these disorders. This does not mean that all psychiatric diagnoses are invalid; rather, the methods used to establish the validity of today's psychiatric diagnoses are still relatively crude and largely based on clinical criteria proposed by Eli Robins and Sam Guze in the early 1970s. These include clear descriptions of symptoms that cluster together, the ability to delimit one disorder from another, the consistency of the syndrome over time, and family history, the latter reflecting the fact that these syndromes tend to run in families. Up to the present time, tools have not been available to verify if these defined syndromes are consistent with specific brain pathology, dysfunction in specific brain systems, or specific biomarkers. On the other hand, the clinical definitions of syndromes such as dementia of the Alzheimer's type (DAT) and behavioral variant frontotemporal dementia (FTD) appear to correlate with pathology in specific brain networks, and it is becoming increasingly likely that clinicians will be able to combine clinical descriptions with functional brain imaging and clinically relevant biomarkers to aid in the diagnosis of these disorders. Whether this will be true for traditional psychiatric disorders is more speculative.

The problem of establishing validity for psychiatric disorders has been pushed to the forefront by advances in genetics and neuroimaging. Studies in these disciplines highlight considerable overlap among current syndromes. Compounding this, it is not clear that many current diagnostic categories have natural boundaries that separate them (so-called "zones of rarity" between the disorders). As we argued earlier in this book, major psychiatric disorders affect all aspects of mind, and thus shared neural circuitry is to be expected. This, however, does confound the ability to use neuroimaging to delimit disorders, although this still remains possible. These considerations and others have led some to champion the idea of diagnostic "utility" rather than validity. In the words of Robert Kendell and Assen Jablensky, a diagnosis has utility "if it provides nontrivial information about prognosis, likely treatment outcomes and/or testable propositions about biological and social correlates." In this sense many, but not all, current psychiatric diagnoses are useful but not necessarily valid. Advances in biology may be the only ticket out of this conundrum.

We want to end this brief discussion about diagnosis with a few comments about the importance of understanding the longitudinal course of psychiatric disorders. As noted already, the long-term course of illness (consistency over time) is one of the major criteria currently used to validate a disorder. Some illnesses, such as schizophrenia, tend to have a chronic life-long course; although there may be periods of symptom remission, the disorder rarely, perhaps never, "goes away." Other disorders, particularly many of the mood disorders, tend to be more episodic, meaning that they exhibit discrete periods of weeks or longer when symptoms are significant separated by periods when symptoms are in remission. This waxing and waning course describes the longitudinal pattern of many psychiatric disorders. Alcoholism is a good example. Even when not drinking, an alcoholic is considered to be in "recovery," not well or cured. The mechanisms and vulnerabilities underlying the person's alcoholism have not disappeared. We emphasize these points because we believe they are relevant to understanding the brain mechanisms that produce illness. Once a psychiatric disorder has developed, the ICNs involved in the disorder often remain impaired or at least vulnerable for life. We don't know why this is the case, but deciphering the responsible mechanisms could go a long way toward devising more effective treatment and prevention strategies. We would also emphasize that having a preexisting psychiatric disorder often makes an individual vulnerable to other disorders and that the presence of a preexisting psychiatric disorder colors the clinical picture and course of the second disorder. For example, an individual with alcoholism is at risk for major depression and vice versa. Furthermore, an alcoholic who subsequently develops major depression likely has a form of depression that differs from an individual who has experienced only episodes of depression (Chapter 2).

These points are important to consider when investigating the underlying brain mechanisms contributing to illness in a given individual and for disentangling the biology of one disorder from another. We would also emphasize that the recurrent and sometimes chronic nature of psychiatric disorders suggests that the neural circuitry involved in these disorders becomes more complex over time. This is most clearly seen in the substance-abuse disorders (Chapter 5), but we believe it is also the case in other psychiatric illnesses. Early in substance-abuse syndromes, the abused drugs attack a specific neural system (the dopamine motivation/reward system). Over time, however, symptoms become more complex and result in a "neurocognitive" disorder. The evolution of more complex circuitry involving a widening collection of ICNs over time is a likely driver of the fact that there is so much shared neural circuitry among psychiatric disorders. For this reason, we believe it is important to understand the earliest manifestations of a particular patient's illness and the progression of symptoms and dysfunction over time. From a research standpoint, we believe that the best hope for disentangling the circuits involved in psychiatric disorders will come from studies done very early in the course of illness, before brain plasticity and network interactions have had a chance to make things extremely complicated. This includes a focus on antecedents arising in childhood and adolescence.

CURRENT USE OF LABORATORY AND IMAGING PROCEDURES

In current psychiatric practice, the primary use of laboratory tests and imaging procedures is to determine whether medical or neurological conditions are contributing to psychiatric symptoms. Because the biological "cause" of any primary psychiatric disorder has yet to be defined, laboratory and imaging procedures are used to rule in or rule out potential non-psychiatric causes of the symptoms. For example, it is fairly routine practice to evaluate thyroid function in patients with new onset of anxiety and/or depressive symptoms. If a person has markedly elevated thyroid function, then the psychiatric disorder may be a result of the hyperthyroidism. In such a situation, a psychiatrist would likely refer the patient to a primary care physician and follow the patient in collaboration with the internist or endocrinologist while the thyroid illness is being treated. Depending on the severity of the depression, a decision may be made to treat the psychiatric symptoms while the abnormal thyroid function is brought under control. Often, but not always, anxiety or depressive symptoms remit as hyperthyroidism is effectively treated. Psychiatrists use a variety of laboratory tests to help evaluate medical causes of psychiatric symptoms; examples of such tests are found in standard psychiatry textbooks.

Psychiatrists may also use imaging tests and x-rays to help rule out medical or neurological causes of psychiatric symptoms. Computed tomography (CT) scans or nuclear magnetic resonance imaging (MRI) scans are done to determine whether disorders such as strokes, brain tumors, or other structural brain changes are associated with the behavioral changes elicited in the clinical examination. In general, these procedures are not performed to rule in a primary psychiatric illness; rather, they are done to exclude a neurological or medical disorder that may underlie the symptoms. Parallel statements can be made about the use of electroencephalograms (EEG) and procedures such as lumbar punctures (LP) and evaluation of cerebrospinal fluid (CSF).

Many imaging procedures being studied today have potential to be useful to psychiatrists in the future. These include functional imaging procedures such as BOLD (blood oxygen level dependent) functional MRI (fMRI), functional connectivity MRI (fcMRI), diffusion tensor imaging (DTI), magnetic resonance spectroscopy (MRS), positron emission tomography (PET) imaging, single photon emission computerized tomography (SPECT), and receptor imaging. At the current time, these procedures are used only in psychiatric research and have not yet found their way into clinical practice.

CURRENT USE OF PSYCHOLOGICAL TESTING

A large array of psychological tests can be performed to help clarify diagnostic issues or to aid clinicians in obtaining a better understanding of their patients. These procedures do not substitute for careful diagnostic interviews; rather, they provide supplemental information that can help identify, and at times quantify, aspects of a patient's symptoms. For example, cognitive testing can help establish the functional defects that may occur in various forms of dementia or other cognition-impairing disorders. Such testing may include evaluations of declarative memory, working memory, executive function, language, and attention. Examples of tests used to screen for cognitive dysfunction include brief instruments such as the Mini-Mental Status Examination (MMSE) and the Short Blessed Test. More extensive tests include the Wechsler Adult Intelligence Scale (WAIS), the Halstead-Reitan Battery, and the Luria Nebraska Battery. These latter tests, particularly the Halstead-Reitan and Luria batteries, are generally administered and interpreted by neuropsychologists and can be used to help localize cognitive deficits to regions of the brain and to specific neural networks.

Certain psychological tests, such as the Minnesota Multiphasic Personality Inventory (MMPI), may help determine whether a person is malingering. This type of test also may provide supportive information about various personality traits and may help to support diagnostic impressions. Typically, consultation with a psychologist skilled in interpretation of the MMPI is necessary to obtain maximal benefit from this test. Similarly, there are several personality inventories that provide information about personality traits. Cloninger's Temperament and Character Inventory (TCI) or Costa and McCrae's revised NEO (neuroticism, extroversion, and openness) Personality Inventory are two examples. These inventories provide information that may help a psychiatrist better understand the personality characteristics of a patient;

for instance, the results may aid in predicting how a person copes with stressors or how a patient may react to various treatments. Although they can supply helpful information, psychological and personality tests are not substitutes for careful clinical interviews.

We have described tests that have been studied extensively in large groups of individuals and have reasonable reliability and validity. Not all psychological tests have undergone such evaluation, however, and there are many tests that have poor reliability and validity, and fall into the realm of pseudoscience. Examples include projective tests such as the Rorschach Inkblot Test, the Thematic Apperception Test, and some of the tests designed to elicit histories of sexual abuse. Clinicians who use psychological testing should become very familiar with the tests they use and understand the degree to which they are reliable and valid. Consultation with experienced psychologists and neuropsychologists can be extremely helpful in dealing with these issues.

FUTURE APPROACHES TO DIAGNOSIS

We hope that, at some point in the foreseeable future, advances in systems neuro-sciences will provide psychiatrists with the ability to diagnose disorders based on symptoms that are understood at the level of malfunctioning brain systems. In addition, with the aid of illness- or symptom-specific biomarkers, psychiatrists will likely be better able to determine biological mechanisms contributing to malfunc-tioning brain systems that are responsible for the primary psychiatric disorder. Advances in areas such as pharmacogenetics, neurocognitive testing, and personality measurement have the potential to lead to the development of improved personalized treatment plans, taking into account an individual patient's likelihood of therapeutic response to specific treatments and relative risk of side effects.

We are optimistic about the future in part because of the rapid progress being made in understanding Alzheimer's disease at the level of systems and molecular neuroscience. Based on studies using functional connectivity MRI and PET to examine the distribution of amyloid in the brain, it is now known that the earliest symptoms of Alzheimer's disease likely involve malfunctioning of the default-mode ICN (Chapter 2). Amyloid plaques and neurofibrillary tangles accumulate in key major hubs of this network, including retrosplenial cortex, precuneus, and medial temporal lobe. It is important to note, however, that the build-up of plaques and tangles represents only one pathological process leading to the clinical syndrome called DAT. Other pathological insults may also cause malfunctioning of the default system and lead to symptoms that would be diagnosed as DAT based on clinical presentation. For instance, a combination of hippocampal sclerosis and micro-vascular lesions in the default network may produce a clinical picture consistent with DAT. Thus, two very different molecular/pathological processes could both lead to the same phenotypic picture because they both target functioning of the default system. The specific treatments of the clinical syndrome resulting from these two causes are likely to be different, however. In the first example, therapies that interfere with the formation or turnover of the beta-amyloid and *tau* proteins involved in the pathogenesis of plaques and tangles would be appropriate. In the second instance, minimizing or reversing the processes that lead to microvascular lesions would be appropriate. This might be accomplished by treating hypertension, diabetes, or hyperlipidemias, and possibly by utilizing strategies to enhance cerebral blood flow. Rehabilitative therapies aimed at ameliorating cognitive and behavioral deficits would be helpful in either case because such therapies can help the brain find ways to work around the malfunctioning system. Some rehabilitative strategies are likely to be nonspecific. For instance, physical exercise, environmental enrichment, and a healthy nutritional program would likely benefit patients with either pathology. Some rehabilitative approaches may specifically take advantage of knowledge of the default system and possible ways to circumvent specific defects in cognitive function. These approaches may utilize behavioral or computer-based strategies to compensate for the loss of function associated with damage to specific brain regions. The important point is that rehabilitative strategies will likely be similar for the two causes of dementia described here, whereas the treatment of the underlying cause would be different and based on molecular biomarkers and pathophysiology. Importantly, we believe that both specific mechanism-based therapies and personalized rehabilitative approaches will likely be required to achieve optimal outcomes. Similar strategies will likely be important for primary psychiatric disorders.

Advances in personalized medicine will also be important in maximizing therapeutic approaches. For example, it should be possible in the near future to measure an individual's pharmacogenetic profile. This information will be useful in selecting appropriate medications and in avoiding side effects and drug interactions. With respect to Alzheimer's disease, some persons have one or two copies of apolipoprotein E4 (apoE4), whereas others have copies of either apolipoprotein E3 or E2. Persons with one or especially two copies of apoE4 are at increased risk of developing late-onset Alzheimer's disease. It is possible that treatments will be developed that target the problems created by apoE4, and such treatments would be effective only in those persons carrying an apoE4 gene.

Based on this discussion, we envision a future diagnostic approach that would include illness phenotype, cause, and personalized information. For instance, using the two examples of phenotypic Alzheimer's disease just discussed, the categorization might be something like the following:

Case 1

Illness phenotype (clinical presentation): DAT

Cause (pathophysiology): Accumulation of amyloid visualized on PET neuroimaging using Pittsburgh Compound B or similar marker; abnormal levels of amyloid and *tau* in cerebrospinal fluid (CSF).

Personalized information: Apolipoprotein E4 (two copies) present; patient is also a slow metabolizer of drugs using the P450 2D6 liver enzyme.

Therapeutic approach: Gamma secretase inhibitors to diminish plaque formation coupled with immunotherapy to remove existing plaques. Rehabilitative efforts including a cognition-enhancing drug coupled with strategies and cognitive exercises to improve declarative memory formation, working memory, and attentional processing. Additional strategies would include a program of physical activity, enhanced socialization, and diet.

Case 2

Illness phenotype: DAT

Cause: Hippocampal sclerosis and microvascular pathology as determined by high-resolution MRI studies combined with quantitative volumetric measurements; plaque accumulation not observed on PET studies using Pittsburgh Compound B or similar marker.

Personalized information: Apolipoprotein E4 negative; hypertension and diabetes positive; high inflammatory factor profile.

Therapeutic approach: Treat hypertension and control diabetes mellitus. Anti-inflammatory strategies to diminish lesion extension. Rehabilitative efforts similar to Case 1, but personalized to the individual's level of function.

These examples assume that current research using PET scans to image amyloid deposition will prove to be reliable and valid. In addition, they assume that research demonstrating decreased CSF levels of amyloid and increased CSF levels of phosphorylated tau in persons with amyloid plaque accumulation is found to be reliable and valid. Although research involving these biomarkers is highly promising, measuring their levels as part of normal clinical practice is currently premature. We expect this to evolve rapidly over the next decade. Furthermore, advances in drug development will be required before we can provide targeted strategies to diminish plaque and tangle formation and to limit microvascular changes. None of these strategies is outside the realm of possibility, however, and drugs directed toward these aims are currently in development.

FUTURE TRENDS RELATED TO PSYCHIATRIC DIAGNOSES

As we have stated repeatedly, we believe that systems neuroscience and elucidation of the operations of ICNs in healthy persons and those with various psychiatric and neurological illnesses will help to establish which brain systems malfunction to cause specific symptoms. This is one of the results that could emerge from the Human Connectome Project, which will capitalize on evolving methodologies to identify and map the distribution and function of ICNs in healthy individuals. Armed with this information, it may be possible to identify connectivity phenotypes in individuals with a variety of neuropsychiatric disorders. Results from this type of research may lead to new diagnostic criteria based on symptom groupings that are most compatible with dysfunction of defined ICNs. Genetics research may also be useful in fine-tuning the criteria for various diagnoses. Disorders such as schizophrenia and bipolar disorder are classified as distinct illnesses in DSM-IV. As more is learned about overlapping genetic risks and, possibly, shared abnormalities in certain ICNs, there may be reasons to redefine these illnesses in a manner that is more compatible with the underlying pathophysiology. As more is learned about the relationship of ICNs to particular symptoms of psychiatric disease, including psychotic symptoms, cognitive symptoms, motivational symptoms, and various emotional symptoms, we should be able to develop a better understanding of symptom combinations and the comorbidity problem that currently plagues the field. It may turn out that the current phenotypic breakdown is fairly accurate for many illnesses. Evidence suggests this is the case for Alzheimer's disease and behavioral variant FTD. On the other hand, it may turn out that some disorders, including psychotic disorders and personality disorders, will undergo substantial modifications of diagnostic criteria. There is also interest in determining whether our current categorical approach to psychiatric diagnosis is appropriate or whether we should begin to consider at least some disorders from a dimensional perspective in which traits running in the population may influence and color the presentation of other disorders and even the definition of a disorder. The evolution of meaningful quantitative endophenotypes, including those derived from neuroimaging, could help push this forward.

The technologies that are currently used to define ICNs involve functional imaging procedures such as BOLD fMRI together with high-resolution structural MRI scans. These imaging methods provide high degrees of anatomical resolution along with the ability to analyze correlated oscillations in BOLD signals across brain regions, which are the basis for fMRI-based connectivity maps. To enhance the ability to study higher-frequency oscillations in neural activity across brain regions and networks, it should be possible to combine neuroimaging with high-resolution EEG and magnetoencephalography (MEG). The latter two methods provide enhanced temporal resolution, although the spatial resolution of subcortical structures is more limited. All of these techniques require advanced mathematical and statistical analyses to determine which parts of the brain work in concert to accomplish certain tasks. It is possible that advances in brain imaging and clinical electrophysiology will be combined with more sophisticated measures of other physiological parameters such as cardiac output, skin conductance, muscle tone, and regional cerebral blood flow to provide a more comprehensive analysis of brain and body physiology.

It is likely that certain brain regions of disease-specific interest will be discovered based on abnormal structure or function. Functional deficits may be determined by the demonstration of performance deficits on highly specific cognitive and emotional-processing paradigms. Examples of this include the use of functional imaging to detect changes in brain activity as humans interact with one another while participating in socioeconomic games. These complex games provide an opportunity for more sophisticated understanding of information processing in "real-world" settings and potential problems that arise from mental dysfunction. Such studies have already highlighted social-processing defects in subjects with borderline personality disorder, substance-dependence disorders, and autism. Specific brain regions pinpointed in these studies can be used as the seeds or pivot points for functional connectivity studies to determine how specific networks function in health and illness. Importantly, such strategies have the potential to produce more sophisticated conceptualizations of illnesses and more constructive rehabilitative strategies to help individuals cope with deficits in specific types of processing. For example, in some individuals with borderline personality disorder, defects in social reciprocity and emotional reactivity become most prominently manifest when cooperation with others breaks down. Such a finding could become the focus for therapeutic interventions targeting specific brain networks that process social and emotional information under specific circumstances. Importantly, viewing a personality disorder as an alteration in brain networks rather than a "character flaw" could go a long way toward diminishing the stigma, derision, and inappropriate treatments sometimes associated with these diagnoses.

Functional connectivity studies can also be performed in monozygotic and dizygotic twins who are concordant or discordant for the symptoms/syndromes of interest. Such paradigms would allow for more detailed understanding of connectivity changes that underlie specific symptoms versus connectivity abnormalities that reflect a genetic diathesis for developing symptoms or that are unrelated to symptoms. The combination of functional and structural imaging techniques with various types of cognitive neuroscience based challenge studies provides a powerful tool to elucidate malfunctioning brain systems.

Biomarkers may also be discovered that correlate with specific symptoms or illnesses. In Alzheimer's disease, abnormal CSF levels of amyloid and phosphorylated *tau* have strong potential to serve as biomarkers of plaque and tangle pathology and as ways to track the progression of illness. A variety of chemical and functional biomarkers that correlate with the cause of malfunctioning of various ICNs are likely to be discovered in the future. Efforts to develop meaningful biomarkers to track the function of specific neurotransmitter systems such as the glutamate, GABA, or dopamine systems are important steps in this regard.

We believe that tools are becoming increasingly available that will allow psychiatry to make a transformational leap from a field where diagnosis is based on symptom clusters derived from clinical interviews to a field where symptoms can be clustered based on an understanding of the underlying brain dysfunction. Such a transformation should provide the basis for discovering causes of the specific malfunctioning of brain systems. This, in turn, will provide the groundwork for the development of therapies directed specifically toward those causes. Progress down this pathway would be facilitated by training increased numbers of clinicians and researchers in the fields of clinical psychiatry and systems neurosciences.

Points to Remember

Current diagnostic categories are based on descriptions of symptoms that cluster together, the ability to delimit one disorder from another, the consistency of the syndrome over time, and family history. This approach to diagnostic criteria has proved valuable in developing a diagnostic system that has a high degree of reliability. The ability to confirm that many current clinical categories are valid diagnostic entities from a neuroscience perspective has suffered from the lack of understanding of brain mechanisms involved in symptoms and disorders.

As more is learned using functional neuroimaging to study various disorders, some current diagnostic categories are likely to be redefined based on knowledge of specific malfunctioning of neural systems. As knowledge of specific ICNs helps to redefine the diagnostic landscape, opportunities to develop ICN-specific treatments are likely to arise.

SUGGESTED READINGS

Kishida, K. T., King-Casas, B., & Montague, P. R. (2010). Neuroeconomic approaches to mental disorders. *Neuron, 67,* 543–554.

Lilienfeld, S. O., Lynn, S. J., & Lohr, J. M. (Eds.). (2003). *Science and pseudoscience in clinical psychology.* New York: The Guilford Press.

Sadock, B. J., Sadock, V. A., & Ruiz, P. (Eds.). (2009). *Kaplan & Sadock's comprehensive textbook of psychiatry* (9th ed.). Philadelphia: Lippincott Williams & Wilkins.

Zorumski, C. F., & Rubin, E. H. (2010). *Demystifying psychiatry—A resource for patients and families.* New York: Oxford University Press.

OTHER REFERENCES

Buckner, R. L., Snyder, A. Z., Shannon, B. J., LaRossa, G., Sachs, R., Fotenos, A. F., et al. (2005). Molecular, structural and functional characterization of Alzheimer's disease: Evidence for a relationship between default activity, amyloid and memory. *Journal of Neuroscience, 25,* 7709–7717.

Chiu, P. H., Kayali, M. A., Kishida, K. T., Tomlin, D., Klinger, L. G., Klinger, M. R., et al. (2008). Self responses along cingulate cortex reveal quantitative neural phenotype for high-functioning autism. *Neuron, 57,* 463–473.

Cloninger, C. R. (2004). *Feeling good: The science of well-being.* New York: Oxford University Press.

Costa, P. T., Jr., & McCrae, R. R. (1985). *The NEO personality inventory manual.* Odessa, FL: Psychological Assessment Resources.

Craig-Schapiro, R., Fagan, A. M., & Holtzman, D. M. (2009). Biomarkers of Alzheimer's disease. *Neurobiology of Disease, 35,* 128–140.

Davis, P. G., Morris, J. C., & Grant, E. (1990). Brief screening tests versus clinical staging in senile dementia of the Alzheimer's type. *Journal of the American Geriatric Society, 38,* 129–135.

Folstein, M. F., Folstein, S. E., & McHugh, P. R. (1975). "Mini-mental state." A practical method for grading the cognitive state of patients for the clinician. *Journal of Psychiatric Research, 12,* 189–198.

Fox, M. D., & Raichle, M. E. (2007). Spontaneous fluctuations in brain activity observed with functional magnetic resonance imaging. *Nature Reviews Neuroscience, 8,* 700–711.

Johansen-Berg, H., & Rushworth, M. F. S. (2009). Using diffusion imaging to study human connectional anatomy. *Annual Review of Neuroscience, 32,* 75–94.

Kendell, R., & Jablensky, A. (2003). Distinguishing between the validity and utility of psychiatric diagnoses. *American Journal of Psychiatry, 160,* 4–12.

King-Casas, B., Sharp, C., Lomax-Bream, L., Lohrenz, T., Fonagy, P., & Montague, P. R. (2008). The rupture and repair of cooperation in borderline personality disorder. *Science, 321,* 806–810.

Raichle, M. E. (2008). A brief history of human brain mapping. *Trends in Neurosciences, 32,* 118–126.

Raichle, M. E. (2009). A paradigm shift in functional brain imaging. *Journal of Neuroscience, 29,* 729–734.

Robins, E., & Guze, S. B. (1970). Establishment of diagnostic validity in psychiatric illness: Its application to schizophrenia. *American Journal of Psychiatry, 126,* 983–987.

Seeley, W. W., Crawford, R. K., Zhou, J., Miller, B. L., & Greicius, M. D. (2009). Neurodegenerative diseases target large-scale human brain networks. *Neuron, 62,* 42–52.

12

Why Do Some Psychiatric Disorders Become Chronic Problems?

The past century has witnessed major progress in the treatment of psychiatric disorders. Medications targeting psychosis, anxiety, mood, cognitive function, and substance abuse are now readily available. In addition, significant advances have been made in psychotherapy, including the advent of structured therapies with documented efficacy in treating a variety of disorders. Cognitive behavioral therapy (CBT), interpersonal psychotherapy (IPT), and some of their derivatives are clear examples. Brain-stimulation methods have advanced more slowly, but the past decade has witnessed significant progress in the use of electroconvulsive therapy (ECT), repetitive transcranial magnetic stimulation (rTMS), vagus nerve stimulation (VNS), and, most recently, deep brain stimulation (DBS). All of these treatments are being examined in well-designed clinical trials, providing much firmer footing for evidence-based practice. Psychosocial approaches are also increasingly recognized as important and effective ways to improve the outcomes of an array of psychiatric disorders. These approaches include support groups, clubhouse rehabilitative models, employment training for persons with chronic illnesses, and lifestyle interventions that target exercise, diet, and sleep hygiene. In addition, increasing knowledge about defects involving brain systems in various psychiatric illnesses is leading to computer-based treatments that attempt to modify or rectify some of the specific deficits of a particular illness.

Despite these advances, a significant percentage of patients with major psychiatric disorders fail to achieve remission. Large-scale effectiveness trials of antipsychotic medications (e.g., the CATIE and CUtLASS projects), antidepressants (e.g., STAR*D and the Texas Medication Algorithm Project), and mood stabilizers (e.g., STEP-BP) have evaluated psychotropic medications in "real-world" settings. The results have been sobering and lead us to conclude that current psychiatric medications are good but not great. In this chapter, we will consider some of the reasons why patients do not respond to current treatments and what might be done to improve response rates. Initially, we will discuss some aspects of current treatments and practice; then we will focus on how advances in brain sciences can help us understand why some illnesses may remain refractory to traditional interventions.

PROBLEMS WITH CURRENT TREATMENTS AND PRACTICE

A major problem with current treatments is that they likely have little to do with the mechanisms causing illness. Using antidepressants as an example, almost all available medications target the same monoamine transmitter systems (serotonin, norepinephrine, and perhaps dopamine). In terms of neurotransmitter targets, little has changed since the introduction of monoamine oxidase inhibitors (MAOIs) and tricyclic antidepressants (TCAs) in the 1950s. While side effects and toxicity have generally been reduced with some of the newer antidepressants, it is not clear that effectiveness has improved. Recent meta-analyses highlight this problem and indicate that currently available antidepressants produce little benefit beyond what is observed with placebo in individuals with mild to moderately severe depressions. This likely reflects limitations of current medications as well as the complex and highly heterogeneous nature of the "depression" diagnosis (Chapter 2). It does appear, however, that antidepressant medications have their greatest impact on individuals with the most severe depressions. Thus, while antidepressants are not as effective as we would like against the broad spectrum of depressive illnesses, they do work and have a clear place in clinical practice. Compounding these efficacy/heterogeneity problems, definitive evidence indicating that changes in monoamine neurotransmitter systems are the cause of any psychiatric disorder is lacking, and thus current pharmacologic treatments are mostly symptomatic and syndromic. This is not necessarily bad; symptomatic treatments are the norm for many common diseases in medicine and neurology and can be highly beneficial. Nonetheless, the lack of agents with unique and complementary mechanisms of action limits pharmacologic options. A few of the available agents have interesting and perhaps somewhat different properties that could be exploited in drug development. Bupropion and perhaps mirtazapine might be examples, but even here monoamines are likely the principal targets.

The same limitations apply to antipsychotic medications. With antipsychotics, it is even less clear that newer medications have much benefit over agents developed in the 1950s. The one clear exception is clozapine, a first-generation agent that has been shown to benefit patients who are resistant to other classes of antipsychotics. Unfortunately, attempts to create a "new" and safer clozapine have not met with much success, and this drug may be the only truly "atypical" antipsychotic medication available. With regard to mood stabilizers, the routine use of anticonvulsants like valproate has been a significant advance, but even here it is not clear that the newer agents match what can be achieved with lithium, despite lithium's side effects.

The current goals of psychiatric treatment are to minimize symptoms and to help patients reach a state of clinical remission (meaning that they have few or no residual symptoms). Compelling evidence indicates that patients with only partially remitted psychiatric disorders (called "responders") have a high probability of relapse over relatively short periods of time (months to a year or so). With all current treatments, the fundamental mechanisms responsible for illness are likely unaltered, and it is clear that current psychiatric medications don't "cure" any illness. Studies examining the use of medications in conjunction with various forms of psychotherapy or other rehabilitative strategies indicate that a combination of medications and therapy usually results in better outcomes than either strategy alone. Even when pharmaco-therapies and psychotherapies are combined and the patient is actively participating in treatment, the goal of achieving complete and long-lasting remission is met far less often than one would hope. In other words, there are significant limits to our treatment capabilities even when intensive clinical resources are available and utilized by the patient.

A second problem that contributes to poor treatment outcomes involves the fact that there are simply not enough psychiatrists and other highly trained mental health professionals to provide the skilled care that is needed. The administration of psychotropic medications, brain-stimulation methods, and psychotherapies requires well-trained and experienced practitioners. Psychiatry is a medical shortage field: there are not enough psychiatrists to provide the needed services. This short-age is even more dramatic in certain subspecialties, such as child and adolescent psychiatry and geriatric psychiatry. As we described in our earlier book *Demystifying Psychiatry*, the shortage of psychiatrists will substantially increase in the future, given the aging of currently practicing psychiatrists in the United States, the rate at which new psychiatrists are entering the field, and the likelihood of increasing demands for services as the U.S. population ages.

To minimize the problem created by this shortage, psychiatry as a field must develop more effective collaborative care arrangements with primary care providers (PCPs) and other mental health professionals in order to provide cost-efficient care to more patients. Besides the economic problems involved with providing adequate reimbursement for services in a collaborative model, two significant person-power issues would need to be addressed. First, PCPs have little if any formal training in psychiatry. Thus, while they can sometimes handle uncomplicated psychiatric ill-nesses, PCPs have difficulties dealing with the more severe and refractory disorders. Ways to overcome this problem might include models of care involving a combina-tion of time-limited on-site psychiatric consults in primary care settings and off-site phone, Internet-based, or video consultations. The development of telepsychiatry as a viable care-delivery strategy seems imperative, particularly for rural and inner-city populations that are grossly underserved at present.

The second issue impeding the development of collaborative care models involves the limited availability of high-quality, well-trained, non-physician, mental health professionals, including psychologists, social workers, case managers, and coun-selors. The most effective forms of psychotherapy, including CBT and IPT, require substantial formal training and supervision. Most therapists are well intentioned, but they do not have rigorous training in current state-of-the-art methods. Thus, they are not using the most advanced evidence-based methods in the care that they deliver. Tom Insel, Director of the National Institute of Mental Health (NIMH), noted that less than half of all clinical training programs in psychology and social work emphasize the most advanced evidence-based therapies. Compounding this problem, many areas of the country, again largely rural and inner-city, have shortages of all mental health professionals. The net result is that the level of care currently being provided for many individuals with psychiatric disorders is inadequate or even inappropriate. We would also point out that most therapy and rehabilitative strategies used in treating psychiatric disorders have little grounding in the advances in systems neurobiology that we have highlighted in this book and that we believe form the basis for the future of the field.

BRAIN MECHANISMS CONTRIBUTING TO REFRACTORY ILLNESSES

We now want to shift our focus to consider brain mechanisms that may contribute to the chronicity and refractoriness of some psychiatric disorders. At the outset, it is important to remember that the human brain is highly plastic and capable of experience-dependent change. Indeed, neural plasticity is the basis for learning and memory. Plasticity is a two-edged sword, however, and over time we learn not only things that are beneficial but also things that are not useful or are even harmful. Fear conditioning to inappropriate stimuli is a clear example of learned behavior that can be detrimental. The repetitive use of synapses and brain circuits is the basis for much, if not all, of this plasticity. When circuits are used repeatedly, they undergo long-lasting changes that enhance the likelihood that those same circuits will be functionally connected in the future.

When a person becomes ill with a psychiatric (or neurological) disorder, there are changes in specific brain networks that either produce or accompany the illness. As the illness progresses, aberrant circuits continue to transmit defective information, and over time, these aberrant circuits can increasingly become the "norm" for certain brain functions. For example, an initial set of panic attacks could expand into a more pervasive and disabling agoraphobia with or without major depression.

The underlying brain pathology (structural and functional) that initially caused symptoms may also progress over time and reinforce aberrant circuits, making matters even worse. Consequently, there are two major problems: the initial cause of the illness may progress, and the results of the illness may lead to altered pathways that increasingly reinforce abnormal function over time. This predicts that the longer someone is ill with a brain disorder, the more difficult it will be to reverse the disorder. Thus, prolonged periods of untreated illness, poor compliance with treatment, or poor response to treatment likely make brain illnesses more difficult to treat. This principle is not unique to psychiatry. For example, repeated focal seizures are notorious for generating "mirror" or secondary foci in the brain, making it increasingly difficult to treat some forms of epilepsy. This may reflect a "kindling" type of phenomenon. Kindling can be observed in rodents by repeated (daily) administration of an initially subconvulsive electrical stimulus in the limbic system (usually amygdala or hippocampus). Eventually, the subconvulsive stimulus results in full-blown generalized seizures. Clinically, this phenomenon is seen most often in partial complex epilepsy, and it is likely one reason for the now almost routine necessity for neurosurgical interventions in refractory patients. The dementing disorders, especially Alzheimer's disease, provide other examples of the principle that continued illness progression is related to more serious and refractory symptoms. In part because of the neuronal loss associated with these disorders, the best hope for effective intervention comes early in the illness course; the longer these illnesses progress, the lower the probability that they can be reversed, particularly in the adult brain.

It is not clear how directly these principles pertain to all psychiatric disorders, but lessons from the large-scale STAR*D clinical effectiveness trial indicate that many people with depression, particularly those who are refractory to treatment, share several characteristics: an early age of onset (childhood or teens), chronic symptoms, and a high degree of comorbidity with other psychiatric and medical disorders. Similarly, although more controversial, there is evidence that prolonged periods of untreated psychosis correlate with more difficulties in the management of schizophrenia and perhaps other psychotic disorders. For example, individuals with delusional disorder often do not come to treatment until later in their course of illness. These individuals can be very difficult to treat with currently available medications, although we don't know if their symptoms would be more responsive if they had been treated earlier in the course of their illness. The use of anticonvulsants for bipolar disorder arose from the hypothesis that a "kindling-like" (or behavioral sensitization) phenomenon was occurring in many patients with this disorder. This idea was partially based on data suggesting that the frequency of episodes of illness increased over time and that the severity of the episodes increased with repeated bouts of illness. The effectiveness of certain anticonvulsant drugs in preventing limbic system kindling in animal models served as the basis for their initial trial in bipolar disorder.

The possibility that longer durations of untreated illness predict increased treatment refractoriness makes it important that psychiatric disorders are recognized as early as possible and that the most effective treatments are used aggressively early in the course of treatment. For example, some are now advocating first-line use of clozapine, perhaps the most effective antipsychotic available, early in the course of schizophrenia, before the illness becomes crystallized and chronic. Some evidence suggests that this strategy may improve the mortality rate in schizophrenia, and clozapine is one of the few treatments that appear to diminish suicide associated with this disorder. Other treatments that may decrease the risk of completed suicide include lithium and possibly ECT. Some psychiatrists have asked whether we should consider earlier use of ECT in mood and psychotic disorders, given the high degree of effectiveness of this treatment. Although more controversial, it may be possible to target individuals at very high risk for illness for earlier interventions. Such individuals would certainly include adolescents and young adults, but might also extend to children with high genetic load and/or prodromal symptoms, including social withdrawal, odd thinking, and/or cognitive impairment. The recent preliminary study showing beneficial effects of long-chain omega-3 fatty acids in individuals at ultra-high risk for psychosis is an early proof-of-concept for this type of approach. The development of meaningful biomarkers for illnesses would help this effort.

Numerous ethical issues must be considered in any early intervention program, especially when geared toward children or adolescents. Importantly, early interventions need not necessarily be medications, and psychosocial interventions in children and adolescents may be effective and appropriate for some disorders.

CONNECTIVITY NETWORKS, BRAIN MECHANISMS, AND REFRACTORY DISORDERS

Our emphasis throughout this book has been on understanding the involvement of brain networks in psychiatric disorders with the belief that this level of analysis has the highest likelihood of influencing clinical thinking and practice. We also believe that several principles derived from work on neural networks can help us understand why some patients are refractory to treatment. In deference to Eugen Bleuler and his 4 A's of schizophrenia (ambivalence, affective flattening, autistic thinking, and associational loosening), we will frame our discussion around what we call the "5 A's" of refractoriness (Table 12-1). Some but not all of these reflect the current 5 A's of negative symptoms in schizophrenia (blunted affect, avolition, asociality, anhedonia, and alogia). We believe that the five factors of refractoriness discussed below reflect aspects of how brain dysfunction contributes to psychiatric illness. While this discussion is speculative, we believe that it is based on reasonable principles of brain function and highlights features that can be targets for therapeutic and rehabilitative efforts aimed at improving overall function and outcomes. At the minimum, the points raised here merit further research attention.

Anosognosia

Psychiatrists often are confronted with patients who don't realize that anything is wrong with them and who don't want treatment. A variety of terms are used to describe this behavior, including "denial" and "lack of insight." While these can be useful descriptors, we are struck by the idea that denial is likely a product of brain dysfunction and that misinformation within brain networks contributes to distortions and

Table 12-1 The "5 A's" of Refractoriness

Anosognosia (disconnection problem)
    Attention problem ("denial")
Anergia (energy problem)
    Obesity, low fitness, poor sleep
Amotivation (goal problem)
    Alcohol/drugs/"bad ideas"
Aplasticity (plasticity problem)
    Intellect vs. education
Asociality (social network problem)
    Chronic social stress, social isolation

---

cognitive errors. In the hemineglect syndrome outlined in Chapter 1, damage to the right cerebral cortex results in left-sided weakness and sometimes a defect in the left visual field. The left hemisphere becomes overactive and, in order to make sense of ambiguous and defective information, it makes up excuses for the defect, resulting in the afflicted person's failure to recognize the left side of space or to identify body parts as belonging to himself or herself. This phenomenon is sometimes called "anosognosia." In his book *The Insanity Offense: How America's Failure to Treat the Seriously Mentally Ill Endangers Its Citizens*, E. Fuller Torrey discussed schizophrenia and severe mental disorders from this perspective and concluded that the failure of many patients to recognize their abnormal thinking or their illness state is a form of anosognosia. It is not simply a psychological defense mechanism but a manifestation of brain pathology, perhaps reflecting a form of inattention.

We think this concept has considerable merit. It helps define a problem that leads to much misunderstanding and finger-pointing in a more scientifically and perhaps therapeutically tractable manner. Results from studying the contribution of brain networks to the neurological syndrome of hemineglect are instructive in this regard. In particular, it appears that attention and reorienting networks in the nondominant hemisphere are impaired, which leads to problems in focusing attention on the defect. An imbalance in processing between the two cerebral hemispheres also seems to play a significant role. Similar, though less profound, defects in focusing attention could contribute to denial in psychiatric disorders. We have already discussed recent findings regarding inattention and the default network in major depression (Chapter 7), but there is also evidence that subjects with schizophrenia, and perhaps anxiety states, have problems shifting attention from default-mode processing. This likely results in excessive focus on an internal world that is error-laden at the expense of more realistic and probabilistic appraisals of the external environment. Recent data linking poor insight to structural changes in the posterior cingulate gyrus and right precuneus (parts of the default system) in subjects with new-onset psychosis provide tentative support for this idea.

Although more speculative for psychiatric disorders than nondominant hemisphere strokes, thinking about defects in reorienting networks and attention might lead to novel ways to help patients gain insight or, at a minimum, improve compliance with treatment. We would argue that someone who cannot recognize that his or her thinking or mood is a problem has little hope of following through with treatment recommendations or other interventions. Interestingly, there is evidence that rebalancing the two cerebral hemispheres can improve symptoms of hemineglect, at least transiently. Early attempts used applications of warm water to the right ear to heat and thus "activate" the injured right hemisphere or cold water to the left ear to inhibit the overactive left hemisphere. Both approaches resulted in transient improvement. Recent efforts have involved either stimulating the damaged right hemisphere or inhibiting the overactive left hemisphere with different frequencies of rTMS. Interestingly, rTMS targeted to prefrontal regions enhances gamma-frequency rhythms that contribute to cortical organization across brain regions; such effects could help to reset connections among cortical regions.

Anergia

The brain's ability to correct errors often involves top-down processing in which higher cognitive centers in prefrontal cortex (PFC) override defects in cognition, emotion, and motivation. This type of processing also involves the hippocampus as an integrator that evaluates current thinking relative to stored cognitive maps, initiating corrections in thinking and navigation. From cellular and network perspectives, such processing is energy-intensive. The brain routinely uses about 20% to 25% of cardiac output to sustain its function, and communication over longer distances (such as from PFC to subcortical structures) is more energy-demanding than local intraregional processing. Furthermore, energy utilization is not distributed equally across brain regions, and networks increase and decrease their metabolism and blood flow depending on their involvement in specific processing tasks. This is the basis for functional neuroimaging. Thus, illnesses or conditions that impair efficient energy use can have adverse effects on the brain's ability to monitor and correct problems in perceptions.

Why is this important in psychiatry? Many individuals with serious psychiatric disorders have difficulty maintaining a healthy lifestyle and overall physical fitness. Poor fitness is associated with fatigue and inefficient use of energy. Conditions associated with some psychiatric disorders include obesity, diabetes mellitus, and hyperlipidemias. In some cases, these metabolic problems result from a sedentary and withdrawn lifestyle, but they can be compounded greatly by weight gain induced by psychotropic medications, particularly antipsychotic drugs and mood stabilizers. Obesity, diabetes, and hyperlipidemias, along with heavy cigarette use, are major factors contributing to the observation that individuals with chronic mental disorders die an average of 20 to 25 years earlier than expected based on population norms. At a minimum, this is a serious public health problem. We would argue that these metabolic problems may also influence the brain's ability to utilize energy efficiently and, as a result, create problems with effective top-down processing.

Adding to problems involving energy use is the fact that many psychiatric disorders are associated with varying degrees of sleep disturbance. The function of sleep is not completely understood, but it appears to play roles in the restoration of glial energy stores and in memory consolidation (including perhaps synaptic resetting). Glucose, the main fuel of neurons, is stored in limited amounts via glycogen accumulation in glia. Neurons contain virtually no glycogen, and glia send metabolic intermediates, including glucose, lactate, and perhaps pyruvate, to neurons to help fuel neuronal processing in addition to using their glycogen stores to support their own functions, such as ionic homeostasis. Glial glycogen stores are depleted during wakefulness and replenished during sleep. Even when insomnia is corrected pharmacologically, normal sleep cycles often are not fully restored. Most psychotropic drugs alter REM and/or non-REM (particularly deep) sleep phases. Decreased sleep or an imbalance in sleep architecture can interfere with learning and can contribute further to problems with top-down processing and error correction. Importantly, poor physical fitness, obesity, and insomnia are potential targets for intervention, and many leading centers now emphasize lifestyle variables as part of psychiatric rehabilitative efforts.

Amotivation

The brain systems involved in setting goals use dopamine input from the ventral tegmental area to regulate activity in the nucleus accumbens, PFC, hippocampus, and other regions. This system is intimately entwined with reward processing in the brain and is critical for reinforcement-based learning. Clinical improvement in many psychiatric disorders is highly dependent upon the motivation of patients to accept and follow treatment recommendations. This can be a major problem because networks involved in motivation are part of the malfunctioning circuitry underlying the disorders. Thus, factors that usurp this circuitry can be devastating for implementing and adhering to an effective treatment plan. This is most obvious when patients are abusing drugs or alcohol. Almost all addictive drugs, including alcohol, initially target the dopamine reward system, and over time these agents can hijack the function of this system. In effect, abused drugs become major motivating factors in patients' lives and have major adverse effects on clinical outcomes, including worsening symptoms of primary psychiatric disorders. Mood and psychotic disorders are often accompanied by varying degrees of substance abuse, which typically include alcohol and marijuana abuse at a minimum but can also involve cocaine and other stimulants and opiates such as heroin. Nicotine dependence is common and may afflict 80% or more of individuals with schizophrenia. Nicotine is interesting in this regard. While it clearly affects the dopamine/motivational system, it is less clear that it produces the same long-term adverse neurocognitive effects as other addictive drugs, although some evidence suggests that nicotine dependence may predispose individuals to mood and other addictive disorders. Other evidence suggests that nicotine may be used by schizophrenics as a way to self-medicate and improve defects in attention. Nonetheless, the long-term adverse health effects of nicotine dependence are unequivocal.

On their own, substance-abuse disorders are typically chronic conditions associated with repeated relapses. When combined with mood, anxiety, and psychotic disorders, the relapsing and remitting course of substance abuse becomes even more problematic, and it is a common contributor to noncompliance, morbidity, and mortality. It goes without saying that there is little hope for lasting improvement in any psychiatric disorder as long as an individual is abusing drugs or alcohol. For these reasons, the archaic practice inflicted by some regulatory and third-party agencies to separate treatment for "addictive" and "mental" disorders (e.g., "psychiatric" vs. "chemical dependence" units) makes absolutely no sense.

An intriguing aspect of the human mind that complicates issues involving motivation is that abstract human thought can be a motivator and/or reward in itself. We noted this earlier when we discussed "altruistic" forms of suicide in which an individual is willing to give up life for an abstract religious or political belief.

Humans can become seduced by their own thinking, and this can create major problems with treatment compliance and motivation. This problem is most apparent with psychotic thinking, where abnormal abstract thoughts are considered to be true even in the face of substantial and at times overwhelming evidence to the contrary. Similarly, certain forms of obsessional preoccupation have a motivating and seductive quality, despite the associated anxiety. Examples include persistent ruminations about certain people or places as well as major preoccupations with sexual themes. Personality traits also contribute to problems with motivation when individuals become convinced that they are correct and the rest of the world is wrong, a hallmark of the personality disorders. Interestingly, the brain systems underlying the temperament traits of novelty seeking, harm avoidance, reward dependence, and persistence share neural circuitry with the motivation and habit systems.

A better understanding of how to modulate motivational systems would be beneficial in helping patients follow through with treatment recommendations. If the motivational system is usurped by abused drugs in patients with other psychiatric disorders, it is important to address the substance-abuse disorders early and aggressively. This serves two purposes: first, eliminating the abused substance gradually allows motivational systems to become more available to assist with treatment of the primary psychiatric disorder, and second, effective strategies used to address substance abuse might also have beneficial effects on the primary psychiatric disorder. An example of the latter would be the benefits associated with motivational interviewing strategies commonly used to treat substance abuse. At a minimum, elimination of abused drugs would be expected to have a positive impact on underlying psychopathology.

Aplasticity

Psychiatric treatments and rehabilitative strategies depend upon the plasticity of the human brain and its ability to learn, remember, and correct itself as a result of experience. Factors that limit or impair this plasticity have adverse effects on the outcome of psychiatric disorders. While intelligence *per se* does not protect against major psychiatric disorders, individuals with lower general intelligence, including limitations in areas of higher-order cognitive function such as planning, foresight, decision making, and abstraction, are at higher risk. In some cases, cognitive dysfunction is associated with impulse-control problems and difficulties with top-down processing. Often, it can be difficult to determine the temporal sequence of cognitive problems, including whether preexisting cognitive difficulties predisposed a person to the development of a psychiatric disorder or whether the psychiatric illness caused cognitive dysfunction as one of its manifestations. What is clear is that cognitive impairment hinders mental flexibility and is one of the major drivers of disability and poor long-term outcome.

Despite this, all human brains are plastic and all humans are capable of learning. This fact provides reason for optimism. To the extent that behavioral and mental problems reflect defects in knowledge or education, there is hope of intervention and improvement. Strategies such as social skills training, stress management, reinforcement learning, and vocational restructuring are important components of psychiatric care and form a base for rehabilitative efforts in individuals with chronic mental disorders. These approaches are often used very effectively in clubhouse models that target psychosocial interventions to the person's level of illness while building self-esteem and working toward social competence and independence. Variants of these approaches are also important in treating milder psychiatric disorders.

One of the major difficulties in dealing with people suffering from severe psychiatric disorders is the lack of cognitive flexibility that can accompany these illnesses. This sometimes reflects preexisting or illness-associated cognitive impairment. In some cases, it reflects stereotyped (habitual) thinking and behavior—a tendency to employ a limited and relatively rigid repertoire of approaches to deal with problems, particularly in ambiguous situations. This problem cuts across psychiatric (and some neurological) diagnoses and is often associated with lack of insight. For example, individuals with psychotic disorders tend to have fairly rigid interpretations of events occurring around them, often reflecting their delusional ideas about the world. Similarly, stereotyped and rigid thinking can accompany mood, anxiety, and personality disorders. In mood and anxiety disorders rigid thinking often reflects the underlying emotional state, while in personality disorders it reflects long-standing habitual approaches to dealing with others. The tendency to use habitual responses as a default mode of responding is natural for the human brain and is an efficient energy and time saving mechanism compared to the slower and more demanding processing required for goal-directed behaviors. Effective forms of psychotherapy, particularly CBT, IPT, and dialectical behavioral therapy, often target inflexible thinking and serve as critical components of treatment strategies dealing with these issues.

Asociality

Humans are inherently social animals, and this is reflected in the way our brains work. While genetics clearly plays a role in brain function, much of our mental development has an epigenetic basis and evolves as we interact with others and the environment. Numerous studies have highlighted the influence of culture and social interactions on brain activity and growth. Social aspects of our lives occupy a great deal of our mental effort. For example, it is estimated that about 70% of human conversations are about other humans; some refer to this as "gossip." These conversations are a way that we assess our own lives and make decisions about how we should behave and with whom we should interact. There is evidence that when given advice from a friend, we will typically use that advice to make decisions but will discount its importance—that is, input from others influences us greatly, but we don't necessarily recognize that it does. As pointed out by Steven Quartz and Terry Sejnowski in their book *Liars, Lovers and Heroes*, the quality of a person's social relationships is one of the best predictors of overall life satisfaction. Humans don't do well in social isolation, yet about 25% of the population lives alone. This isolation seems to be worse for men than women, particularly as people age. Retirement, including the loss of meaningful activities and social interactions, is a challenging time for humans.

One of the tragic aspects of major psychiatric disorders is that they isolate their victims. Almost regardless of diagnosis, there is a tendency for those with serious illness to retreat from contact with others. This can result from delusional thinking associated with psychotic disorders, amotivation or low energy associated with mood disorders, social fears and avoidance behaviors associated with anxiety disorders, or a preference for solitary drinking or drug use among those with substance-abuse disorders. In some cases, social stigma associated with psychiatric illness adds to this problem. In other cases, chronic difficulties with social interactions, noncompliance with treatment, and inappropriate behavior compound these issues, leading to even greater degrees of isolation. The result is that many persons with psychiatric disorders are deprived of their social network and in effect lose one of their major lifelines for improvement. A number of recent studies have documented the importance of social networks in determining overall health, including whether one will become obese, lose weight, or smoke. This goes further, and the small-world nature of human social networks often determines whether a person is employed or finds work if unemployed. Here our local social cluster can be helpful in some aspects, but as shown by Mark Granovetter in the 1970s, the weak ties that link our close social network to other less familiar groups may be an even bigger help with certain aspects of our lives, such as finding a new job.

Social networks depend on developing trust and cooperation among members of a group. This might be particularly difficult for people with certain psychiatric disorders. The development of trust and social cooperation is an interesting phenomenon from an evolutionary standpoint, and it has been the topic of considerable research. One interesting approach over the past decade has involved efforts to perform functional neuroimaging while individuals, including persons with psychiatric disorders, engage socially while playing certain types of interactive economic games. For example, Read Montague and colleagues used this technique to study individuals with borderline personality disorder (BPD) while they participated in a multi-round economic exchange game. These studies found that persons with BPD have difficulties perceiving social gestures and are impaired at re-establishing cooperation when trust is broken during the course of a game. Interestingly, the behavioral observations correlated with changes in brain activity, particularly in the anterior insula, a region that helps to process interoceptive and autonomic nervous system data. In control subjects, insular activity showed a strong linear relationship with both the amounts of money offered and received during the game. Subjects with BPD showed increased insular activity only in response to payments given out; they did not respond to offers received. While it is unclear whether this type of defect in social reciprocity reflects illness cause, effect, or correlation, this work has important implications for thinking about the social processing defects in BPD and in designing strategies to help individuals with this disorder. It also highlights the role that neural processing defects may play in determining some of the interpersonal problems that individuals with personality disorders exhibit.

The point of this discussion is to emphasize that efforts to improve the quality of human social networks can have a major impact on the outcome of psychiatric disorders, including compliance with treatment and degree of disability. Various therapeutic communities can help with this by providing group support, educational opportunities, employment training, social skills training, and group exercise facilities. Partnerships with community organizations, including the National Alliance on Mental Illness (NAMI), faith-based organizations where appropriate, and recovery-based groups such as Alcoholics Anonymous and derivatives, can also be helpful.

HOW CAN PSYCHIATRY TAKE ADVANTAGE OF SYNAPTIC PLASTICITY?

Psychiatric symptoms and disorders involve dysfunctions of brain networks and are not simply cellular, synaptic, or molecular problems. Nonetheless, studies of synaptic plasticity and neurogenesis point to significant opportunities for improving the outcome of individuals with psychiatric disorders via molecular and synaptic mechanisms. We have already alluded to several of these in this chapter and will summarize them here briefly. Although often overlooked by modern medicine, we believe these variables, which include lifestyle and social interventions, should form the basis for thinking about rehabilitative strategies in psychiatry. While it is unlikely that cures for psychiatric disorders are coming in the foreseeable future, improvement in symptoms and function should be the clinical expectation. Some of the following points are derived from comments made by Steven Quartz and Terry Sejnowski in describing "how to build a better brain."

The Brain Needs to Learn

The brain needs exposure to lifelong learning opportunities and the chance to work on interesting problems. Current evidence suggests that individuals who remain mentally engaged in work or in playing cognitive games age more successfully than those who spend time passively watching television or surfing the Internet. This presents easy targets for interventions.

The Brain Needs Novelty

Over time, humans gravitate to habitual and stereotyped behaviors. For example, think about where you park your car at work: it is highly likely that it will be found within a very small radius each day. Fixed and habitual behaviors can be helpful and reassuring, particularly when we are stressed, but they are not necessarily good for mental flexibility. The ability to engage in complex and novel, but not overly stressful, activities can help cognitive function. Even rodents do better when exposed to novel environments that they can explore in an unthreatened fashion.

Social Interactions Are Important

Humans require positive interpersonal contact. Such interactions provide not only opportunities for learning and novelty but also sources of social support and a sense of well-being. This has an impact on brain function. Again, even rodents do better when housed in non-stressful groups. The key is that the social contact is positive: being in a dominated or threatened position is as unhelpful for humans as it is for rodents. Older literature on social factors involved in psychiatric disorders emphasized this need for positive contact and found that high degrees of "expressed emotion" in a living situation, particularly negative comments in face-to-face interactions with family members, often predicted relapse in psychotic illnesses.

Lifestyle Variables Can Have Huge and Non-Linear Effects on Outcomes

Diet, exercise, sleep, and stress reduction are good for neurogenesis and have an impact on brain function, self-esteem, and feelings of self-control. Recent studies support this contention and indicate that subjects with schizophrenia enrolled in an exercise training program exhibit significant increases in hippocampal volume and short-term memory function over a 3-month period. Elimination of nicotine (and probably caffeine), coupled with no more than moderate use of alcohol, is a corollary of this. Interestingly, moderate alcohol use appears to be better than abstinence, perhaps pointing to its role as a social lubricant, in addition to other potential health benefits. Other abused drugs do not appear to carry this benefit.

Points to Remember

Many psychiatric disorders are chronic problems. They can be remitting and relapsing, but often by the time individuals present for psychiatric care, they are in it for the long haul. Even if active symptoms partially or fully remit, there are social consequences from the earlier symptoms that can lead to distress and diminish the ability to achieve goals. Understanding the long-term course of psychiatric illnesses and their consequences is critical, and it is imperative that psychiatrists target interventions toward factors that drive poor compliance, morbidity, and mortality early in treatment. The longer someone remains ill and delays treatment, the lower the probability of a good outcome.

Research that targets a better understanding of the brain mechanisms underlying specific psychiatric symptoms and psychiatric disorders will be helpful in providing knowledge that will diminish the stigma associated with these disorders and aid in the development of interventions that can make a difference in long-term outcomes.

For psychiatric treatments to work, brain plasticity is required. Thus, psychiatrists must become experts in interventions that influence and enhance this plasticity. These can include medications, brain-stimulation methods, and traditional psychotherapies, but should also involve lifestyle and social network variables. New approaches based on brain-retraining techniques that are derived from knowledge of abnormal brain systems also have substantial potential for future therapeutic directions.

SUGGESTED READINGS

Montague, R. (2006). *Why choose this book? How we make decisions.* New York: Dutton Press.

Quartz, S. R., & Sejnowski, T. J. (2002). *Liars, lovers and heroes: What the new brain science reveals about how we become who we are.* New York: William Morrow.

Zorumski, C. F., & Rubin, E. H. (2010). *Demystifying psychiatry—A resource for patients and families.* New York: Oxford University Press.

OTHER REFERENCES

Amminger, G. P., Schafer, M. R., Papageorgiou, K., Klier, C. M., Cotton, S. M., Harrigan, S. M., et al. (2010). Long-chain omega-3 fatty acids for indicated prevention of psychotic disorders: A randomized, placebo-controlled trial. *Archives of General Psychiatry, 67,* 146–154.

Christakis, N. A., & Fowler, J. H. (2007). The spread of obesity in a large social network over 32 years. *New England Journal of Medicine, 357,* 370–379.

Christakis, N. A., & Fowler, J. H. (2008). The collective dynamics of smoking in a large social network. *New England Journal of Medicine, 358,* 2249–2258.

Famy, C., Streissguth, A. P., & Unis, A. S. (1998). Mental illness in adults with fetal alcohol syndrome or fetal alcohol effects. *American Journal of Psychiatry, 155,* 552–554.

Fournier, J. C., DeRubeis, R. J., Hollon, S. D., Dimidjian, S., Amsterdam, J. D., Shelton, R. C., et al. (2010). Antidepressant drug effects and depression severity—a patient-level meta-analysis. *Journal of the American Medical Association, 303,* 47–53.

Fratiglioni, L., Paillard-Borg, S., & Winblad, B. (2004). An active and socially integrated lifestyle in late life might protect against dementia. *Lancet Neurology, 3,* 343–353.

Gabbard, G. O., & Kay, J. (2001). The fate of integrated treatment: Whatever happened to the biopsychosocial psychiatrist? *American Journal of Psychiatry, 158,* 1956–1963.

Gilbert, D. T., Killingsworth, M. A., Eyre, R. N., & Wilson, T. D. (2009). The surprising power of neighborly advice. *Science, 323,* 1617–1619.

Granovetter, M. (1973). The strength of weak ties. *American Journal of Sociology, 78,* 1360–1380.

Insel, T. R. (2009). Translating scientific opportunity into public health impact. *Archives of General Psychiatry, 66,* 128–133.

King-Casas, B., Sharp, C., Lomax-Bream, L., Lohrenz, T., Fonagy, P., & Montague, P. R. (2008). The rupture and repair of cooperation in borderline personality disorder. *Science, 321,* 806–810.

Koenen, K. C., Moffitt, T. E., Roberts, A. L., Martin, L. T., Kubzansky, L., Harrington, H., et al. (2009). Childhood IQ and adult mental disorders: A test of the cognitive reserve hypothesis. *American Journal of Psychiatry, 166,* 50–57.

Lieberman, J. A. (2006). Comparative effectiveness of antipsychotic drugs. *Archives of General Psychiatry, 63*, 1069–1072.

Marshall, R. S. (2009). Rehabilitation approaches to hemineglect. *Neurologist, 15*, 185–192.

Morgan, K. D., Dazzan, P., Morgan, C., Lappin, J., Hutchinson, G., Suckling, J., et al. (2010). Insight, grey matter and cognitive function in first-onset psychosis. *British Journal of Psychiatry, 197*, 141–148.

Newcomer, J. W., & Hennekens, C. H. (2007). Severe mental illness and risk of cardiovascular disease. *Journal of the American Medical Association, 298*, 1794–1796.

Pajonk, F.-G., Wobrock, T., Gruber, O., Scherk, H., Berner, D., Kaizl, I., et al. (2010). Hippocampal plasticity in response to exercise in schizophrenia. *Archives of General Psychiatry, 67*, 133–143.

Redgrave, P., Rodriguez, M., Smith, Y., Rodriguez-Oroz, M. C., Lehericy, S., Bergman, H., et al. (2010). Goal-directed and habitual control in the basal ganglia: Implications for Parkinson's disease. *Nature Reviews Neuroscience, 11*, 760–772.

Rush, A. J. (2007). STAR*D: What have we learned? *American Journal of Psychiatry, 164*, 201–204.

Tiihonen, J., Lonnqvist, J., Wahlbeck, K., Klaukka, T., Niskanen, L., Tanskanen, A., et al. (2009). 11-year follow-up of mortality in patients with schizophrenia: A population-based cohort study (FIN11 study). *Lancet, 374*, 620–627.

Torrey, E. F. (2008). *The insanity offense: How America's failure to treat the seriously mentally ill endangers its citizens.* New York: W.W. Norton & Company.

Van den Heuvel, M. P., Stam, C. J., Kahn, R. S., & Hulshoff Pol, H. E. (2009). Efficiency of functional brain networks and intellectual performance. *Journal of Neuroscience, 29*, 7619–7624.

13

Approaches to Treatment

Psychiatrists use a wide range of treatments to manage patients with mental disorders. Today's treatments, although far from perfect, are better than past treatments in terms of clinical benefits and certain side effects. While it is beyond the scope of this book to review all available treatments for psychiatric disorders, we have designed this chapter to be an introduction to a neural systems approach to thinking about treatments in psychiatry. We will expand on themes developed in earlier chapters and raise questions about the possible influence of various treatments on the function of brain networks. Based on the current state of the art, some of the points we discuss are more firmly rooted in science than others. Nonetheless, we hope that this overview provides a guide for conceptualizing psychopharmacology, brain-stimulation methods, psychotherapies, and lifestyle-based therapies.

At the outset, there are several concepts about psychiatric treatments that we would emphasize:

1. The mechanisms of action of current psychiatric treatments are not fully understood. Current research is leading us closer to understanding how these treatments may improve symptoms; however, the information is far from being complete or scientifically satisfying.
2. Available treatments are not specific for any single illness or group of illnesses. For instance, although we call a group of drugs "antidepressants," these drugs influence brain systems that have substantial effects on depression, anxiety, obsessive thinking, compulsive behaviors, and pain states. This overlap largely reflects the organization of brain systems underlying the human mind and the fact that available drugs affect neurotransmitter systems that act diffusely throughout the central nervous system (CNS) to modulate function.
3. Psychotropic drugs vary in their mechanisms of action and side effects, but ultimately they act on parallel but overlapping circuits underlying cognition, emotion, and motivation. For instance, benzodiazepines have substantially different mechanisms of action than antipsychotics, but both can calm agitated patients. Similarly, although SSRIs (selective serotonin reuptake inhibitors) and NRIs (norepinephrine reuptake inhibitors) sound as though they have different effects on brain function via different neurotransmitter systems, they actually work in a manner that is more similar than their names suggest. Again, this reflects not only a lack of complete selectivity in their actions but also the diffuse and overlapping nature of these transmitter systems.

4. Psychotherapies may be helpful as a result of both nonspecific and specific mechanisms. Nonspecific mechanisms involve the general benefits of interacting with a concerned therapist and learning strategies for stress reduction. Specific mechanisms may involve the influence of a therapeutic approach on activity within brain pathways involved in a disorder, such as learning to desensitize to fear and anxiety.

5. Brain-stimulation (device-mediated) treatments can be very effective when used for appropriate indications. Electroconvulsive therapy (ECT) is the most effective treatment available for severe depression. Other brain-stimulation methods, including repetitive transcranial magnetic stimulation (rTMS), vagus nerve stimulation (VNS), and deep brain stimulation (DBS), have significant potential, but they are in their infancy and not ready for general use in psychiatry at this time.

6. Some treatments are rehabilitative; that is, they train healthy parts of the brain to "work around" brain regions that are not functioning effectively. Other treatments may directly affect malfunctioning brain regions and, therefore, influence the problems that arise from the specific causes of illness. As the underlying causes of disorders are better understood and the specific neural systems involved are better defined, more specific treatments can be developed to reverse the underlying defects. Even with more specific treatments, however, we believe that psychiatry would benefit from a greater emphasis on rehabilitative strategies that target improved overall functioning of the human mind. The goal of these strategies is to improve function to the maximum extent possible in the face of illnesses that are episodic at best, and chronic and deteriorating at worst.

PSYCHOPHARMACOLOGY

There are many excellent psychopharmacology texts. These describe the wealth of information that is known about therapeutic drugs—perhaps too much information to remember or keep at one's fingertips. How should clinicians approach thinking about medications? We suggest that understanding basic principles is key: basic principles underlying mechanisms of drug actions, basic principles of pharmacokinetics, and basic principles about how to start, continue, and discontinue a drug. In addition, practicing good medicine includes being aware of and on the lookout for side effects and informing patients about them. In the ensuing discussion, we will focus on mechanisms of action of drugs and will emphasize how drugs may influence specific brain systems.

Mechanisms of Action

Psychotropic medications work by influencing multiple brain systems. Some drugs belong to categories that reflect proposed mechanisms of action. SSRIs and SNRIs (serotonin and norepinephrine reuptake inhibitors) are two such classes of drugs.

Although we understand how certain psychiatric drugs influence specific transmitter systems, we do not fully understand how the effects on these transmitter systems lead to symptomatic improvement. This lack of knowledge is highlighted further when considering how the known acute effects of a drug (e.g., serotonin uptake inhibition) result in therapeutic effects that take weeks or longer to develop. Acute drug actions for most psychoactive drugs are only the beginning of much more complicated cellular, synaptic, and network stories. We encourage students and clinicians to stay up to date with current hypotheses but to remember that such hypotheses are works in progress and limited in scope. In this book, we have encouraged readers to think about illnesses at the level of systems neurosciences, and we will continue this theme by discussing the ways medications may correct aberrant function within brain circuits. We will examine several categories of medications and suggest some of the questions that we hope will be answered by future research.

Antidepressants

Many categories of antidepressants, including the SSRIs, SNRIs, and tricyclic antidepressants, inhibit proteins that transport norepinephrine and/or serotonin from the extracellular space back into presynaptic terminals. As described in Chapter 10, this effect occurs rapidly; however, these drugs typically take days to weeks to produce maximal benefits. While most therapeutic effects of antidepressants take weeks or months to become manifest, recent findings with the NRI reboxetine suggest that even a single dose of medication can influence certain symptoms. Intriguingly, it appears that some of the excessive negative bias associated with depression can begin to change with the first dose(s) of medication. However, patients don't recognize these early effects, and they don't report any benefits of the medication until changes in mood and other symptoms occur weeks later. The early effects on emotional bias highlight the importance of conceptualizing depression as a "neurocognitive" disorder that involves dysfunction within and across brain networks involved in emotion, motivation, and cognition. Consistent with this, other recent studies have examined neurocircuitry predictors of acute antidepressant responses to infusions of the NMDA receptor antagonist, ketamine. Interestingly, subjects showing the greatest acute response to ketamine exhibited the least engagement of the subgenual anterior cingulate cortex during a working memory task and a negative correlation between subgenual cingulate and amygdala activity. It remains to be seen whether these types of findings translate into clinical use, but the ability to identify early predictors of treatment response would be a significant step forward.

These findings also raise the possibility that certain psychiatric symptoms can be selectively targeted for therapeutic purposes. Consistent with this idea, a recent study in healthy control subjects suggests that SSRIs and NRIs acutely alter activity in different brain regions following administration of a single dose. Reboxetine increases activity in the medial thalamus and prefrontal cortex (PFC), suggesting early effects on attention and arousal, while citalopram, an SSRI, enhances function in dorsal striatum, midbrain, insula, and PFC, suggesting early effects on executive and emotional control systems. If these latter findings are replicated in subjects with depression, they raise the possibility of targeting subtypes of symptoms, perhaps based on initial neuroimaging and cognitive profiles.

It is also important to understand that inhibition of transmitter reuptake is only the first step in a cascade of therapeutic events. The subsequent production of second messengers and growth factors initiates cellular events that result in an increased density of dendrites and increased connections between cells. Ultimately, the effects of these drugs involve changes in gene expression and protein synthesis that affect neural connectivity and plasticity. These later changes affecting longer-term neuronal structure and function appear to be most germane to lasting therapeutic effects, but they are the least understood aspects of drug action. For example, it is uncertain whether effects within specific brain regions are the critical changes. Similarly, it is not known how regional changes alter network dynamics across brain regions. These issues can likely be addressed by functional connectivity brain-imaging studies and sophisticated electrographic methods such as magnetoencephalograhy and perhaps electrocortography.

This is the current state of knowledge regarding the proposed mechanism of action of several types of antidepressants. But what does this really tell us about how these medications improve symptoms? Why should enhanced connections within a brain region and across brain regions lead to improvement in depressive symptoms? As we understand more about the brain systems involved in depression (Chapters 6 and 7), it will be important to determine how antidepressant-enhanced growth of cellular connections corrects the intrinsic connectivity networks (ICNs) that are malfunctioning during depression. To understand this process, it will be helpful to know more about the regional and cellular specificity of the effects of these drugs. It is likely that these medications influence many (perhaps most) regions of the brain; yet only certain regions are involved in depression. How does an effect that broadly influences the brain lead to improvement in a specific group of symptoms while not being detrimental to other ICNs that regulate other processes? We hypothesize that defective processing within specific ICNs benefits from new connections, whereas normally functioning systems may benefit from, but are at least not disrupted by, new growth. What is happening in the depressed brain that enables this specificity in drug action? We don't yet know; however, answers to these types of questions could go a long way to developing more targeted treatments.

Other antidepressants may work a bit differently. Monoamine oxidase inhibitors block the breakdown of norepinephrine, dopamine, and serotonin. The resulting increased levels of these transmitters then are likely to trigger similar cascades of events discussed for reuptake inhibitors. Do MAO inhibitors have differential effects on specific brain systems and lead to different patterns of dendritic growth and connectivity than the SSRIs and NRIs? Currently, we don't know why MAO inhibitors may be helpful to patients who fail to respond to other categories of medications.

Bupropion may influence dopamine, among other effects. This raises the possibility that this drug may act a bit differently from other antidepressants, perhaps having more prominent effects on motivation, attention, and working memory. Bupropion also can be effective in helping patients abstain from cigarettes, and it may do this by influencing the central reward ICN. Does bupropion's influence on dopamine contribute to its antidepressant effects? If so, how are the effects on the central reward ICN related to its influence on depression-related ICNs? Bupropion's antidepressant effects take weeks to develop fully, suggesting again that long-term changes in cellular function and connections are likely to be occurring. Most antidepressants can have negative effects on sex drive, enjoyment, and performance. Bupropion is somewhat different in this regard. Why is there a relationship between antidepressant efficacy and sexual side effects for most, but not all, antidepressants? The answer to this question will require a better understanding of the relationship between ICNs controlling mood and those controlling pleasure or procreation, including both central and peripheral effects.

Most antidepressants are also effective in treating anxiety. They can help patients with a variety of anxiety disorders, including panic disorder, generalized anxiety disorder, posttraumatic stress disorder, and obsessive-compulsive disorder. Similar to the time it takes for antidepressant efficacy, these drugs require several weeks to alleviate anxiety symptoms. Why should drugs that help depression also help anxiety disorders? Although anxiety and depression frequently occur together, these drugs can lessen anxiety even in persons who do not have concurrent depression. As discussed in Chapter 5, brain systems underlying different anxiety states appear to overlap with depression-related ICNs; however, there also may be ICNs that are more specific to anxiety states. Does the increased cellular connectivity triggered by antidepressants also repair circuits that are malfunctioning in anxiety disorders, or do other mechanisms contribute? What are the anatomic and functional specificities of these effects? Do medication-induced changes in cellular connectivity help repair whatever malfunctioning circuits are within reach of the adrenergic and serotonergic systems, or do benefits ultimately accrue from widespread brain changes, reflecting the broad distribution of monoaminergic systems within the brain? Many antidepressant drugs also help patients with chronic pain. Are chronic pain circuits within the sphere of influence of these broadly distributed transmitter systems and thus do they benefit from the growth-inducing changes that the antidepressants initiate?

This discussion is obviously not meant to be a review of the mechanisms of action of antidepressants; rather, it is meant to demonstrate that we have much to learn before we understand what complex drugs like antidepressants actually do. Simple explanations based on acute effects of drugs on single transmitter systems provide some insight, but they are unlikely to account entirely for the changes leading to clinical benefits. It is also critical to understand that all drugs, even those called "selective," are sloppy. Redundancy in the structure of neurotransmitter receptors, transporters, and other proteins ensures that all drugs do more than one thing. For example, some SSRIs affect the synthesis or metabolism of neurosteroids, which are powerful endogenous neuromodulators that can enhance GABAergic inhibition. How and whether these effects contribute to clinical actions is uncertain. The point here is that we can be fooled into believing we understand more than we do when considering drug actions. Only when we understand the ICNs involved in illness and the dynamics of these neurocircuits in healthy and disordered brains will we begin to unravel how drugs actually work.

Anxiolytics

We have already mentioned that many antidepressant agents are also effective anxiolytics. Benzodiazepines are also very effective at treating certain anxiety disorders, and, as noted earlier, they work quickly: they immediately enhance the ability of the neurotransmitter GABA to inhibit neurons when certain types of GABA-A receptors are activated. GABA-A receptors are ligand-gated ion channels (ionotropic receptors) and consist of five protein subunits. Benzodiazepines bind to a site that is formed by adjacent alpha and gamma subunits. Many types of GABA-A receptors contain both of these subunit types; those that do not contain both subunits do not respond to benzodiazepines. Gamma subunits help to target GABA-A receptors to synapses; thus, benzodiazepines are likely to have greater effects on synaptic than extrasynaptic GABA receptors, given that many extrasynaptic receptors do not express gamma subunits. Understanding the importance of extrasynaptic receptors in modulating brain function is a rapidly advancing area in neuroscience and one with potential for new drug development. In addition to gamma subunits, there are six subtypes of alpha subunits, and these differ greatly in their responsiveness to benzodiazepines. Receptors containing alpha 1, 2, 3, and 5 subunits are enhanced by anxiolytic benzodiazepines, whereas those expressing alpha 4 or alpha 6 subunits are insensitive. Based on work in rodents, it appears that different effects of benzodiazepines depend on the particular type of alpha subunit expressed. Receptors containing alpha 1 subunits mediate sedation, while those expressing alpha 2, or alpha 3 subunits may produce anti-anxiety effects. These intriguing findings offer hope for developing drugs with greater specificity and perhaps fewer side effects. Furthermore, they may help to explain some of the questions regarding specificity raised earlier. In fact, zolpidem is an agent that acts selectively at benzodiazepine sites on receptors expressing alpha 1 subunits and is an effective sleep medication with little apparent anxiolytic action.

Anxiety involves, at least in part, a network in which the extended amygdala, including the amygdala itself and the bed nucleus of the stria terminalis, plays a major role. It is likely that actions within the amygdala or its major connections have a lot to do with the beneficial effects of benzodiazepines. What is it about the functional anatomy of the GABAergic system that allows benzodiazepines to quell the amygdala without having severely incapacitating side effects? Benzodiazepine-responsive GABA receptors are widely distributed throughout the brain. One might think that augmenting the major fast inhibitory transmitter found throughout the brain would have profound effects on all aspects of brain function. It is true that these drugs can enhance sleep, help with seizure control, and, at high doses, help muscles relax; nonetheless, at anxiolytic doses, they don't stop the brain from functioning.

Does this suggest that the circuits malfunctioning in anxiety disorders are susceptible to repair at drug concentrations that are low enough that they don't strongly dysregulate normally functioning brain systems? To address this issue, it is important to understand how GABA acts within the amygdala and limbic system. GABA is typically a local circuit transmitter. Unlike neurons using monoamines as their transmitter, GABAergic interneurons use their synaptic contacts to act rapidly within a local brain region to keep the principal excitatory (output) neurons under control. By making GABA more effective, benzodiazepines make interneurons more powerful in regulating the output of the excitatory neurons, in this case diminishing outputs that drive stress and flight responses. Specificity may arise by virtue of the types of GABA-A receptors expressed on the principal neurons and where those receptors are expressed. For example, alpha 2-containing receptors may be particularly important in dampening spike firing by the excitatory output neurons, diminishing their ability to influence downstream targets. Dampening the firing of output neurons may also diminish their participation in forms of learning associated with anxiety disorders, such as fear conditioning.

The molecular mechanisms underlying the acute effects of benzodiazepines are fairly well understood, but extrapolating this knowledge to a system level remains a challenge. Unlike the antidepressants, these drugs work rapidly, and, therefore, their influence is likely to involve immediate receptor effects rather than growth of new connections. Benzodiazepines are also sometimes used to help chronic anxiety disorders such as generalized anxiety disorder (GAD). In these circumstances, are the beneficial effects the result of changes in brain ICNs that take a while to occur or the result of repeated exposures to the short-term effects of the medication? It is true that a person may develop a recurrence of symptoms if he or she misses a dose or two of a short-acting benzodiazepine; what isn't always clear is whether these symptoms represent the underlying anxiety state or a drug withdrawal phenomenon.

Benzodiazepines are among the most selective drugs used in psychiatry. They are very good at influencing specific types of GABA-A receptors while having little direct effect on other transmitter systems. Nonetheless, these drugs, like other psychotropic medications, also have off-target actions that complicate their use. For example, most benzodiazepines not only act at the sites on GABA-A receptors described above (called "central" benzodiazepine receptors), but they also cross cell membranes and bind a class of receptors on mitochondria (sometimes called "peripheral" benzodiazepine receptors), influencing mitochondrial function and enhancing the synthesis of GABAergic neurosteroids. Benzodiazepines vary in their ability to activate the mitochondrial receptors; clonazepam has little effect, while diazepam, alprazolam, and the anesthetic midazolam have significant effects. Thus, benzodiazepines are not all alike, and this may contribute to differences in clinical actions, including side effects.

Antipsychotics

A large number of drugs help patients suffering from hallucinations, delusions, and formal thought disorders. These drugs can diminish the positive psychotic symptoms that occur in many illnesses, including major depression, bipolar disorder, schizophrenia, delirium, dementias, and drug abuse. However, the effectiveness and safety of these medications vary depending on the nature of the illness. For instance, psychosis in dementia is less responsive than psychosis in schizophrenia; there are also more side effects as well as more dangerous side effects in elderly patients with dementia than in younger patients with schizophrenia.

Psychotic symptoms, independent of the illness with which they are associated, are thought to involve changes in the dopamine system and are the product of aberrant cognition. Antipsychotic drugs appear to work by blocking certain types of dopamine receptors; D2 receptor blockade is associated most commonly with antipsychotic efficacy. Unfortunately, D2 blockade in the striatum is also associated with movement related side effects. Newer antipsychotics have been developed that block certain serotonin (5HT2) receptors in addition to D2 receptors. This combination of dopamine and serotonin receptor blockade can minimize movement related side effects while maintaining antipsychotic efficacy. The serotonergic blockade is thought to increase release of dopamine in the striatum without increasing dopamine release in limbic regions to the same extent. This allows D2 blockade in limbic and cortical regions but minimizes D2 blockade in the striatum. D2 blockade in the striatum likely accounts for movement-related side effects (e.g., Parkinsonism, dystonia), while dopamine receptor blockade in limbic and cortical regions is more likely involved in modulating cognitive and emotional symptoms. ICNs involved in producing psychotic symptoms likely include both limbic and cortical areas, and dopamine clearly influences these ICNs. Dopamine receptor blockade also influences emotional processing and the ability of prefrontal cortex to determine important versus extraneous inputs.

While the D2 hypothesis of antipsychotic action has been helpful as a way to think about psychosis and the effects of medication, it is an oversimplification of the mechanisms contributing to psychosis. Importantly, the function of the ICNs involved in psychotic symptoms can't be understood purely in terms of D2 receptor blockade. For example, clozapine is extremely effective in treating psychotic symptoms even in patients resistant to the effects of other antipsychotics, but it is not as effective at blocking D2-type receptors as many other antipsychotics. Clozapine does bind D2 receptors, but it exits the receptor at a faster rate than most other drugs, leading to less time that the receptor is actually blocked. Similar and even faster off-rates are seen with quetiapine, another antipsychotic medication. These findings raise important questions about how long and to what degree D2 receptors must be blocked in order to produce antipsychotic effects. These considerations have led to the development of aripiprazole, a drug that is a partial agonist at D2 receptors. This means that aripiprazole occupies D2 receptors and prevents dopamine from binding but also has some intrinsic ability to do what dopamine does, although less effectively than dopamine itself. Thus, while aripiprazole dampens dopamine's actions at D2 receptors, it does not completely eliminate dopamine activity like a pure antagonist would. This is an example of how knowledge about the acute effects of a drug can lead to new ideas for drug development. It is not certain whether clozapine, the only antipsychotic that may truly be "atypical" (i.e., helps patients that other antipsychotic medications do not), has other properties that give it unique actions. It does influence other dopamine receptors (e.g., D4 receptors) as well as several other transmitters. How does clozapine work and why is it effective in treating psychotic symptoms in patients who do not respond to other antipsychotics? Does it have different effects on dopamine systems and their interaction with ICNs associated with psychoses, or does this drug work in a manner independent of dopamine? Antipsychotics usually take days to weeks to work fully, and, therefore, it is likely that long-term changes in cellular connectivity are involved.

There are many questions regarding psychosis and antipsychotics that should keep researchers busy and clinicians interested. For example, dopamine is involved in many brain functions including cognitive, motivation, and reward mechanisms; how do antipsychotics alleviate psychotic symptoms without disrupting other brain functions? Or do they? What is the relationship between the ICNs involved in psychosis and those involved in reward behaviors? Are there other approaches to treat psychoses that don't directly target dopamine? Interestingly, early proof-of-concept studies suggest that targeting the glutamate system via metabotropic glutamate receptors or the GABAergic system via specific subtypes of GABA-A receptors may provide alternative or complementary strategies for treating psychotic symptoms. Are there more effective strategies for treating psychotic disorders beyond targeting acute positive symptoms—strategies that would more effectively deal with the cognitive and motivational components of the illnesses (the so-called "negative" symptoms of schizophrenia)? These symptoms contribute greatly to disability, and present medications are largely ineffective against them. The various roles of dopamine within cognitive, emotional, and motivational systems preclude simple conceptualizations of psychosis as a state of altered dopamine function. In fact, present evidence suggests that dopamine function may be increased within striatal systems while being depressed in cortical cognitive systems in subjects with psychosis.

Mood Stabilizers

Mood stabilizers are typically used to dampen mood swings in persons with bipolar disorder. Three categories of mood stabilizers currently exist: lithium, anticonvulsants, and antipsychotics. How these different types of medications help persons with mania, bipolar depression, or mixed mood states is unknown. In particular, it is unclear why antipsychotics have mood-stabilizing properties. Certainly, their effects on dopamine receptors in emotion and motivation pathways in the amygdala, hippocampus, and nucleus accumbens could contribute. On the other hand, lithium is a simple element that can influence brain activity in a variety of ways that differ from the antipsychotics. Lithium can inhibit the process of cellular apoptosis (programmed cell death) and can help protect neurons against a variety of insults. These effects likely result from increases in the production of the anti-apoptotic protein BCL-2, or inhibition of glycogen synthase kinase-3β (GSK), an enzyme involved in cell death pathways. Lithium also has effects on the production of inositol phosphate second messengers via inhibition of inositol-1-phosphatase. Lithium also promotes the growth of new neurons in the dentate gyrus and has cellular effects that differ from the growth-enhancing effects of antidepressants. It is interesting to note that lithium is one of the few treatments in psychiatry that actually appear to diminish the risk of completed suicide. Valproate, a mood-stabilizing anticonvulsant, shares some neuroprotective properties with lithium, but valproate has other effects that are distinct from lithium (e.g., anticonvulsant actions). Whether these various effects are responsible for mood stabilization remains unknown, although other anticonvulsants (e.g., carbamazepine) are also used as mood stabilizers. It is thought that lamotrigine, another mood-altering anticonvulsant, has stronger antidepressant properties in patients with bipolar disorder than other mood stabilizers. If this is true, what is the mechanism? Many people are moody individuals. Do mood stabilizers affect normal moodiness, or are they effective only for mood instability resulting from the pathological state of bipolar disorder? As we better understand the neurocircuitry involved in bipolar disorder, we should learn more about the mechanisms of action of these drugs and be able to develop different and better types of medications.

Anti-dementia Agents

Substantial progress is being made in understanding the molecular causes of dementia of the Alzheimer's type (DAT). However, at the current time, there are no treatments that directly attack the causes of this disorder. Two classes of drugs are currently used to help delay deterioration: cholinesterase inhibitors and an NMDA receptor antagonist. How do cholinesterase inhibitors work? We know that these drugs increase acetylcholine levels and that cholinergic systems in the brain facilitate learning and memory. Of course, many other transmitter systems also influence memory. We know that central cholinergic systems are damaged in DAT; however, many other transmitter systems are also damaged in DAT, and, in fact, the cholinergic system is not among the first systems involved. Why does augmenting cholinergic function slow disease progression? Does augmenting acetylcholine levels lead to preservation of function in damaged ICNs and therefore decrease the rate of deterioration?

The beneficial effects of the cholinesterase inhibitors in DAT are instructive for psychiatry. In DAT, the key pathological events involve the production of amyloid plaques and neuritic tangles. Furthermore, the default ICN appears to be a major target for early dysfunction (Chapter 2), perhaps reflecting the high degree of synaptic activity and energy use in this system. Thus, in contrast to major psychiatric disorders, much is currently understood about the pathophysiology of DAT. Yet, treatment with cholinesterase inhibitors is much like other treatments in psychiatry: these agents have little (or nothing) to do with the primary pathology of the illness and may not even target the ICN of primary interest. It is also unclear whether these drugs slow illness progression by enhancing the function of the defective ICN or by allowing unaffected ICNs to work around defects in the default system. Similarly, it seems likely that the psychopharmacologic treatments outlined earlier in this chapter are also palliative in nature and may help defective networks reset or work around the problem that causes psychiatric dysfunction.

Memantine is a relatively weak noncompetitive antagonist of NMDA-type glutamate receptors, the receptors that play a critical role in synaptic plasticity and learning and memory. This drug appears to slow the deterioration of cognition and functional status in persons who are at moderate stages of dementia. Such individuals are highly symptomatic, and families are often beginning to consider nursing home care for their loved ones. How can a drug that blocks key receptors involved in memory formation help an illness in which memory problems are a prominent feature? Memantine's effects in DAT may result from its ability to protect cells from glutamate-mediated excitotoxicity but at the same time not produce sufficient inhibition of NMDA receptors to disrupt synaptic plasticity and cause learning defects. Alternatively, memantine may help overcome certain forms of NMDA receptor-mediated metaplasticity that impair the synaptic plasticity required for memory formation (Chapter 6).

Memantine shares biophysical mechanisms with ketamine and phencyclidine (PCP); all of these drugs cause a block of NMDA ion channels in which the blocking molecule binds in the open channel. So why doesn't memantine cause psychosis or marked memory impairment like ketamine and PCP? While the answer is not completely clear, differences in how memantine interacts with NMDA channels may contribute. Memantine appears to bind to two sites within the ion channel: a superficial (non-trapping) site and a deep (trapping) site. Ketamine occupies only the deep site. By occupying the superficial site, some memantine is able to exit the channel quickly and thus not produce the same dense block as ketamine. This subtle difference in mechanisms may result in huge differences in clinical effects. Recent data also suggest that memantine preferentially blocks extrasynaptic NMDA receptors, leaving the receptors involved in synaptic plasticity unaffected. On the other hand, it remains unclear whether memantine works strictly via the glutamate system. Memantine is most helpful during the moderate stage of DAT, a stage at which a lot of neuronal damage has already occurred. Its clinical effectiveness is also fairly limited. Why would a weak NMDA receptor antagonist slow the progression of DAT at the moderate stage of illness but not have a more powerful effect earlier in the disorder?

The more we understand the mechanisms underlying the brain destruction that occurs during DAT, the more we might understand how to intervene. Imaging and biomarker studies are now raising the possibility of diagnosing DAT before clinical symptoms become apparent. Simultaneously, medications are being developed that interfere with the life cycle of the putative causative agents: beta amyloid (plaques) and hyperphosphorylated *tau* protein (tangles). If DAT could be diagnosed prior to the onset of clinical symptoms, it might be possible to utilize effective neuroprotective treatments and prevent the onset of this illness or at least markedly slow its progression at very early stages of symptoms. This type of progress is a great example of the convergence of basic sciences, translational research, and therapeutics, and it serves as a model for what might be possible in primary psychiatric disorders.

Stimulants

Stimulants are frequently prescribed to treat attention-deficit/hyperactivity disorder (ADHD). People with this disorder have significant difficulties focusing and maintaining attention. Stimulants such as methylphenidate or amphetamines increase synaptic concentrations of dopamine by blocking its reuptake and/or enhancing its release from presynaptic terminals. Why do these drugs have a major behavioral action specifically on concentration and attention even though they influence wide regions of the brain?

Stimulants may influence certain cognitive systems even when these systems are not broken. For instance, college students without ADHD sometimes take these drugs to give themselves a perceived competitive edge in studying longer and perhaps more efficiently. In such situations, effects on cortical ICNs involved in working memory and attention may be particularly important, as are effects on arousal. A better understanding of the functioning of ICNs related to attention and the influence of stimulants on these ICNs should provide a better understanding of the use and misuse of these drugs.

Some stimulants have marked addictive and abuse potential, particularly when taken intravenously. When administered in a manner that results in rapid spikes in brain concentrations, the effects of these prescription drugs are similar to those of cocaine. Here, effects on the midbrain ventral tegmental area–nucleus accumbens motivational system may be particularly important (Chapter 5).

Drugs of Abuse

There are several categories of abused and addictive drugs, including alcohol (ethanol) and other sedatives, nicotine, stimulants, opiates, and cannabinoids. All strongly affect the ICN involved in the behavioral reward system in which dopamine is a key transmitter. Drugs of abuse activate this system by influencing overlapping parts of the network via different mechanisms. This characteristic is leading to the development of treatments for substance abuse that take advantage of the central reward ICN as a portal of entry. For instance, the opiate antagonist naltrexone is proving to be helpful in treating patients addicted to alcohol, even though effects on opiate receptors are not a principal mechanism of action for alcohol.

Many abused drugs seem to exert their influence by interacting with drug-specific receptors that affect the central reward ICN. These receptors include dopamine receptors, nicotine receptors, cannabinoid receptors, and opiate receptors. All of these receptors are natural components of the brain, and each responds to specific endogenous agonists. For example, an endogenous cannabinoid system that is involved in the effects of marijuana has been discovered. Cannabinoid 1 (CB1) receptors are metabotropic receptors and are among the most common receptors found in the brain. Several endogenous CB1 agonists derived from membrane lipids have been discovered over the past decade. Studies examining the effectiveness of cannabinoid antagonists in treating persons with addictions to marijuana and to other substances of abuse are in progress. Marijuana's effects on the endogenous cannabinoid system highlight the recurring theme that drugs of abuse typically overrun the operation of normal brain systems.

Drugs of abuse have the potential to reset the central reward ICN in a manner that requires the presence of the abused drug for normal function. When the drug is absent, specific pathways are activated that lead to drug-seeking behavior and to negative emotional states (depression, irritability, and anxiety). One effect of becoming addicted to these drugs is that the connectivity between dorsolateral prefrontal cortex, an area that plays a key role in working memory (Chapter 4), and the reward system becomes functionally diminished. The prefrontal cortex also helps us to moderate and control our behaviors. Without the intervention of the prefrontal cortex, a person has extreme difficulty in performing the executive processing required to avoid drug-seeking behaviors. The need to relieve anxiety and to find the next "fix" can become overwhelming. There are obvious differences among drug groups in the power of this addictiveness. For example, heroin is extremely addictive. Alcohol and nicotine, both legal agents, also have powerful addictive properties. Cannabinoids, although capable of substantial abuse, do not lead to as aggressive a drive for repeated drug use as some of the other drugs.

It is interesting to note that social networking is currently among the most powerful approaches in treating drug abuse and addictions. There is also evidence that a person's social network has a lot to do with whether the person becomes addicted to nicotine or quits smoking. Similarly, social networks influence the likelihood of obesity. While medications can facilitate a person's ability to resist drug use, social network groups such as Alcoholics Anonymous (AA) or group-mediated therapies are also very helpful. Social networks and social support can, at times, prove to be powerful enough to negate the drive for continued drug use. Social networking may serve as a form of cognitive rehabilitation that helps to reconnect prefrontal control systems to the reward ICN. Even with a strong social network, persons with addiction who have been "clean" for years or even decades consider themselves to be in a constant state of "recovery." They realize that they can quickly relapse should they return to use of the drug. It may take decades for brain networks to return to normal. In fact, we don't know if these networks ever fully return to normal; hence, the effects of addiction on brain circuitry may be life-long. The social aspects of drug abuse and their potential impact on brain function highlight a major reason we included "asociality" among our "5 A's" leading to chronic mental dysfunction (Chapter 12).

BRAIN-STIMULATION METHODS

Electroconvulsive Therapy

ECT is a powerful treatment when used for appropriate indications. It is most commonly used for patients with severe depression. Such patients have often failed to respond to multiple courses of antidepressant medications and psychotherapies.

A series of ECT treatments often leads to substantial or full remission of symptoms. ECT is typically administered as a course of about 6 to 12 treatments at a rate of 2 or 3 treatments per week. While initial clinical benefits can occur faster than with antidepressant medications, maximal clinical improvement typically takes about 2 to 3 weeks. Once ECT is discontinued, symptoms are likely to return unless other maintenance treatments are added. The high degree of relapse following ECT discontinuation is similar to the relapse observed when other antidepressant treatments are abruptly or prematurely discontinued. Patients with severe depression who respond to a course of ECT can be continued on a gradually tapering course of longer-term ECT (maintenance ECT) together with continuation treatment with medications. Although severe major depression is the most common indication for ECT, this treatment also can be beneficial for acute psychosis resulting from a variety of causes, catatonia, mania, and even the motor symptoms of Parkinson's disease. It is largely ineffective against personality disorders, substance-abuse syndromes, and chronic psychotic symptoms, particularly negative symptoms.

ECT is administered with unilateral (nondominant hemisphere, usually stimulating the right side of the head in the frontotemporal and parietal regions) or bilateral (bitemporal or bifrontal) electrode placement. Unilateral treatments, when administered properly in terms of electrical dose, can be as effective as bilateral treatments and have a lower incidence of certain cognitive side effects (confusion and verbal memory loss). ECT treatments involve the administration of a brief electric current. The administered charge (charge = current × time) must be large enough to cause a generalized electrical seizure in the brain, and the characteristics of the electrical stimulus also have an impact on clinical outcome. These electrical factors include how far above seizure threshold the stimulus is (for unilateral ECT) and perhaps the duration of the current pulses administered (particularly for bilateral ECT). Why characteristics of the electrical stimulus play a role in the benefits of ECT is not clear. What is clear is that all electrically induced seizures are not equal when it comes to producing clinical improvement.

Why repeated seizures have antidepressant efficacy is also not known. It is known that ECT treatments can influence various brain regions and alter the way those brain regions interact with each other. Repeated ECT-induced seizures have anticonvulsant effects; that is, repeated seizures help neurons become more resistant to subsequent seizures, perhaps through homeostatic mechanisms. How or whether this anticonvulsant effect contributes to therapeutic effects is unknown. In animals, ECT triggers a large number of neurochemical and receptor changes. We would suggest that ECT works by helping the brain networks reset from dysfunction associated with psychiatric illness, ultimately improving the function and perhaps connectivity between specific ICNs. The treatment may also diminish aberrant connectivity within and across networks. Consistent with these speculations, imaging studies provide some evidence that a successful course of ECT dampens activity in regions of prefrontal cortex, including the subgenual anterior cingulate cortex (ACC), that are overly active in depression. We would also note that the effectiveness of ECT across a variety of psychiatric disorders and its propensity to produce significant cognitive (memory) side effects are strong indications that its actions are not specific for any given ICN or brain region.

ECT does not correct the underlying causes of depression or any other psychiatric disorder; it temporarily alters the function of brain circuits. It is hoped that once reset by ECT, the circuits may be more receptive to stabilization by continued treatments that are less invasive. At times, patients can maintain a state of good mental health on treatment regimens that include medications and psychotherapies; at other times, the only treatment that seems to help is maintenance ECT. Here, the frequency of treatments is slowly decreased over a several-month period while the patient's symptoms are monitored carefully. In many ways, maintenance treatment with ECT is no different than maintenance treatment with medications or perhaps even psychotherapy. Considerable clinical literature indicates that stopping treatment for depression or other psychiatric disorders soon after the onset of clinical improvement carries a very high risk of relapse. The reasons why this is true are not well understood, but it is safe to say that effective treatment does not eliminate the cause of network dysfunction leading to illness.

As we learn more about the ICNs influenced by ECT, new approaches to treatment that are less costly and perhaps less invasive with fewer side effects will likely be developed. In addition, ECT technology may advance and allow more focal treatments. For instance, devices may be developed that stimulate certain regions of brain while inhibiting others (see rTMS section below). If this type of specificity can be achieved, electrical treatments could become useful in treating a broader range of psychiatric disorders, perhaps with fewer side effects than convulsive therapy.

Vagus Nerve Stimulation

VNS involves chronic intermittent stimulation of the vagus nerve. It has been used for more than 15 years in patients with refractory epilepsy and, more recently, has shown promise in helping some patients with severe, treatment-resistant depression. Interestingly, its effectiveness in depression may increase over time, with maximal benefits taking 6 months or longer to develop fully. Based on anecdotal observations, beneficial effects may last for years with continuous stimulation.

VNS requires a surgical procedure in which a stimulating electrode is positioned on the vagus nerve and is used to activate afferent fibers that connect to centers in the brain stem. These vagal afferents influence the nucleus tractus solitarius (NTS), a key brain-stem area that participates in processing inputs from the autonomic nervous system. The NTS is connected to brain regions that are likely involved in the circuitry underlying depression, including the anterior insular cortex, a region that seems to play a major role in processing interoceptive information. Why should chronic stimulation of vagal afferents over periods of months lead to clinical improvement? The answer is not known. However, as imaging technology advances, it is likely that longitudinal studies involving functional imaging will lead to a much better understanding of how this treatment influences ICN function. Preliminary studies suggest that successful VNS alters neural activity in brain regions that are abnormal during depression, including the subgenual ACC. Because VNS also has anticonvulsant properties, there is interest in determining whether it has mood-stabilizing properties in bipolar disorder. Although preliminary data suggest that this might be the case, the evidence is far from compelling at the present time.

Transcranial Magnetic Stimulation

Repetitive TMS (rTMS) uses an electromagnet to generate electrical fields over specific regions of the head in order to induce currents in the upper layers of the brain. Such stimulation can excite or inhibit cortical neurons. Neuronal changes depend on the frequency of stimulation and the location of the stimulating magnet. Stimulation at higher frequencies (10 Hz) appears to excite cortical neurons, while lower frequencies (1 Hz) inhibit underlying cortical regions. Interestingly, the effects on cortical neurons as a function of stimulus frequency are consistent with what is observed in the induction of long-term potentiation (LTP) and long-term depression (LTD) in cortex and hippocampus; the same number of pulses administered at higher frequencies result in LTP, while lower-frequency stimulation produces LTD.

rTMS appears to help some patients with depression, but it probably isn't as effective as ECT in highly refractory patients using current stimulation protocols. Importantly, unlike ECT, rTMS does not involve either general anesthesia or the induction of a seizure. Similar to ECT, however, rTMS does involve a course of treatments usually administered once a day, five days per week over a several-week period. Over a course of treatments, functional changes in brain structures that are part of the limbic system are indirectly induced. Optimal treatment parameters, such as the frequency and strength of stimulation as well as the location of the magnets, are being studied but have not yet been worked out in nearly as much detail as the electrical stimuli used for ECT. Since rTMS can be done in an outpatient office, it has the potential to be widely used by psychiatrists. Therefore, it is important that the stimulation parameters are defined in greater detail and that the clinical conditions that respond to this treatment are well understood before rTMS is made available for wide-scale use.

rTMS may provide a means of altering cortical activity much more focally than other treatments in psychiatry. This is an intriguing aspect of rTMS that is relevant to thinking about the brain regions involved in mood and information processing. In effect, rTMS and derivative methods could offer the potential to modulate specific ICNs, such as cortical attention circuits and working memory circuits, for therapeutic purposes. Efforts are also being made to use more powerful magnetic fields to replace electrical stimulation as a way to induce therapeutic generalized seizures. This is called magnetic seizure therapy (MST). There is hope that MST may be able to produce the clinical benefits of ECT with fewer cognitive side effects. Similar considerations motivate efforts to develop more focally administered electrical stimulation to induce seizures (called FEAST).

Deep Brain Stimulation

Electrical stimulation of structures deep within the brain via neurosurgically implanted electrodes has been available for the treatment of severe Parkinson's disease for many years. This approach is now being studied as a potential treatment for highly refractory depression and obsessive-compulsive disorder (OCD). Based on neuroimaging studies implicating the subgenual ACC as a key node in the circuitry of depression, Helen Mayberg and colleagues have been studying the effects of DBS of white matter tracks adjacent to this region. Although the number of patients studied with DBS is small (20 in the published Mayberg studies at the time of this writing), the results are encouraging, with up to 60% achieving substantial relief of symptoms with ongoing and continuous stimulation. This is a remarkable outcome, given the highly refractory and chronic symptoms in these patients. Stimulating certain key convergence zones may provide the ability to reset ICNs in a manner that allows them to return to "normal" or near-normal function. The early results from the Mayberg group are important for a number of reasons, not the least of which is that, to our knowledge, this is the first time that neuroimaging findings have led to a specific therapeutic intervention in psychiatry.

Other research groups are targeting DBS to the nucleus accumbens reward pathway for treatment of refractory depression. Stimulation parameters and locations are likely to become better defined as more research groups actively investigate this procedure. Results are similarly promising for the treatment of severe OCD, where several sites of stimulation, including the anterior limb of the internal capsule, are being evaluated; trials stimulating this region are also underway in refractory depression, again highlighting possible shared circuitry among disorders. By utilizing functional imaging technology together with stimulation paradigms, the ability to accurately define the various functional circuits underlying these illnesses should increase.

It is amazing that artificial stimulation of the brain seems to reset brain systems in a manner that improves psychiatric (and neurological) symptoms. The diversity of methods used to influence brain electrical activity is vast. Stimulating large areas of the brain with ECT or large areas of superficial cortex with rTMS can help some patients. Both of these methods involve several treatment sessions per week and intermittent exposure to electrical or magnetic stimulation. Interestingly, benefits can be observed fairly quickly, particularly with ECT, but maximal response takes a few weeks of treatment. VNS and DBS require more continuous stimulation of vagal afferents or brain regions involved in illness circuitry, but again, maximal benefits may require a significant period of stimulation, particularly for VNS. In fact, with VNS, benefits seem to accrue up to a year or so after initiation of treatment in some patients, and those who improve seem to maintain the benefits with continued stimulation.

To improve these treatments, much more must be learned about the biology of the illnesses, the function of the underlying neural systems in health and illness, and the optimal stimulation parameters for modulating brain function. It is now possible to study the mechanisms of action of these various devices on the functioning of ICNs. For example, recent studies in a rodent model of parkinsonism have attempted to determine how DBS in the subthalamic nucleus (STN) produces therapeutic effects. This work used sophisticated techniques of "optogenetics" in which the expression of light-activated ion channels is used to probe neural circuitry and behavior. These studies found that the effects of DBS may result from stimulation of axons entering the STN and not from direct effects on STN neurons themselves. This work has implications for the clinical use of DBS in Parkinson's disease. It suggests that other less invasive ways to stimulate the afferent STN axons may also be beneficial, perhaps by targeting more accessible output neurons in primary motor cortex that project to STN. This work also raises the possibility that modulation of axon tracts may be a critical component mediating the benefits of DBS in psychiatric disorders. Toward this end, trials are underway using more focal epidural electrical stimulation of prefrontal cortex in patients with refractory depression.

PSYCHOTHERAPIES

There is compelling evidence that psychotherapies can be helpful in treating many psychiatric disorders. Psychotherapeutic efficacy likely depends on many factors, including the personality and skills of the therapist and the specific type of therapy. Deciphering how various components of psychotherapy play a role in clinical benefits is in some ways parallel to analyzing the similarities and differences of various classes of antidepressants. Available data support the idea that clinical improvement resulting from psychotherapies, medications, or combinations of both is associated with changes in the function of specific brain systems. Based on observed changes in regional metabolism in frontal cortex and the hippocampus, it appears that antidepressant medications, ECT, and cognitive behavioral therapy (CBT) have distinct effects on the circuitry of depression. Medications appear to increase metabolism in frontal cortex while diminishing activity in hippocampus. CBT has the opposite effects, decreasing metabolism in frontal cortex and increasing activity in the hippocampus, while ECT diminishes metabolism in both regions. These intriguing observations suggest that there are distinct, but possibly complementary, ways to reset the neural systems involved in psychiatric illnesses. Interestingly, the enhanced hippocampal metabolism observed with CBT may reflect the learning associated with this form of treatment, while the enhanced metabolism in frontal cortex seen with medications may give clues about the role of monoamines in modulating cortical function, perhaps affecting attention and working memory. Similarly, it is important to disentangle which effects on neural circuitry contribute to clinical benefits, which are therapeutically neutral, and which result in side effects.

In prior sections, we noted the nonspecificity of pharmacologic and device-mediated treatments. It is also important to note that many psychotherapies are also nonspecific in their clinical utility. For example, CBT, the most intensely studied of the psychotherapies, can benefit a wide range of conditions, including mood disorders, anxiety disorders, chronic insomnia, chronic pain, and possibly schizophrenia, at the minimum. To us this highlights the rehabilitative nature of psychotherapy and the power that it may have when combined with pharmacologic or brain-stimulation approaches.

It is increasingly being recognized that using neuroscientific methods to study the effectiveness and underlying mechanisms of psychotherapies is important. The same scientific rigor that is applied to pharmacologic interventions and device-mediated interventions can be applied to all psychotherapies. In recent years, clinicians skilled in psychotherapeutic interventions have become increasingly interested in studying how psychotherapies affect brain function, and clinicians specializing in somatic interventions are increasingly interested in understanding the effects of psychotherapy on brain systems. The tension between psychotherapy and somatic therapy camps has been a significant and misguided part of psychiatry's past, but it is unlikely to play as noticeable a role in psychiatry's future as the two camps converge on understanding neural mechanisms in illnesses and their treatments.

LIFESTYLE INTERVENTIONS

Certain lifestyle activities can have significant beneficial effects on all aspects of health, including mental health. Routine exercise, sleep hygiene, learning, social interactions, balanced diets, weight control, and avoidance of tobacco and excessive alcohol all appear to promote well-being. How these lifestyle factors may prevent or aid in the treatment of psychiatric symptoms is not yet understood, but their mechanisms of action are likely to be diverse. Although these "interventions" are even less specific than the treatments discussed previously, they can and should be studied. For example, the effects of exercise and weight loss can be investigated in terms of their effects on overall health and brain function using both human studies and animal models. At the present time, it suffices to emphasize that heart-healthy behaviors coupled with appropriate social interactions are, in general, good for people. The specificity and mechanisms of these effects are exciting areas for future work.

REHABILITATIVE VERSUS ETIOLOGIC THERAPIES

In considering the beneficial effects of talk therapy, Samuel Guze suggested that various psychotherapies represent forms of medical rehabilitation. In other words, psychotherapies can help patients function at higher levels even in the presence of ongoing symptoms; however, these treatments are not curative and their effectiveness is independent of the etiology of the symptoms. At the time he championed this concept, Guze sought to refute the notion that psychodynamic therapy specifically corrects the cause of symptoms. Importantly, treatments do not have to be directed at the mechanisms underlying an illness in order to be effective; current psychotropic medications are good examples of this fact. The rehabilitation analogy is based on the observation that physical, occupational, and speech therapies help patients regain function following strokes or other brain injuries. These therapies do not address the cause of the brain damage and do little to repair dead tissue; rather, they help patients learn methods of adapting to the damage and find other strategies to accomplish tasks such as walking, talking, and activities of daily living. This approach to treatment is different from ones like the use of antibiotics to treat infections. With the correct antibiotic, the actual cause of the illness is eradicated. The use of a combination of syndromic/symptom-based treatments and rehabilitative strategies is not unique to psychiatry; it is the norm in the management of most common illnesses in medicine.

We would extend Guze's concepts and suggest that there is likely to be a continuum between rehabilitative therapies and etiologic therapies when applied to the treatment of neuropsychiatric illnesses. Some aspects of psychotherapies are truly rehabilitative in that resulting changes in behavior may have little to do with the mechanisms underlying the symptoms. Thus, people may begin to feel better after they start to exercise or just become more active, and this "feeling better" may counteract some of the low mood that an underlying depression is causing. This is the essence of the "behavioral" component of CBT for depression. Certain therapies, however, may target brain systems that are directly involved in the underlying disorder. People with phobias, for example, can be successfully treated with exposure and desensitization therapy. Repeated controlled exposure to spiders may allow a person to become less fearful of spiders, and gradual exposure to heights may help a person to control a fear of heights. In fact, recent research suggests that administering a drug such as D-cycloserine, an agent that improves learning and enhances the function of gluta-mate synapses via effects on NMDA receptors, speeds the rate of improvement with exposure/desensitization therapies. This new learning may correct the abnormal function of fear circuits driving the phobia. Given advances in understanding how specific forms of learning are processed in the brain, it is possible that certain psy-chotherapies could be designed to target neural systems involved in the genesis of certain symptoms, even though they do not alter molecular or synaptic defects.

We believe that psychotherapies can be considered as falling at different places along a rehabilitative–etiologic continuum depending on the therapy and the disor-der. Most psychotherapies are rehabilitative, while other psychotherapies may par-tially target etiology or at least target specific brain systems relevant to the etiology. Studying psychotherapies from this perspective offers hope of devising even more effective approaches going forward. The work with D-cycloserine is an early proof-of-concept that targeting the synaptic machinery of learning and memory may be a way to enhance the effectiveness of certain psychotherapies. However, we would strongly caution against drawing conclusions about the mechanisms underlying any illness based on the effects of any psychotherapy. Psychiatry has pursued this path in the past, resulting in scientifically naïve statements about the "causes" of illnesses based on the effects of a therapy or the theory underlying a therapy. The more that psychotherapy research is rooted in modern brain science, including sophisticated neuroimaging, the higher the likelihood that treatments can be devised to influence aberrant circuitry.

What about psychotropic medications? Again, while these agents may have both direct and indirect effects on the ICNs that underlie illness, it is unlikely that medica-tions target the molecular etiologies of symptoms. Naturally, different medications may be more or less specific in terms of addressing actual causality. The acute actions of benzodiazepines may directly affect stress pathways that are on overdrive during an anxiety-producing situation. Although they do not prevent the stimuli associated with the stress response, they are effective in blocking or dampening that response. Antidepressants and antipsychotics are likely to have direct and indirect effects on the ICNs that underlie mood and psychotic symptoms, but these agents are unlikely to have any effect on the primary cause of the disorders. Thus, these drugs may fall midway on the rehabilitative–etiologic spectrum.

Cholinesterase inhibitors may improve some pathways that are harmed by the brain destruction associated with DAT. Although they don't reverse etiology, these drugs do directly influence specific pathways and can delay progression of clinical symptoms for 6 to 12 months. Medications are being developed that are designed to block the formation of beta-amyloid, the putative causative toxic protein that accumulates in DAT. These types of agents may be closer to drugs that interfere with the actual etiology of an illness. Similarly, antibody therapies designed to decrease or eliminate toxic accumulations of amyloid may target a process that is closely related to the etiology of the disorder. The key point is that the etiology of a disorder must be understood before it is possible to define etiology-based therapies. It also remains to be seen how well etiology-based therapies reverse symptoms after an illness has developed. It is possible, perhaps even likely, that once an illness has become manifest, wide-ranging degenerative and plastic changes in the brain will obviate the effectiveness of even highly specific etiology-based treatments. Indeed, recent findings suggest that amyloid deposition has both local and longer-range effects on brain function. In this case, a combination of etiology-based treatment and rehabilitative strategies may be required for optimal clinical outcomes.

What about ECT? Although it is one of the most effective treatments in psychiatry and perhaps all of medicine, its effects persist for only a limited time following the last treatment in an acute course. The efficacy of ECT suggests that it influences illness pathways but does not eliminate the cause. Furthermore, its ability to reset ICNs involved in illness is only temporary. It is not clear why the beneficial effects of ECT are time-limited, although the need for ongoing maintenance treatment is not unique to ECT and is found with psychotropic medications and other brain-stimulation methods. Interestingly, effective evidence-based psychotherapy may result in some of the more enduring therapeutic effects in psychiatry, perhaps reflecting the power of learning on the human brain.

It is important to realize that no matter where treatments fall along this rehabilitative–etiologic spectrum, they can be very helpful. Physical rehabilitation following a stroke or injury is often the most effective way to restore function partially or completely. Similarly, the rehabilitative effects of exercise on mood and general well-being may be as helpful as, or perhaps even more helpful than, medications for mild depression. Changing the behaviors of caregivers of patients with DAT can be more beneficial to the patient than a cholinesterase inhibitor, and the combination of both cholinesterase inhibitors and educational intervention may work synergistically.

THE ROLE OF THE PATIENT AND OTHERS
IN TREATMENT

As is true for many common illnesses, treatment of psychiatric illnesses can benefit from the involvement of family, friends, and support systems. We address this topic in our prior book *Demystifying Psychiatry*. When considering rehabilitative strategies in psychiatry, it is important to consider the role of social networks in determining clinical outcomes. Isolation and loneliness are unhealthy and bad for brain function. The rehabilitative role of social ties is visible in most aspects of life. Support from social networks such as small groups for alcoholics (Alcoholics Anonymous), club-house models of assisting persons with illnesses such as schizophrenia, and cancer support groups can be very effective at helping people feel that others care, that they are not alone, and that they have self-worth. For many disorders, support systems that address the family's needs as well as those of the patient can be very valuable. For example, the Alzheimer's Association provides many support services for caregivers, who can easily become stressed and depressed. Their tiered level of support can be highly effective in providing the psychological and physical resources to help a family keep the patient at home instead of moving him or her to a nursing home. Similar approaches are found in Al-Anon for families of alcoholics and in the National Alliance on Mental Illness for families struggling with other mental disorders.

Although we have focused on the neuroscience of psychiatric illness in this book, we do not believe that neuroscience will provide all the answers going forward. On the other hand, ignoring neuroscience will greatly delay progress in addressing the causes of these disorders and in developing new and innovative ways to manage psychiatric disorders. Once we understand molecular and synaptic causes and the ways these causes lead to phenotypic presentation via neural network changes, we will be better able to develop treatments that are targeted to specific aspects of aberrant brain function. Even when we understand much more about the brain mechanisms underlying psychiatric disorders, it is likely that rehabilitative and social support efforts will remain important in clinical practice. This is not unique to psychiatry; it is true in the treatment of almost all common chronic disorders in medicine and neurology.

Points to Remember

As knowledge is gained about the pathophysiologies of psychiatric illnesses, the effects of medications on brain systems will be better understood.

Understanding the influence of medications on transmitters and receptors is useful, but understanding the influence of medications on brain systems that malfunction in psychiatric disorders will be more useful in terms of developing new and more effective approaches to treatment.

Some medications work quickly, while others take weeks to become effective. This difference in time course likely indicates that some medications lead to long-term changes in connectivity of various ICNs. The dimension of time is important to consider when examining how treatments work.

Psychotherapies can be very effective. Research methods are now available that will allow better understanding of the influence of various therapies on brain systems.

Lifestyle changes can help prevent and possibly treat certain medical and psychiatric illnesses. The mechanisms underlying the efficacy of lifestyle changes are an area for future research.

Various treatments for psychiatric disorders lie on a continuum from nonspecific to highly specific with regard to their mechanisms for influencing brain pathways.

Humans are social animals and do better in handling chronic illnesses when they and their caregivers become involved in appropriate support networks.

SUGGESTED READINGS

Krishnan, V., & Nestler, E. J. (2008). The molecular neurobiology of depression. *Nature, 455,* 894–902.

Ressler, K. J., & Mayberg, H. S. (2007). Targeting abnormal neural circuits in mood and anxiety disorders: from the laboratory to the clinic. *Nature Neuroscience, 10,* 1116–1124.

Schatzberg, A. F., & Nemeroff, C. B. (Eds.). (2009). *The American Psychiatric Publishing textbook of psychopharmacology* (4th ed.). Washington, DC: American Psychiatric Publishing.

Zorumski, C. F., & Rubin, E. H. (2010). *Demystifying psychiatry—A resource for patients and families.* New York: Oxford University Press.

OTHER REFERENCES

Bezprozvanny, I., (2009). Amyloid goes global. *Science Signaling, 2,* 1–3.

Breiter, H. C., Gollub, R. L., Weisskoff, R. M., Kennedy, D. N., Makris, N., Berke, J. D., et al. (1997). Acute effects of cocaine on human brain activity and emotion. *Neuron, 19,* 591–611.

Bruhl, A. B., Kaffenberger, T., & Herwig, U. (2010). Serotonergic and noradrenergic modulation of emotion processing by single dose antidepressants. *Neuropsychopharmacology, 35,* 521–533.

Clark, L., Chamberlain, S. R., & Sahakian, B. J. (2009). Neurocognitive mechanisms in depression: Implications for treatment. *Annual Review of Neuroscience, 32,* 57–74.

Drevets, W. C., Price, J. L., & Furey, M. L. (2008). Brain structural and functional abnormalities in mood disorders: Implications for neurocircuitry models of depression. *Brain Structure and Function, 213,* 93–118.

George, M. S., & Aston-Jones, G. (2010). Noninvasive techniques for probing neurocircuitry and treating illness: Vagus nerve stimulation (VNS), transcranial magnetic stimulation (TMS) and transcranial direct current stimulation (tDCS). *Neuropsychopharmacology, 35,* 301–316.

Giacobbe, P., Mayberg, H. S., & Lozano, A. M. (2009). Treatment resistant depression as a failure of brain homeostatic mechanisms: Implications for deep brain stimulation. *Experimental Neurology, 219,* 44–52.

Grunder, G., Carlsson, A., & Wong, D. F. (2003). Mechanism of new antipsychotic medications. *Archives of General Psychiatry, 60,* 974–977.

Hallett, M. (2007). Transcranial magnetic stimulation: A primer. *Neuron, 55,* 187–199.

Harmer, C. J., O'Sullivan, U., Favaron, E., Massey-Chase, R., Ayres, R., Reinecke, A., et al. (2009). Effect of acute antidepressant administration on negative affective bias in depressed patients. *American Journal of Psychiatry, 166*, 1178–1184.

Hollon, S. D., Stewart, M. O., & Strunk, D. (2006). Enduring effects for cognitive behavior therapy in the treatment of depression and anxiety. *Annual Review of Psychology, 57*, 285–315.

Jeste, D. V., Blazer, D., Casey, D., Meeks, T., Salzman, C., Schneider, L., et al. (2008). ACNP white paper: Update on use of antipsychotic drugs in elderly persons with dementia. *Neuropsychopharmacology, 33*, 957–970.

Kapur, S. (2004). How antipsychotics become anti-psychotic—from dopamine to salience to psychosis. *Trends in Pharmacological Sciences, 25*, 402–406.

Kapur, S., & Seeman, P. (2001). Does fast dissociation from the dopamine D2 receptor explain the action of atypical antipsychotics?: A new hypothesis. *American Journal of Psychiatry, 158*, 360–369.

Kotermanski, S. W., Wood, J. T., & Johnson, J. (2009). Memantine binding to a superficial site on NMDA receptors contributes to partial trapping. *Journal of Physiology (London), 587*, 4589–4603.

Kovacsics, C. E., Gottesman, I. I., & Gould, T. D. (2009). Lithium's antisuicidal efficacy: Elucidation of neurobiological targets using endophenotype strategies. *Annual Review of Pharmacology and Toxicology, 49*, 175–198.

Manji, H. K., Moore, G. J., & Chen, G. (1999). Lithium at 50: Have the neuroprotective effects of this unique cation been overlooked? *Biological Psychiatry, 46*, 929–940.

McKernan, R. M., Rosahl, T. W., Reynolds, D. S., Sur, C., Wafford, K. A., Atack, J. R., et al. (2000). Sedative but not anxiolytic properties of benzodiazepines are mediated by the GABA$_A$ receptor alpha1 subtype. *Nature Neuroscience, 3*, 587–592.

Raina, P., Santaguida, P., Ismaila, A., Patterson, C., Cowan, D., Levine, M., et al. (2008). Effectiveness of cholinesterase inhibitors and memantine for treating dementia: Evidence review for a clinical practice guideline. *Annals of Internal Medicine, 148*, 379–397.

Salvadore, G., Cornwell, B. R., Sambataro, F., Latov, D., Colon-Rosario, V., Carver, F., et al. (2010). Anterior cingulate desynchronization and functional connectivity with the amygdala during a working memory task predict rapid antidepressant response to ketamine. *Neuropsychopharmacology, 35*, 1415–1422.

Simpson, E. H., Kellendonk, C., & Kandel, E. R. (2010). A possible role for the striatum in the pathogenesis of the cognitive symptoms of schizophrenia. *Neuron, 65*, 585–596.

Tokuda, K., O'Dell, K. A., Izumi, Y., & Zorumski, C. F. (2010) Midazolam inhibits hippocampal long-term potentiation and learning through dual central and peripheral benzodiazepine receptor activation and neurosteroidogenesis. *Journal of Neuroscience, 30*, 16788–16795.

Xia, P., Chen, H.-S. V., Zhang, D., & Lipton, S. A. (2010). Memantine prefentially blocks extrasynaptic NMDA receptor currents in hippocampal autapses. *Journal of Neuroscience, 30*, 246–250.

14

The Future of Psychiatry

Psychiatry is at an important point in its history. Over the next few years, two major initiatives with relevance to the field will come to fruition: the fifth edition of the *Diagnostic and Statistical Manual of the American Psychiatric Association* (DSM-5) and the Human Connectome Project. The former will expand upon DSM-IV and introduce a diagnostic system with updated concepts and criteria for classifying mental disorders. The latter is a scientific initiative by the National Institutes of Health that will use brain imaging and neurophysiological methods to map the connectivity and function of brain regions and networks. Although we are intrigued by both efforts, we wonder which will have a greater impact on the future of psychiatry. Given the current state of science, we would argue that the connectome project has the potential to change radically how we think about psychiatric disorders and their treatment, and thus it is likely to have a much greater long-term influence on the field. We view DSM-5 as only a small step forward, given the current state of science. Furthermore, we believe that work on DSM-6 should not proceed until the findings from the connectome project and advances in behavioral genetics are fully digested and can be incorporated into the process.

One of our major goals in writing this book is to highlight the tremendous potential of psychiatry as a branch of clinical neuroscience and to illustrate the ways in which a deeper understanding of brain network biology is becoming increasingly relevant to understanding psychiatric illnesses. This is work in progress, and how the field will evolve is open to speculation, including ours. What seems clear, however, is that psychiatric disorders are not the result of defects in one or even a few neurotransmitter systems, or one or several genes. These disorders do not result from changes in isolated brain structures. The key to understanding psychiatric illnesses lies in determining how brain networks function, which networks are involved in which illnesses, and how abnormal processing results in the signs and symptoms of mental disorders. Understanding how the human brain interacts with its environment is a critical component of this. The explosion of information about how the human brain processes information and makes decisions is advancing rapidly, but it is only in its infancy. Methods for imaging and studying brain function will become increasingly sophisticated in the future, as will the ability to couple human studies with cellular, molecular, and synaptic studies in animals. Animal models that are much more relevant to human illnesses than our current models will be developed. Advances in fields such as optogenetics that use the expression of light-activated proteins and signaling molecules to probe neural systems in animals are revolutionizing how we think about network neuroscience. Optogenetic studies also offer the possibility of providing innovative ways to alter network function in a variety of neuropsychiatric illnesses, perhaps by using light-activated molecules as a way to manipulate activity in specific brain systems. Proofs-of-principle for these concepts are already being found in animal models and are moving forward in other fields, such as cancer biology. Of particular relevance to psychiatry have been recent efforts to manipulate specific basal ganglia pathways in rodent models of Parkinson's disease using optogenetic methods. These studies have demonstrated a dissociation of two striatal pathways, with stimulation of the "indirect" pathway (the path that uses D2 dopamine receptors) producing motor dysfunction and stimulation of the "direct" pathway (using D1 receptors) improving motor function. This work highlights the importance of understanding how specific neural pathways, even within the same network, are involved in clinical dysfunction and can possibly be manipulated for therapeutic purposes.

Research in systems neuroscience offers hope for deciphering how neural circuits function and how they go awry in a broad range of disorders. Similarly, advances in human genetics are beginning to unravel how genes and their products contribute to complex brain illnesses. It is now easy to envision how the power of human neuroimaging and genetics can be combined to unravel the activities of human brain systems. This includes recent multi-center studies that demonstrate the feasibility of mapping brain networks using large numbers of subjects. Large sample sizes will likely be required to unravel variation in connectivity networks, the involvement of connectivity networks in illnesses, and the contribution of specific genes to network functions. This work will serve as an underpinning for advances in cellular and molecular neuroscience that will provide potential new targets for therapeutic interventions. It has become clear that many psychiatric disorders, like most (if not all) common chronic medical conditions, involve many genes that each contribute only a small amount to the heritability of the disorder. The potential importance of understanding the roles of rarer, more recent mutations that lead to changes in gene copy number is only beginning to be appreciated, but this holds potential for describing how signaling cascades contribute to illnesses. Drawing analogies from what is being learned about common metabolic disorders such as diabetes and obesity, we expect that each genetic finding will be only one small step forward in helping to understand mechanisms, refine diagnoses, and target new treatments. Results from genetic studies may help to subclassify monolithic syndromes, however, and this can have an impact on therapeutic strategies. For example, individuals with different subtypes of maturity-onset diabetes of the young (MODY) require different approaches to control their glucose levels depending, in part, on whether they have mutations in the glucokinase gene and, if so, how the mutations affect enzyme kinetics. This is an exciting example of how genetics can drive personalized medicine. Also, genetic findings have led some scientists to conclude that some forms of obesity may be best conceptualized as brain and neurobehavioral disorders that have strong genetic and environmental contributions. This will undoubtedly be true of all psychiatric disorders.

Psychiatry finds itself at a crossroads. One branch of the field embraces the advances in science and is looking for ways that those advances can affect clinical practice. Another branch holds to more traditional views and emphasizes a humanistic focus on individuals, families, and society, sometimes viewing progress in neuroscience as antithetical (or at least irrelevant) to clinical care. Both sides have points to make, but we believe the dichotomy is both false and destructive to the field. The two views do not necessarily conflict and are not mutually exclusive. By applying clinically significant neuroscientific and genetic advances to the care of patients and their families, we hope to advance the ability of psychiatrists to help individuals more effectively. At a minimum, understanding psychiatric disorders as brain dysfunctions can relieve a lot of the guilt and stigma still associated with these illnesses.

We believe that in order to remain viable and pertinent as a medical discipline, psychiatry must redefine itself and take advantage of progress in multiple scientific and clinical domains, including a broad array of neurosciences and genetics. In addition, the field must pay closer attention to new information coming from the fields of public health and health-care economics—information that should have a major impact on how psychiatry is conceptualized and practiced. Unfortunately, much of current clinical practice is divorced from the advances in science, and many (if not most) psychiatrists treat the brain as a "black box." In our opinion, future trainees must become comfortable with the concepts discussed in this book and how these concepts evolve as science moves forward. Familiarity with neurosciences and genetics is the path to enhancing the translation of modern science into clinical practice.

PSYCHIATRY AND CLINICAL NEUROSCIENCE

It is of prime importance that psychiatry systematically views itself as a branch of clinical neuroscience and seeks a closer clinical and scientific relationship with its sibling discipline of neurology, particularly the aspects of neurology that focus on cognition and behavior. Psychiatric disorders are brain disorders, and psychiatrists must learn to think about psychiatric illnesses as manifestations of brain and neural circuit dysfunction. The languages of systems neuroscience and clinical psychiatry must converge. This means conceptualizing symptoms and syndromes in terms of aberrant brain circuitry and function. We would argue that intrinsic connectivity networks (ICNs) in the brain provide an appropriate basis for clinicians to describe signs, symptoms, and disorders. It is at this level that the phenotypic expressions of illness will make most clinical sense. For example, patients exhibiting formal thought disorder (particularly severe forms such as tangentiality, derailment, and incoherence) have marked problems translating their thinking into goal-directed speech. Primary or secondary defects in circuits involving language ICNs are likely contributors. While the mechanisms underlying the defects may not be well understood yet, conceptualizing the problem from an ICN perspective has immediate practical implications for treatment.

Aberrant language function can be a target for cognitive intervention and rehabilitation, perhaps using methods already developed for individuals with certain forms of aphasia. Such a rehabilitative approach can pay dividends, as shown by recent advances in dyslexia, where principles derived from neuroscience are strongly influencing educational efforts. Intensive remedial instruction in reading has been shown to modify brain structure and connectivity in a positive way. Recent data indicate that in persons with dyslexia, behavioral measures (i.e., clinical assessments) of language function are poor predictors of improvement in reading abilities following educational efforts. Rather, activation patterns in right prefrontal regions during a reading task, together with white matter integrity in the right superior longitudinal fasciculus (including the arcuate fasciculus), are predictive of improvement. These studies highlight the potential utility of brain imaging in the rehabilitative process. We would also note recent research examining the influence of literacy on brain function. These studies demonstrated significant changes in the way language is processed in the left (dominant) hemisphere with literacy, even when literacy was achieved in adulthood. These changes included greater engagement of the entire language processing network by written sentences as well as enhanced phonological processing in the planum temporale region. Interestingly, learning to read is also accompanied by a decrease in facial perception in the left hemisphere, suggesting compensatory or competition effects.

Similarly, individuals with schizophrenia have been shown repeatedly to have defects in working memory that are, arguably, the most reliable cognitive hallmark of the disorder. These defects can be targets for therapeutic interventions, particularly ones centered on social and occupational rehabilitation. Just as in patients with traumatic brain injuries, it may not be possible to correct the primary defects, but strategies to work around the defects, particularly those that focus on applications to real-world problems, can be developed that could improve the ability of individuals to lead more productive lives. Recent work using learning strategies to enhance cognitive control in individuals with schizophrenia is a hopeful step in this direction. Studies of the default network in several psychiatric illnesses have demonstrated that individuals with schizophrenia, major depression, and possibly anxiety disorders have defects in their ability to refocus attention from interoceptive to exteroceptive worlds while doing specific cognitive tasks. These problems, which are reminiscent of defects observed in neglect syndromes in neurology, could represent a form of "inattention" and likely contribute to what psychiatrists refer to as "denial" and "lack of insight." It is not hard to imagine that a person who has a problem shifting between internal and external worlds might also have a problem recognizing a defect in thinking. The fact that defects in focusing task-oriented attention (conceptualized in systems neuroscience and not psychiatric terms) cut across psychiatric disorders might also explain the repeated observation that cognitive behavioral therapy is effective in a wide range of disorders. It is inappropriate to ignore these defects as simply being untreatable manifestations of illness. Serious efforts are underway to develop pharmacologic treatments for cognitive impairment based on principles learned from research on synaptic plasticity, and such treatments could be important adjuncts to psychotherapeutic, behavioral, and educational efforts. Also, the evolving work on fear conditioning in animals is leading to potentially novel psychotherapeutic approaches to extinguish stress-induced learning in humans based on the ability of memory networks in the brain to rewrite emotional memories during the process of memory reconsolidation. Here a combination of targeted pharmacology and sophisticated cognitive and behavioral interventions may prove to be most effective, as evidenced by studies demonstrating the utility of β-blockers to diminish autonomic arousal during emotional memory retrieval and extinction. Other strategies using targeted brain stimulation methods, including transcranial magnetic stimulation and transcranial direct current stimulation, are also possible approaches for manipulating aberrant ICNs.

PSYCHIATRIC DIAGNOSIS AND TREATMENT

In Chapter 5, we raised the possibility of reconceptualizing psychiatric illnesses along the dimensions of cognitive, emotional, or motivational networks, thus aligning illnesses more closely with the functional operations of the human mind. We believe this scheme has practical implications for how we think about diagnosis and treatment. For example, we have emphasized that individuals with the diagnosis of "major depression" are markedly heterogeneous (Chapter 2) and that failure to take this heterogeneity into account results in diagnostic imprecision, which can result in less effective treatment. When it comes to treating depression, one size definitely does not fit all. At a minimum, we would argue that non-psychotic major depression in the absence of another psychiatric disorder (called "primary" depression in an older diagnostic system) is different from major depression with psychosis or major depression arising in the context of a preexisting motivational disorder (e.g., substance-abuse or personality disorder), emotional disorder (e.g., social anxiety disorder), or cognitive disorder (e.g., dementia, traumatic brain injury, or obsessive-compulsive disorder). Although antidepressant medications may be used to treat all of these subtypes of depression, their effectiveness is likely to differ across subtypes and to vary with illness severity. Other pharmacologic and rehabilitative approaches will often be needed to address the preexisting and comorbid dysfunctions, which are likely to color the outcome of any treatment.

Beyond this approach to thinking about diagnosis, we wonder whether psychiatry will eventually be able to use results from structural and functional neuroimaging studies to devise more effective treatment strategies. For example, some but not all patients with major depression have changes in hippocampal volume, changes in the size of the subgenual anterior cingulate cortex, and/or thinning of neocortex. Are different subtypes of depression associated with different subsets of structural changes? How do these structural changes affect brain networks and responses to various treatments? Can these changes be detected reliably and validly in individual patients? Research demonstrating the clinical usefulness of such approaches seems warranted and timely. At present, these considerations are missing from diagnostic and therapeutic approaches. Similarly, we wonder about the implications of changes in default network function that are observed in patients with depression. Do all depressed patients have these changes? How do structural brain changes affect default network function? What do these changes mean for therapeutic strategies, and can problems of "inattention" (failure to shift out of default mode) be targets for treatment? We cannot answer these questions today, but we think that they are important for future understanding of psychiatric disorders and their treatment.

The preceding discussion demonstrates that rethinking psychiatric dysfunction, perhaps along the lines of what we propose in this book, is needed. As noted by Paul Holtzheimer and Helen Mayberg, the "syndrome" of depression (the collection of symptoms) may be the wrong place to focus clinically; the real problem is more likely a defect in how mood states are regulated as neural rhythms. While we have focused on major depression in this discussion, similar considerations can be raised for other psychiatric illnesses, as outlined earlier in this book.

PSYCHIATRY AND REHABILITATIVE MEDICINE

A direct corollary of the preceding discussion is that psychiatry must begin to see itself as being much more closely aligned with the approaches and goals of rehabilitative medicine, particularly cognitive rehabilitation. It is unlikely that we will see "cures" for psychiatric disorders in the foreseeable future. We don't take this to be particularly negative or even unusual, but rather see it as the norm for almost all common disorders in medicine, including epilepsy, diabetes, and many cardiovascular illnesses. Despite the inability to offer cures, psychiatrists have a variety of tools that can alleviate symptoms and function, and these tools will improve over time, particularly if the field takes advantage of advances in neurorehabilitation. As we view it, a major goal of psychiatric treatment is to minimize symptoms and optimize function in the face of illnesses that are recurrent at best and chronic, even deteriorating, at worst. Treatment should include efforts not only to improve symptoms to the maximum extent possible but also to help patients and families cope with deficits. Strategies to accomplish the latter include much of what is done in the practice of psychotherapy, where the emphasis must be on using state-of-the-art evidence-based methods to enhance function. Psychiatry has a variety of such tools available, including cognitive behavioral therapy (CBT), interpersonal therapy, dialectical behavioral therapy, specific behavioral therapies, and others. There is little doubt that newer therapies with evidence-based support will evolve in the future and will find their way into practice. In addition to these approaches, better partnering with professionals in rehabilitative medicine, occupational therapy, and perhaps physical therapy can also help to improve function, particularly with regard to the cognitive impairment associated with many major psychiatric disorders. We also note the potential of less invasive brain stimulation techniques, particularly transcranial magnetic stimulation, as a way to alter neurocircuits for rehabilitative purposes.

We would also emphasize the benefits of what some call "TLC" ("therapeutic lifestyle changes")—interventions that target diet, activities of daily living, sleep hygiene, social interactions, exercise, and environmental enrichment. These interventions are good for both the body and the brain, and they can have significant impact on overall well-being. Diet and activity levels are of clear importance. Obesity is a major problem in the United States and exhibits a bidirectional relationship with depression, increasing the risk of depression and being an outcome of having depression. There is also evidence suggesting that physical and motor fitness have significantly positive effects on cognition as humans age. Lifestyle changes can thus be critical contributors to the rehabilitative process and have potential to form the basis for prevention programs, particularly when coupled with efforts to eliminate cigarette and illicit drug use and minimize alcohol consumption.

As we learn more about the neural system defects in various syndromes, more specific rehabilitative strategies can be developed. Some of these strategies may involve computer-based technologies to help patients learn ways to bypass malfunctioning brain systems. An early example of this approach is the use of Internet-based CBT for treating chronic insomnia. An additional advantage of such technology-based methods is that they may provide access to care for a broader array of patients. This is especially important given current and projected limitations in the availability of therapists with expertise in state-of-the-art treatments. CBT has one of the best research-based track records in treating chronic insomnia, yet it is grossly underutilized, often in lieu of simpler to implement but, at times, sloppy pharmacologic approaches. The paucity of well-trained therapists and limited reimbursement contribute significantly to this underutilization. Internet-based approaches may be one of the most cost-effective ways out of the conundrum, if these approaches can be shown to be effective. Chronic insomnia is highly relevant to both brain function and psychiatric outcomes: severe insomnia is associated with shrinkage in the dentate gyrus and CA3 region of the hippocampus, and with worse outcomes in the treatment of depression, particularly in individuals with medical comorbidities.

We would emphasize that individual psychiatrists probably won't administer all rehabilitative strategies on their own. Thus, collaborative practice arrangements with professionals in other disciplines will be important. These include traditional partners such as psychology, social work, and various types of counseling services. Improved partnerships and collaborative practice arrangements with physicians in primary care medicine, neurology, and rehabilitative medicine, as well as their associated allied health disciplines, will also be increasingly important.

PSYCHIATRY AND PRIMARY CARE

The relationship of psychiatry to primary care medicine warrants special attention for several reasons. Obesity, diabetes, hyperlipidemias, and nicotine and alcohol dependence are major problems for many patients with psychiatric disorders and adversely affect psychiatric outcomes and life expectancy. Contributors to these problems are multifactorial and include genetics, effects of illness, lifestyle variables, and side effects of psychotropic medications. These factors play significant roles in the observation that individuals with chronic psychiatric disorders die many years earlier than expected (20 to 25 years on average, according to some estimates from population-based studies and public databases). For these reasons, psychiatrists must engage much more directly in primary care aspects of care. This has not traditionally been a focus of psychiatric practice, but because of the denial and stigma associated with psychiatric disorders, psychiatrists may be the only physicians involved in the care of certain patients. Many patients are unlikely to follow through with additional physician appointments even when referred by their psychiatrists; it is often difficult enough to get these patients to return regularly for psychiatric care. Because of the increasing shortage of psychiatrists, we believe it is important to develop models where primary care teams provide higher-quality psychiatric care with the assistance of psychiatrists. We applaud efforts in community health centers where psychiatrists and primary care physicians are working jointly to provide services—a type of one-stop shopping for patients and their families. These models must be expanded to become the norm in practice. Recent work examining the benefits of collaborative care for patients with depression and chronic medical conditions provides support for this idea. Also, better models for consultation and telepsychiatry must be developed in order to reach underserved rural and inner-city populations and deliver specialized support for front-line care providers.

PSYCHIATRY AND PUBLIC HEALTH

Psychiatric disorders are important public health problems, accounting for substantial disability and death. In Western economies, psychiatric disorders, including the dementing illnesses, account for nearly 50% of all disabilities. Over the next 10 to 20 years, it is estimated that major depression will become the second leading cause of disease burden worldwide, after cardiac illnesses. The relatively early age of onset and persistence of many major psychiatric disorders is a significant contributor to the disability and high economic costs associated with these disorders. It appears that the cognitive impairment associated with psychiatric illnesses is a key factor contributing to dysfunction, particularly in illnesses such as schizophrenia and severe mood disorders. Again, this makes rehabilitative efforts aimed at improving or minimizing cognitive dysfunction all the more important. To focus solely on mood, anxiety, or active psychotic symptoms is no longer tenable if we hope to alter the public health impact of psychiatric illnesses.

As noted previously, severe psychiatric disorders play a significant role in mortality as well. Suicide is clearly a major factor, but it is not the only contributor. Suicide claims more than 30,000 lives per year in the United States; this puts it near the top ten causes of death among adults, and it is much higher on the list for adolescents. Mood disorders, substance-abuse disorders, and schizophrenia are the major disorders associated with suicides, but anxiety disorders and personality disorders also contribute to suicide risk, particularly when accompanied by depression or substance abuse. Violence associated with psychiatric disorders, often with psychiatric patients being victims, is also a significant factor in increased mortality. Substance use in the context of violent acts and accidental deaths compounds the mortality burden. Comorbid psychiatric disorders, particularly depression, worsen the outcomes of many primary medical disorders, including heart disease, diabetes, cancer, AIDS, and others. It is important to emphasize that depression in the context of major medical illnesses is not simply a "reaction to illness," but rather a marker of illness severity that confers its own risks and, at times, serves as an antecedent increasing risk for other illnesses. Thus, psychiatry has a major role to play in general and specialized internal medicine and surgery. Many of the leading medical causes of death in the United States are directly the result of drug dependence—in particular, dependence on nicotine and alcohol. Together, these two legal drugs account for more deaths than any other cause cited in top ten lists. Yet, both, particularly nicotine dependence, are largely ignored in medical practice or, if not ignored, are among the disorders with the worst reimbursement rates from third-party payers, making them low priorities in medical management.

The impact of psychiatric disorders on public health makes it imperative that psychiatrists direct their clinical efforts toward understanding and diminishing the factors contributing to disability and death. Here, the most effective strategies will likely involve early detection and prevention. As we noted earlier, brain disorders get worse or become more refractory over time when left untreated. Thus, treatment efforts are most effective when implemented early in the course of illness, perhaps at the prodromal or high-risk stage. For example, epidemiological studies suggest that once a person has smoked 100 cigarettes, he or she has a high probability of being nicotine-dependent and a long-term (if not life-long) smoker. Put another way, five packs of cigarettes are enough to hook many people for life. Because smoking and drinking typically begin during early adolescence, intervention at the elementary or early high school level is critical. On a positive note, there is evidence that anti-smoking campaigns involving children and adolescents have been effective in decreasing the smoking rate in the population. Even though smoking rates appear to have stabilized at about 20% to 25% of the population (down from nearly 50%), these findings serve as an important proof-of-concept that large-scale prevention efforts can be relatively successful. The fact that at least 20% of the population still smokes implies that the efforts are still not successful enough, however. Other hopeful projects involve efforts that target environmental enrichment programs toward children at risk for antisocial behavior. Here, findings suggesting that diminished fear conditioning in childhood is associated with criminal behavior in adulthood suggest potential avenues for interventions. Some prevention or early intervention strategies may not require face-to-face contact with psychiatrists or therapists. For example, efforts are underway to develop Internet-based methods of providing treatments directed at insomnia and eating disorders. Such interventions, coupled with follow-up visits with mental health professionals, may be appropriate for some individuals. In particular, more effective strategies, including non-pharmacologic approaches, for improving sleep are needed, given the fact that sleep disturbances accompany all major psychiatric disorders and contribute to emotional instability, cognitive dysfunction, and defects in top-down processing.

The development of effective forms of CBT for chronic insomnia is a hopeful step forward. This is an area that requires much more research.

The findings with nicotine dependence and antisocial behaviors also highlight the importance of viewing adult psychiatric problems from a developmental perspective as well as the importance of child and adolescent psychiatrists in prevention efforts. Many adult psychiatric disorders may best be understood from a developmental perspective. Mood or prodromal psychotic symptoms often first appear during childhood or adolescence. Similarly, individuals who develop schizophrenia often first demonstrate cognitive defects during elementary school, including problems with verbal reasoning, working memory, and attention. These manifestations of illness offer the potential for early recognition and perhaps preventive intervention. Such approaches are already underway in psychotic disorders, as exemplified by the PACE (Personal Assessment and Crisis Evaluation) program in Australia and similar programs in other countries. A recent study using CBT for adolescents at high risk for depression also provides an early attempt at such efforts in non-psychotic disorders. It is less clear at what point pharmacologic interventions should be implemented, but clinicians will have to keep abreast of advances in prevention research and carefully weigh the risk/benefit ratio. Empirical studies examining the best approaches for prevention and early intervention are needed, and we would strongly emphasize that pharmaceuticals may need to play a secondary role, particularly given the risks and limitations of current medications in children and adolescents.

Early intervention programs are targeted at individuals at times when the plasticity of the brain is extremely high. Thus, the effects of environmental enrichment, learning, and lifestyle interventions have the potential for great and sustained impact. Because of the nonspecific relationship between childhood adversity and numerous mental disorders, intervention programs must also target the home environment and family dynamics. As noted previously, the effectiveness of early intervention programs in diminishing smoking in the population provides some support for these approaches. The rising rates of obesity among the population, particularly in children and adolescents, is an indicator that lifestyle-based prevention efforts will need to be broad-based to help ward off the ravages of chronic illnesses. Importantly, efforts at early recognition and intervention go hand in hand with the rapidly evolving neuroscience of psychiatry. For example, recent studies highlight the ability to predict the stage of brain network maturity in single individuals based on a 5-minute scan of resting state connectivity. Interpretation of these data is based on a predictable developmental progression from short-range to longer-range network connectivity with maturation. These findings provide a framework for identifying problems in brain connectivity relatively early in development and determining how specific interventions affect connectivity. They also offer the hope of disentangling which networks become dysfunctional at particular stages of childhood and adult psychiatric illnesses. Understanding the development and state of maturity of emotional and motivational circuits relative to cognitive control circuits will likely be important in describing the pathogenesis of a number of mental disorders and in providing explanations about the role of adolescence in the onset of certain illnesses.

TRAINING FUTURE PSYCHIATRISTS

As we think about how to train the next generation of psychiatrists, several trends seem clear. First, the demand for psychiatric services is increasing. The population of the United States is aging. With aging comes increased risk for certain neuropsychiatric disorders, particularly illnesses like Alzheimer's disease that involve neurodegenerative processes. In addition, there is an increasing recognition of severe mental illnesses like mood and psychotic disorders in children and adolescents. Psychiatric disorders are already estimated to affect about one in four to one in three of the population and, when considered from a lifetime perspective, the prevalence may be even higher. Only a small percentage of people with psychiatric disorders actually receive care, and those who do often receive inadequate or inappropriate care. Members of underprivileged or minority groups have an even lower probability of receiving any psychiatric care, much less quality care. Simply stated, there is already an unmet need for high-quality psychiatric services, and this need will increase in the future. A second major trend is that, along with the population in general, the average age of psychiatrists is increasing. There are not enough trainees entering the field to offset the loss of psychiatrists who were trained in the 1960s and 1970s and are now starting to retire. Psychiatry is currently a medical shortage field, and the shortage will deepen over the foreseeable future. Third, the supply of neurologists and primary care physicians available to help deliver care for individuals with mental disorders is inadequate. This conclusion is derived simply from a person-power perspective and does not take into account the fact that most other medical specialists receive little (usually no) formal training in psychiatry during their residencies. There are non-physician mental health professionals helping with care delivery, but their numbers are also inadequate given limitations in the training and expertise of many of these individuals.

These trends make it imperative that future psychiatrists are prepared to deal with complex and highly demanding clinical loads. They will need to be much better versed in clinical neuroscience and its influence on a rapidly evolving landscape of diagnosis and treatment. This can be accomplished, in part, by increasing joint training with neurologists, emphasizing neuroimaging and cognitive neuroscience. It will be important to provide future psychiatrists with training in primary care aspects of psychiatry and experience in collaborative practice arrangements with primary care teams, particularly in situations where psychiatrists provide direct, but time-limited, consultations and interactions, perhaps via electronic methods. We envision clinical practice systems in which psychiatrists partner with primary care physicians and other mental health professionals for the bulk of cases and provide direct services to individuals with severe or highly refractory disorders. This is already happening to some extent, but the lack of formal arrangements and reimbursement models hinders broader applicability. Similarly, psychiatrists should learn to interact more effectively with specialists in rehabilitative medicine as well as occupational and physical therapy in order to take advantage of advances in those fields to help improve the functional outcomes of their patients.

Finally, we reemphasize that psychiatric science is evolving rapidly. A recent editorial in the journal *Nature* highlighted this by calling the current decade "a decade for psychiatric disorders." In this spirit, the next generations of psychiatrists must receive a broad-based education that prepares them for a world of advances in diagnosis and treatment based on neuroscience and genetics. Thus, these fields must be more effectively incorporated into all training programs. Four years of residency training is too short a time to make a person an expert in all aspects of this science, but education in fundamental principles will be critical for careers requiring sophisticated lifelong learning.

Even in the face of major scientific and clinical changes, psychiatry must remain the most patient-centered and humane of medical disciplines. It should never lose this focus because the doctor–patient relationship is, and will remain, critical for all therapeutic and rehabilitative efforts. Thus, psychiatrists must continue to interact with patients as individuals and aid these individuals in achieving the best possible function within their family and social networks. We hope, but don't expect, that psychiatric disorders will become less stigmatized in the future. Thus, in their role as care providers, psychiatrists must also remain advocates for their patients, sometimes serving as voices for individuals who have no effective voice of their own but who deserve to be heard.

SUGGESTED READING

Zorumski, C. F., & Rubin, E. H. (2010). *Demystifying psychiatry—A resource for patients and families.* New York: Oxford University Press.

OTHER REFERENCES

Bassett, A. S., Scherer, S. W., & Brzustowicz, L. M. (2010). Copy number variations in schizophrenia: Critical review and new perspectives on concepts of genetics and disease. *American Journal of Psychiatry, 167,* 899–914.

Biswal, B. B., Mennes, M., Zuo, X.-N., Gohel, S., Kelly, C., Smith, S. M., et al. (2010). Toward discovery science of human brain function. *Proceedings of the National Academy of Sciences (USA), 107,* 4734–4739.

Casey, B. J., Duhoux, S., & Cohen, M. M. (2010). Adolescence: What do transmission, transition and translation have to do with it? *Neuron, 67,* 749–760.

Censor, N., & Cohen, L. G. (2011). Using repetitive transcranial magnetic stimulation to study the underlying neural mechanisms of human motor learning and memory. *Journal of Physiology (London), 589,* 21–28.

Chen, A. J.-W., & D'Esposito, M. (2010). Traumatic brain injury: From bench to bedside to society. *Neuron, 66,* 11–14.

Dehaene S., Pegado, F., Braga, L. W., Ventura, P., Nunes Filho, G., Jobert, A., et al. (2010). How learning to read changes the cortical networks for vision and language. *Science, 330,* 1359–1364.

Dosenbach, N. U. F., Nardos, B., Cohen, A. L., Fair, D. A., Power, J. D., Church, J. A., et al. (2010). Prediction of individual brain maturity using fMRI. *Science, 329,* 1358–1361.

Editorial. (2010). A decade for psychiatric disorders. *Nature, 463,* 9.

Edwards, B. G., Barch, D. M., & Braver, T. S. (2010). Improving prefrontal cortex function in schizophrenia through focused training of cognitive control. *Frontiers in Human Neuroscience, 4 (32),* 1–12.

Fisher, M., Holland, C., Merzenich, M. M., & Vinogradov, S. (2009). Using neuroplasticity-based auditory training to improve verbal memory in schizophrenia. *American Journal of Psychiatry, 166,* 805–811.

Gabrieli, J. D. E. (2009). Dyslexia: a new synergy between education and cognitive neuroscience. *Science, 325,* 280–283.

Gao, Y., Raine, A., Venables, P. H., Dawson, M. E., & Mednick, S. A. (2010). Association of poor childhood fear conditioning and adult crime. *American Journal of Psychiatry, 167,* 56–60.

Garber, J., Clarke, G. N., Weersing, V. R., Beardslee, W. R., Brent, D. A., Gladstone, T. R. G., et al. (2009). Prevention of depression in at-risk adolescents: A randomized controlled trial. *Journal of the American Medical Association, 301,* 2215–2224.

Goto, Y., Yang, C. R., & Otani, S. (2010). Functional and dysfunctional synaptic plasticity in prefrontal cortex: Roles in psychiatric disorders. *Biological Psychiatry, 67,* 199–207.

Gradinaur, V., Mogri, M., Thompson, K. R., Henderson, J. M., & Deisseroth, K. (2009). Optical dissection of parkinsonian neural circuitry. *Science, 324,* 354–359.

Green, J. G., McLaughlin, K. A., Berglund, P. A., Gruber, M. J., Sampson, N. A., Zaslavsky, A. M., et al. (2010). Childhood adversities and adult psychiatric disorders in the National Comorbidity Survey Replication I: Associations with first onset of DSM-IV disorders. *Archives of General Psychiatry, 67,* 113–123.

Hecht, D., Walsh, V., & Lavidor, M. (2010). Transcranial direct current stimulation facilitates decision making in a probabilistic guessing task. *Journal of Neuroscience, 30,* 4241–4245.

Hoeft, F., McCandliss, B. D., Black, J. M., Gantman, A., Zakerani, N., Hulme, C., et al. (2011). Neural systems predicting long-term outcome in dyslexia. *Proceedings of the National Academy of Sciences (USA), 108,* 361–366.

Holtzheimer, P. E., & Mayberg, H. S. (2011). Stuck in a rut: Rethinking depression and its treatment. *Trends in Neuroscience, 34,* 1–9.

Insel, T. R. (2009). Disruptive insights in psychiatry: Transforming a clinical discipline. *Journal of Clinical Investigation, 119,* 700–705.

Katon, W. J., Lin, E. H. B., Van Korff, M., Ciechanowski, P., Ludman, E. J., Young, B., et al. (2010). Collaborative care for patients with depression and chronic illnesses. *New England Journal of Medicine, 363,* 2611–2620.

Keller, T. A., & Just, M. A. (2009). Altering cortical connectivity: Remediation-induced changes in the white matter of poor readers. *Neuron, 64,* 624–631.

Kessler, D., Lewis, G., Kaur, S., Wiles, N., King, M., Weich, S., et al. (2009). Therapist-delivered internet psychotherapy for depression in primary care: A randomized controlled trial. *Lancet, 374,* 628–634.

Kravitz, A. V., Freeze, B. S., Parker, P. R. L., Kay, K., Thwin, M. T., Deisseroth, K., et al. (2010). Regulation of parkinsonism motor behaviors by optogenetic control of basal ganglia circuits. *Nature, 466,* 622–626.

Kroes, M. C. W., Strange, B. A., & Dolan, R. J. (2010). β-adrenergic blockade during memory retrieval in humans evokes a sustained reduction of declarative emotional memory enhancement. *Journal of Neuroscience, 30,* 3959–3963.

Laird, A. R., Eickhoff, S. B., Li, K., Robin, D. A., Glahn, D. C., & Fox, P. T. (2009). Investigating the functional heterogeneity of the default mode network using coordinate-based meta-analytic modeling. *Journal of Neuroscience, 29*, 496–505.

Leshner, A. I., Baghdoyan, H. A., Bennett, S. J., Caples, S. M., DeRubeis, R. J., Glynn, R. J., et al. (2005). National Institutes of Health state of the science conference statement: Manifestations and management of chronic insomnia in adults June 13–15, 2005. *Sleep, 28*, 1049–1057.

Lopez, A. D., & Murray, C. C. J. L. (1998). The global burden of disease, 1990–2020. *Nature Medicine, 4*, 1241–1243.

Luppino, F. S., de Wit, L. M., Bouvy, P. F., Stijnen, T., Cuijpers, P., Penninx, B. W. J. H., et al. (2010). Overweight, obesity and depression: A systematic review and meta-analysis of longitudinal studies. *Archives of General Psychiatry, 67*, 220–229.

McGorry, P. D., Nelson, B., Amminger, G. P., Bechdolf, A., Francey, S. M., Berger, G., et al. (2009). Intervention in individuals at ultra high risk for psychosis: A review and future directions. *Journal of Clinical Psychiatry, 70*, 1206–1212.

Meisenbock, G. (2009). The optogenetic catechism. *Science, 326*, 395–399.

Meltzoff, A. N., Kuhl, P. K., Movellan, J., & Sejnowski, T. J. (2009). Foundations for a new science of learning. *Science, 325*, 284–288.

Mokdad, A. H., Marks, J. S., Stroup, D. F., & Gerberding, J. L. (2004). Actual causes of death in the United States, 2000. *Journal of the American Medical Association, 291*, 1238–1245.

Neylan, T. C., Mueller, S. G., Wang, Z., Metzler, T. J., Lenoci, M., Truran, D., et al. (2010). Insomnia severity is associated with a decreased volume of the CA3/dentate gyrus hippocampal subfield. *Biological Psychiatry, 68*, 494–496.

Ophir, E., Nass, C., & Wagner, A. D. (2009). Cognitive control in media multitaskers. *Proceedings of the National Academy of Sciences (USA), 106*, 583–587.

O'Rahilly, S. (2009). Human genetics illuminates the paths to metabolic disease. *Nature, 462*, 307–314.

Reichenberg, A., Caspi, A., Harrington, H., Houts, R., Keefe, R. S. E., Murray, R., et al. (2010). Static and dynamic cognitive deficits in childhood preceding adult schizophrenia: A 30-year study. *American Journal of Psychiatry, 167*, 160–169.

Scanziani, M., & Hausser, M. (2009). Electrophysiology in the age of light. *Nature, 461*, 930–939.

Schiller, D., Monfils, M.-H., Raio, C. M., Johnson, D. C., LeDoux, J. E., & Phelps, E. A. (2010). Preventing the return of fear in humans using reconsolidation update mechanisms. *Nature, 463*, 49–53.

Tiihonen, J., Lonnqvist, J., Wahlbeck, K., Klaukka, T., Niskanen, L., Tanskanen, A., et al. (2009). 11-year follow-up of mortality in patients with schizophrenia: A population-based cohort study (FIN11 study). *Lancet, 374*, 620–627.

Voelcker-Rehage, C., Godde, B., & Staudinger, U. M. (2010). Physical and motor fitness are both related to cognition in old age. *European Journal of Neuroscience, 31*, 167–176.

Wulff, K., Gatti, S., Wettstein, J. G., & Foster, R. G. (2010). Sleep and circadian rhythm disruption in psychiatric and neurodegenerative disease. *Nature Reviews Neuroscience, 11*, 1–11.

Yung, A. R., McGorry, P. D., Francey, S. M., Nelson, B., Baker, K., Philips, L. J., et al. (2007). PACE: A specialized service for young people at risk of psychotic disorders. *Medical Journal of Australia, 187*, 43–46.

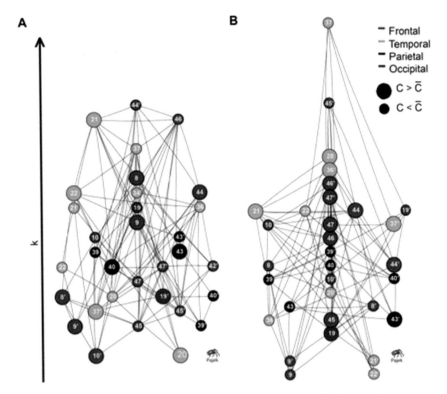

Figure 5-1 Connectivity maps: controls vs. persons with schizophrenia. The diagram depicts differences in cortical connectivity between control subjects (A) and individuals with schizophrenia (B) based on functional MRI data. The diagram shows altered local clustering in frontal cortex and longer path lengths linking cortical regions in individuals with schizophrenia. (Reproduced with permission from Bassett et al., 2008.)

Appendix

Five views of the brain are presented in this Appendix. All abbreviations are listed alphabetically below. These views are adapted with permission from Damasio, H. (2005). *Human Brain Anatomy in Computerized Images* (2nd ed.). New York: Oxford University Press. They provide greater anatomical specificity than the figures in the text and highlight the areas discussed in descriptions of various neural networks.

Abbreviations

2	insula, posterior	MFG	middle frontal gyrus
ac	anterior commissure	mOrbG	middle orbital gyrus
AG	angular gyrus	MTG	middle temporal gyrus
aOrbG	anterior orbital gyrus	OP	occipital pole
bc	body of caudate nucleus	pa	pallidum
bCC, bcc	beak, corpus callosum	PaHG	parahippocampal gyrus
CC, cc	corpus callosum	ParaCG	paracentral gyrus
cerebH	cerebellar hemispheres	pc	posterior commissure
cerebT	cerebellar tonsils	pic	posterior internal capsule
cerebV	cerebellar vermis	po	pars opercularis
CingG	cingulate gyrus	porb	pars orbitalis
Cun	cuneus	pOrbG	posterior orbital gyrus
for	fornix	post CG	postcentral gyrus
FP	frontal pole	preCG	precentral gyrus
FusiG	fusiform gyrus	preCun	precuneus
Grec	gyrus rectus	pt	pars triangularis
HG	Heschl's gyrus	pu	putamen
hip	hippocampus	qpl	quadrigeminal plate
ht	hypothalamus	rSp	retrosplenial area
ic	inferior colliculus	sc	superior colliculus
IFG	inferior frontal gyrus	SC	spinal cord
IPL	inferior parietal lobule	sCC, scc	splenium, corpus callosum
ITG	inferior temporal gyrus	SFG	superior frontal gyrus
LingG	lingual gyrus	SMG	supramarginal gyrus
LOG	lateral occipital gyri	SPL	superior parietal lobule
lOrbG	lateral orbital gyrus	STG	superior temporal gyrus
mb	mammillary body	th	thalamus
med	medulla	TOG	temporo-occipital gyrus
mes	mesencephalon	TP	temporal pole

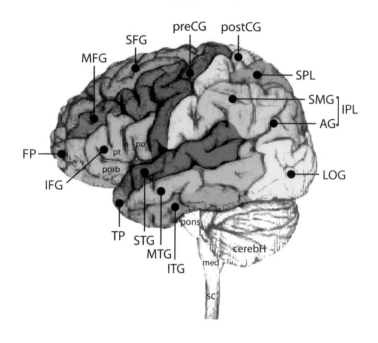

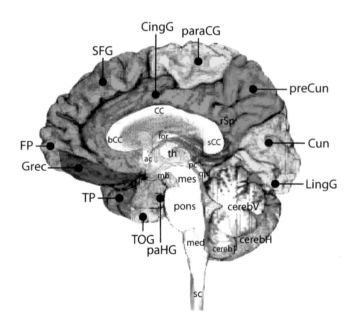

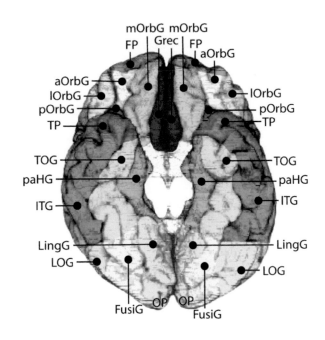

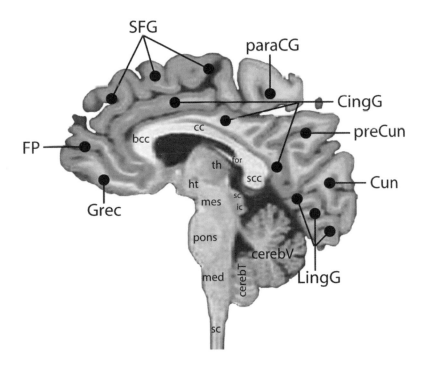

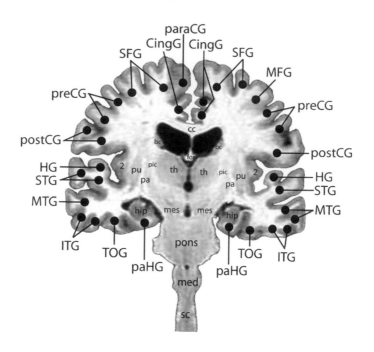

Index

Note: Page numbers followed by "*f*" and "*t*" refer to figures and tables, respectively.

persecutory ideas as, 93

dementia of the Alzheimer's type (DAT)

aerobic glycolysis and, 187–88

age and, 195–96

amyloid plaque and *tau* tangle pathology regarding, 33

anti-dementia agents and, 251–52

categorization of, future approaches to, 220–21

characteristics of, 29–30

cholinesterase and, 251–52

default ICN and, 30*f*, 30–31, 31*t*

diagnosis of, future approaches to, 219–20

fibrillar amyloid burden and, 186–87

genetics and, 166

hippocampal size and, 141

histone acetylation and, 168

NMDA receptor antagonists and, 252

overview, 29

dementias. *See also* behavioral variant frontotemporal dementia; dementia of the Alzheimer's type

overview, 29

systems neuroscience and, 29–34, 30*f*, 31*t*, 32*f*, 32*t*, 33*t*

denial, 231*t*, 231–32

dentate gyrus, 118, 118*f*, 119*f*, 121*f*, 122, 123*f*, 124*t*, 134, 134*f*, 145*f*

depression. *See also* antidepressants; major depressive disorder

bipolar disorder and, 27–28

cocaine addiction and, 26–27

cortical thinning and, 149–50, 150*f*

DBS and, 258–59

default ICN and, 149

familial, 25–26, 149–50, 150*f*

ketamine and, 244

learned safety and, 155

LTD, 126–27, 129–30

medical illnesses and, 274

mental trilogy and, 3–4

neurogenesis and, 154

primary and secondary, 27

rodent swim test and, 145–46

stroke and, 193–94

suicide and, 273

systems neuroscience and, 25–29

thyroid and, 181

TMS and, 257

traumatic brain injury and, 192

treatment and, 28, 101–2, 270–71

types of, 25–28

VNS and, 256–57

developmental abnormalities

environmental challenges and, 184

genetic predisposition and, 183–84

hippocampus influenced by, 143*t*, 143–45, 144*f*

ICNs and, 184–85

nodal structures and, 185

potential treatment of, 185–86

schizophrenia and, 184

diagnosis

biomarkers and, 223

clinical interview and, 214–15

DAT and, 219–20

DSM-IV and, 215

examination, psychiatric, and, 215

future approaches to, 219–21

future trends related to, 221–23

imaging procedures use in, 217–18

laboratory procedure use in, 217

longitudinal course of disorders and, 216–17

MDD and, 270

methods of, 214–17

methods of determining, 214–23

overview regarding, 214

psychological testing used in, 218–19

utility regarding, 216

validity regarding, 215–16

Diagnostic and Statistical Manual of Mental Disorders, Fifth Edition (DSM-5), 266

Diagnostic and Statistical Manual of Mental Disorders, Fourth Edition (DSM-IV), 215

dialectical behavioral therapy, 271

disgust, 16

AIC and, 72

disorders, psychiatric. *See also* abnormalities; *specific disorder*

Printed in the USA/Agawam, MA
December 4, 2023